Every Decker book is accompanied by a CD-ROM.

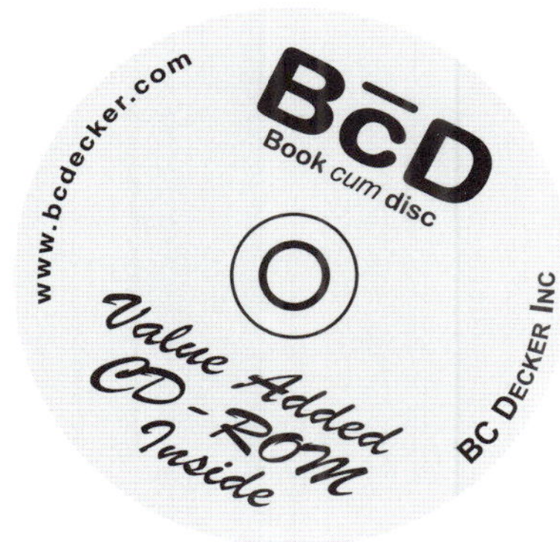

The disc appears in the front of each copy, in its own sealed jacket. Affixed to the front of the book will be a distinctive BC̄D sticker **"Book *cum* disc."**

The disc contains the complete text and illustrations of the book, in fully searchable PDF files. The book and disc are sold *only* as a package; neither is available independently, and no prices are available for the items individually.

BC Decker Inc is committed to providing high-quality electronic publications that complement traditional information and learning methods.

We trust you will find the book/CD package invaluable and invite your comments and suggestions.

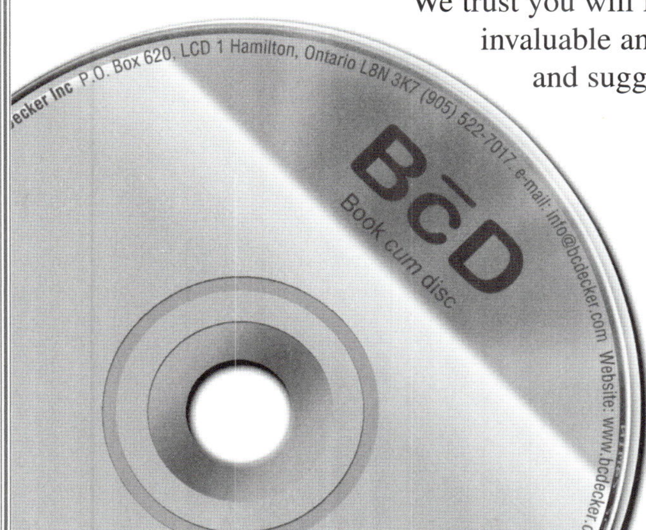

Brian C. Decker
CEO and Publisher

American Cancer Society

Atlas of Clinical Oncology

Published

Blumgart, Fong, Jarnagin	*Hepatobiliary Cancer (2001)*
Cameron	*Pancreatic Cancer (2001)*
Carroll, Grossfeld	*Prostate Cancer (2002)*
Char	*Tumors of the Eye and Ocular Adnexa (2001)*
Clark, Duh, Jahan, Perrier	*Endocrine Tumors (2003)*
Eifel, Levenback	*Cancer of the Female Lower Genital Tract (2001)*
Ginsberg	*Lung Cancer (2002)*
Grossbard	*Malignant Lymphomas (2001)*
Ozols	*Ovarian Cancer (2003)*
Pollock	*Soft Tissue Sarcomas (2001)*
Posner, Vokes, Weichselbaum	*Cancer of the Upper Gastrointestinal Tract (2001)*
Prados	*Brain Cancer (2001)*
Shah	*Cancer of the Head and Neck (2001)*
Silverman	*Oral Cancer (1998)*
Silverman	*Oral Cancer 5th Edition (2003)*
Wiernik	*Adult Leukemias (2001)*
Willett	*Cancer of Lower Gastrointestinal Tract (2001)*
Winchester, Winchester	*Breast Cancer (2000)*

Forthcoming

Droller	*Urothelial Tumors (2003)*
Fuller, Seiden, Young	*Uterine and Endometrial Cancer (2003)*
Raghavan	*Germ Cell Tumors (2003)*
Richie, Steele	*Kidney Tumors (2004)*
Volberding	*Viral and Immunological Malignancies (2004)*
Yasko	*Bone Tumors (2004)*

American Cancer Society

Atlas of Clinical Oncology

Editors

Glenn D. Steele Jr, MD
Geisinger Health System

Theodore L. Phillips, MD
University of California

Bruce A. Chabner, MD
Harvard Medical School

Managing Editor

Ted S. Gansler, MD, MBA
Director of Health Content, American Cancer Society

American Cancer Society

Atlas of

Clinical Oncology

Oral Cancer

Fifth Edition

Sol Silverman Jr., MA, DDS

Professor of Oral Medicine
University of California
School of Dentistry
San Francisco, California

2003
BC Decker Inc
Hamilton • London

BC Decker Inc
P.O. Box 620, LCD 1
Hamilton, Ontario L8N 3K7
Tel: 905-522-7017; 1-800-568-7281
Fax: 905-522-7839; 1-888-311-4987
E-mail: info@bcdecker.com
www.bcdecker.com

03 04 05 / GSA / 9 8 7 6 5 4 3 2 1

ISBN 1–55009–215–4
Printed in Spain

Sales and Distribution

United States
BC Decker Inc
P.O. Box 785
Lewiston, NY 14092-0785
Tel: 905-522-7017; 800-568-7281
Fax: 905-522-7839; 888-311-4987
E-mail: info@bcdecker.com
www.bcdecker.com

Canada
BC Decker Inc
20 Hughson Street South
P.O. Box 620, LCD 1
Hamilton, Ontario L8N 3K7
Tel: 905-522-7017; 800-568-7281
Fax: 905-522-7839; 888-311-4987
E-mail: info@bcdecker.com
www.bcdecker.com

Foreign Rights
John Scott & Company
International Publishers' Agency
P.O. Box 878
Kimberton, PA 19442
Tel: 610-827-1640
Fax: 610-827-1671
E-mail: jsco@voicenet.com

Argentina
CLM (Cuspide Libros Medicos)
Av. Córdoba 2067 – (1120)
Buenos Aires, Argentina
Tel: (5411) 4961-0042/(5411) 4964-0848
Fax: (5411) 4963-7988
E-mail: clm@cuspide.com

Japan
Igaku-Shoin Ltd.
Foreign Publications Department
3-24-17 Hongo
Bunkyo-ku, Tokyo, Japan 113-8719
Tel: 3 3817 5680
Fax: 3 3815 6776
E-mail: fd@igaku-shoin.co.jp

U.K., Europe, Scandinavia, Middle East
Elsevier Science
Customer Service Department
Foots Cray High Street
Sidcup, Kent
DA14 5HP, UK
Tel: 44 (0) 208 308 5760
Fax: 44 (0) 181 308 5702
E-mail: cservice@harcourt.com

Singapore, Malaysia, Thailand, Philippines, Indonesia, Vietnam, Pacific Rim, Korea
Elsevier Science Asia
583 Orchard Road
#09/01, Forum
Singapore 238884
Tel: 65-737-3593
Fax: 65-753-2145

Australia, New Zealand
Elsevier Science Australia
Customer Service Department
STM Division
Locked Bag 16
St. Peters, New South Wales, 2044
Australia
Tel: 61 02 9517-8999
Fax: 61 02 9517-2249
E-mail: stmp@harcourt.com.au
Web site: www.harcourt.com.au

Mexico and Central America
ETM SA de CV
Calle de Tula 59
Colonia Condesa
06140 Mexico DF, Mexico
Tel: 52-5-5553-6657
Fax: 52-5-5211-8468
E-mail: editoresdetextosmex@prodigy.net.mx

Brazil
Tecmedd
Av. Maurílio Biagi, 2850
City Ribeirão Preto – SP – CEP: 14021-000
Tel: 0800 992236
Fax: (16) 3993-9000
E-mail: tecmedd@tecmedd.com.br

Dedication

This textbook, a culmination of more than 40 years of patient care and research, is dedicated to my father, Sol Silverman Esq., my mother, Carolyn Stern Silverman, and my wife, Betty Walden Silverman, for their continual, uncompromising, devoted support for my work in cancer over the span of my professional career.

Contents

Acknowledgment

Sincere appreciation is expressed to the contributing authors whose acknowledged expertise and contributions have made this text an authoritative, state-of-the-art publication and to Priscilla Mayer whose dedicated work with computer processing and editing supported the high-quality product.

Preface

All multicellular animals, and certainly all vertebrates, can develop cancer. The ability to develop cancer is a characteristic of all cells that are capable of reproduction and growth. Cancer, by its very nature—an abnormal, seemingly unrestricted growth of body cells—is distinguished from other forms of illness.

There are many differences in the occurrence of cancer types and sites among human populations: for example, the high incidence of nasopharyngeal cancer among the Chinese compared with other ethnic groups and the low incidence of skin cancer among blacks compared with whites.

Although cancer may occur at any age, it is preponderantly a disease of aging and can be both acute and chronic in its course. More than half of all cancers in the United States occur in persons over the age of 65 years. In this age group, the incidence is 2,261 cases per 100,000 population! Many types of cancer are perceptible only when they are extensive or involve organs difficult to treat, and others may be detected early, treated, and cured.

This complex disease, which is a major cause of morbidity and disability, is second only to heart disease as the leading cause of death among Americans. Approximately one in every three Americans will have cancer in his or her lifetime, and about one in every four deaths is attributable to a malignant tumor.

In the United States, oral cancer accounts for nearly 3% of all cancers and approximately 2% of all cancer deaths. Mortality is high, with 5-year survival rates that approximate only a little more than 50%, in spite of modern treatments that include surgery, radiation, and chemotherapy. However, early detection of mouth cancers (ie, when lesions are less than 3 cm in size and show no evidence of deep invasion or metastasis) dramatically increases the survival rates. Unfortunately, over the past decade there have been only small improvements in early diagnosis of oral cancer: more than 60% of all oral cancers are extensive, late-stage malignancies at the time of diagnosis. Hence, treatment is more aggressive in trying to improve cure rates. This approach, which increases complications of treatments, results in only a slight improvement in survival rates. Therefore, early diagnosis of a lesion during the localized stage, combined with adequate treatment, appears to be the most effective way to further improve oral cancer control.

Recent studies indicate that only a small number of Americans report having been examined for oral cancer. The data varied according to demographic characteristics and the education of the patients, as well as the training and office routines of both the dentists and the physicians. Thus, professional and public education programs are critical in emphasizing the need for routine oral cancer examinations, in addition to teaching the recognition of early signs and symptoms of malignancy. Furthermore, as our knowledge of cancer rapidly increases in the areas of oncogenes, viruses, cellular growth and suppressor factors, and nutritional support, a dramatic reduction in morbidity and mortality and even prevention seem to be realistic goals.

The increased risks arising from the use of tobacco and alcohol are recognized, and more effective cessation programs are being developed. Biomarkers that reflect abnormal cell components are being studied to improve the control and prediction of tissue behavior. Optimal cancer control calls for a diversity of approaches among many health professionals, including prevention programs and diagnostic techniques. The dental profession shares an important responsibility in the management of oral cancer, from diagnosis through rehabilitation. Dentists have a unique opportunity in the routine mouth examination to detect malignant neoplasms while they are still asymptomatic, innocuous, and unsuspected. In addition, the dentist is most often the first clinician consulted for general oral complaints and, therefore, has the initial responsibility of differentiating benign from precancerous and malignant conditions. Furthermore, other health care providers can serve the same purpose by incorporating oral examinations in their procedures, particularly in high-risk individuals, for example, individuals beyond middle age who also smoke and consume alcohol.

Treatment of oral cancer often produces certain dysfunctions and distortions in speech, appearance, mastication, swallowing, saliva flow and consistency, emotional stability, and dental health. Therefore, rehabilitation becomes a major consideration in patient management.

In preparing for their participation in cancer control, health professionals must acquire knowledge of the biologic and epidemiologic aspects of cancer and its prevention, early detection, diagnosis, treatment, and rehabilitation, as well as an understanding of the psychosocial and economic aspects of the disease. The complexities of optimal diagnosis, management, and control require multidisciplinary teams.

This fifth edition of *Oral Cancer* updates the entire problem of oral cancer control: occurrence, etiology, premalignant factors and prevention, diagnosis, treatment, rehabilitation, and survival. It is written in a manner that should serve all clinicians and health professionals as a unique reference that contains both an updated and detailed text along with a generous number of colored figures that additionally provide a "colored atlas" flavor.

The first eight chapters focus mainly on squamous cell carcinoma because it is by far the most common type of oral cancer. In Chapter 2, epidemiology, demographics, and etiology have been updated and expanded to reflect current trends and status. The role of tobacco, nutritional considerations, and viral aspects have been substantially increased to reflect their importance in neoplastic predisposition and risks. The chapter on precancerous oral lesions has been enlarged in both text and figures because of problems in recognizing these lesions (primarily leukoplakias) at risk for malignant transformation. Imaging techniques in Chapter 4 have been expanded significantly in both text and visual images because of their roles in diagnosis, staging, and treatment plans. Treatment has also been enlarged to reflect current attempts in improving survival, which also risk increasing morbidity and oral complications of treatment. Because of problems in survival and quality-of-life issues, material on chemoprevention, modern molecular analysis, and adverse effects of cancer treatments have been substantially expanded. Maxillofacial rehabilitation has progressed dramatically, resulting from advances in patient care and research; therefore, Chapter 8, "Restoration of Palate, Tongue, Mandible, and Facial Defects," has been updated with additional text, tables, and figures.

The etiology, diagnosis, and management of other cancers that involve oral health care providers are covered in the following four chapters. The leukemias and lymphomas have been described by text and illustrations in Chapter 9. These malignancies are treated primarily with immunosuppressive and toxic chemotherapeutic agents that incur oral manifestations requiring special dental management. Chapter 10 covers major and minor salivary gland tumors and emphasizes the special approach needed for the diagnosis and treatment of each type of gland. Sarcomas and other malignancies that affect the jaw bones and sinuses, skin cancers, nasopharyngeal and laryngeal malignancies, melanomas, and pediatric oncology are included in Chapter 11 to complete the overview of head and neck cancers and clinical considerations. Even though malignant melanomas are rare, they are covered in detail because of their poor prognosis and difficulties in differential diagnoses, which include ethnic pigmentation, amalgam tattoos, and focal melanosis. The overview of pediatric oncology citing oral/dental implications has been given attention because of the need to rule out malignancy and management approaches when children present with oral lesions. Human immunodeficiency virus (HIV) infection continues to increase worldwide, with no end in sight. HIV-associated oral malignancies, a major cause of morbidity and mortality in this group, constitute the last chapter. The generous colored illustrations effectively supplement the text, enhancing visual comprehension and practical applications.

In summary, this updated and expanded fifth edition of *Oral Cancer* should serve as a reservoir of both written and visual information to enhance the clinician's role in the prevention, recognition, diagnosis, management, and rehabilitation of malignancies that affect oral and paraoral sites. In turn, this educational resource should aid in reducing the morbidity and mortality associated with cancer.

Sol Silverman Jr., MA, DDS
December 2002

Contributors

JOHN BEUMER III, DDS, MS
Professor
UCLA Department of Dentistry
Los Angeles, California

HERBERT DEDO, MD
Professor and Vice Chairman
Department of Otolaryngology
University of California, San Francisco
San Francisco, California

WILLIAM P. DILLON, MD
Professor
Radiology, Neurology, and Neurological Surgery
Chief of Neuroradiology
Vice Chair
Department of Radiology
University of California, San Francisco
San Francisco, California

DAVID W. EISELE, MD
Professor and Chairman
Otolaryngology Head and Neck Surgery
University of California, San Francisco
San Francisco, California

NANCY J. FISCHBEIN, MD
Assistant Professor in Residence
Department of Radiology
University of California, San Francisco
San Francisco, California

CATHERINE M. FLAITZ, DDS, MS
Interim Dean and Professor
The University of Texas Dental Branch at Houston
Department of Diagnostic Sciences
Oral and Maxillofacial Pathology
Houston, Texas

RICHARD C. K. JORDAN, DDS, PHD
Associate Professor
Department of Stomatology and Pathology
University of California, San Francisco
San Francisco, California

MICHAEL J. KAPLAN, MD
Associate Professor
Otolaryngology Head and Neck Surgery
University of California, San Francisco
San Francisco, California

ALAN M. KRAMER, MD
Associate Clinical Professor of Medicine
University of California, San Francisco
San Francisco, California

NANCY LEE, MD
Assistant Professor
Department of Radiation Oncology
University of California, San Francisco
San Francisco, California

CRAIG S. MILLER, DMD, MS
Professor of Oral Medicine
University of Kentucky College of Dentistry
Department of Oral Health Practice, Oral Medicine
Lexington, Kentucky

DOUGLAS E. PETERSON, DMD, PHD
Professor and Department Chair
University of Connecticut Health Center
Farmington, Connecticut

THEODORE L. PHILLIPS, MD
Professor
Department of Radiation Oncology
University of California, San Francisco
San Francisco, California

Jeanne M. Quivey, MD
Professor
Department of Radiation Oncology
University of California, San Francisco
San Francisco, California

Joseph A. Regezi, MS, DDS
Professor of Oral Pathology
School of Dentistry
University of California, San Francisco
San Francisco, California

Mark M. Schubert, DDS, MSD
Professor
Department of Oral Medicine
University of Washington
Seattle, Washington

Arun B. Sharma, BDS, MSc
Assistant Clinical Professor
School of Dentistry
University of California, San Francisco
San Francisco, California

Sol Silverman Jr., MA, DDS
Professor of Oral Medicine
School of Dentistry
University of California, San Francisco
San Francisco, California

Mark I. Singer, MD, FACS
Professor
Otolaryngology Head and Neck Surgery
University of California, San Francisco
San Francisco, California

Joan S. Thompson, PhD, RD, CD
Associate Professor of Nutrition
Department of Health Promotion and Human Performance
College of Education
Weber State University
Ogden, Utah

Ian M. Zlotolow, DMD
Chief
Dental Service
Memorial Sloan-Kettering Cancer Center
Department of Surgery
New York, New York

1

Epidemiology

SOL SILVERMAN JR., MA, DDS

Epidemiology is the branch of science that studies disease as it appears in its natural surroundings and as it affects a community of people. Epidemiologic studies yield important information such as the origin, relative prevalence, and trends of certain diseases; they can also furnish etiologic clues. By analyzing blood samples, "molecular" epidemiologists are able to assess cancer risks arising from interactions of genes and lifestyles. It may be that inheritance of certain gene variants (polymorphisms) might increase the likelihood of developing cancer, depending on environmental exposures. The data, in turn, aid in determining appropriate and optimal directions of health care services, prevention strategies, research, and resources.

INCIDENCE

Globally, oral and pharyngeal cancer is the sixth leading cancer site.[1] More than 1.2 million new cancers of all sites (excluding skin) will be diagnosed in the United States each year. Cancers of the lips, tongue, floor of the mouth, palate, gingiva, alveolar mucosa, buccal mucosa, and oropharynx will account for approximately 30,000 of these cases (an incidence of about 10 per 100,000). If other head and neck sites (nasopharynx, hypopharynx, larynx, sinuses, and major salivary glands) are included with the oral sites, then cancers of all of these sites combined will account for about 4% of all cancers diagnosed yearly in the United States. Cancer now strikes approximately 1 of every 3 Americans and 3 of every 4 families. It is estimated that more than 85 million Americans now living will some day develop cancer.

HISTOLOGIC TYPES

Carcinomas account for about 96% of all oral cancers and sarcomas for about 4%. The most common type of oral cancer is squamous cell carcinoma, which develops from the stratified squamous epithelium that lines the mouth and pharynx. This form of cancer accounts for approximately 9 of every 10 oral malignancies. Thus, the oral cancer problem primarily concerns the diagnosis, biology, and management of squamous cell carcinoma.

AGE AND SEX

Of all of the factors that may contribute to the development of cancer, age is the factor that confers the highest risk. Oral cancer, like most cancers, is a disease of older age. About 95% of all oral cancers occur in persons over 40 years old, and the average age at the time of diagnosis occurs as individuals approach the age of 65. The importance of this factor in cancer prevalence is augmented because the "over 65" population in the United States now exceeds 36 million, or about 13% of the population.

The "over 65" population is expected to continually increase, possibly reaching 20% of the total US population by 2030. Furthermore, the increase in the population over age 65 has far exceeded that of the rest of the population in the last decade, and, at present, more than one-third of the American people are over the age of 45. The average life expectancy of Americans is at an all-time high, exceeding 74 years, and the age-adjusted death rate is at an all-time low. White women have the longest life expectancy (79 years), followed by black women

(73 years), white men (72 years), and black men (64 years). A past study of 3,535 consecutive autopsied patients over 65 years of age showed that 1,149 (32.5%) had one or more cancers.

Having said all of this, evidence is emerging that oral cancers are occurring more frequently in younger persons (under 40 years).[2] Reports indicate that the tongue is the most common site, and environmental/lifestyle risk factors, for example, tobacco use, disease, and immunosuppression, do not seem to account for these cancers.[3,4] Studies are being designed in an attempt to epidemiologically confirm the incidence and possibly explain a probable genetic-environmental influence.

In the United States, more than 50% of all cancers occur in persons over the age of 65.[5] The older age of cancer patients suggests that a time factor may operate, involving predetermined changes in the biochemical-biophysical processes (nuclear, enzymatic, metabolic, immunologic) of aging cells—changes that may be influenced by chemicals, viruses, hormones, nutrients, or physical irritants. Therefore, programmed cell death (apoptosis) can be modified by factors that may alter cellular production of growth and suppressor proteins. Obviously, over- or underexpression of cell cycle–regulating proteins can cause neoplasia.

Of the more than 1.2 million new cancers occurring in Americans each year, the number in men and women will be about equal. Oral cancer occurs more frequently in males, but the male-to-female ratio, which in 1950 exceeded 6 to 1, is now slightly less than 2 to 1. One possible explanation for this reduced ratio is the great increase in smoking and alcohol consumption among women. In addition, because cancer is an age-related disease, it should be noted that, in the over 65 age group in the general population, the number of women exceeds the number of men by almost 20%.

Data obtained by the National Cancer Institute in its SEER (Surveillance, Epidemiology, and End Results) Program, covering the years 1985 to 1996, demonstrate the age-related distribution of oral and pharyngeal cancers (Table 1–1). During this period, no significant differences have occurred from the previous decade.[6,7] The impact of age is reflected further by the fact that half of all oral cancers occurred in persons over 65 years of age. This is a significant rate of 50 cases per 100,000 population compared with a rate of 14 cases per 100,000 in those aged 40 to 65.

Table 1–1. AGE AND GENDER DISTRIBUTION OF ORAL CANCER (based on 22,449 cases)

Age (yr)	*n*	%	M:F*
< 20	130	< 1	1.0
20–39	1,604	7	2.0
40–49	2,432	11	2.5
50–64	7,163	32	2.4
65+	11,170	50	1.6

Adapted from the National Cancer Institute's SEER (Surveillance, Epidemiology, and End Results) Program. Cancers diagnosed and/or treated during 1985 to 1996 according to biostatistical information from nine population-based registries in Connecticut, Hawaii, Iowa, New Mexico, Utah, Atlanta, Detroit, San Francisco-Oakland, and Seattle-Puget Sound.
*Male-to-female ratio.

SITES

The tongue is the most common site for oral cancer in both American men and women. This is also true of "developed" countries. However, in some developing countries, site prevalences differ, owing to different habits. For example, nasopharyngeal cancer in Southeast Asia and buccal cancer in India are the most common oral and pharyngeal sites. As a matter of fact, oral and pharyngeal cancer is one of the three leading sites of *all* cancers in that area of the world.

Data from the SEER Program also showed that 30% of all oral cancers diagnosed in the United States between 1985 and 1996 occurred in the tongue, followed by the lip and floor of the mouth (Table 1–2). Oral cancer incidence has remained stable, relative to the occurrence of newly diagnosed cancers of all sites, with absolute numbers only slightly increasing each year. The only oral site contrary to this trend was the lip, in which a reduction occurred over the past 10 years. Decades ago, the lip used to be the leading oral site. This trend may reflect public education regarding the dangers of ultraviolet light exposure and the use of sunscreens and hats outdoors. Comparing the past two decades, the greatest increase in oral cancer sites occurred in the tongue (26 to 30%). Oral tongue malignancies (located in the anterior two-thirds) accounted for 53% of tongue cancers. Because 47% occurred in the base of the tongue, the problems

Table 1–2. ORAL CANCER: 3 LEADING SITES

Site	Cases (%)	M:F*	Mean Age
Tongue	30	2.0	61
Lip†	17	5.0	66
Mouth floor	14	2.2	62

Adapted from the National Cancer Institute's SEER (Surveillance, Epidemiology, and End Results) Program, 1985–1996.
*Male-to-female ratio; †94% lower lip.

regarding recognition of the signs and symptoms and early diagnosis are apparent.

Patient profiles are further illustrated by findings in 595 oral cancer patients seen in our oral medicine clinic (Table 1–3). At the time of diagnosis, just over half of the tumors found in the tongue were localized, whereas the greatest number of localized lesions occurred in the lip. However, when the tongue was subdivided into oral and base, a significant difference emerged: 73% of oral-tongue carcinomas were localized, whereas 78% of the malignancies found in the base of the tongue already had regional metastases at the time of diagnosis. These facts again emphasize the importance of accessibility and early diagnosis. When the localized lesions were compared with those associated with lymph node involvement, it was found that the more advanced lesions were associated with a longer delay time before diagnosis. Pain was by far the most frequent first complaint, with the second most common complaint being a "lump."

In the United States, the increased male prevalence of oral cancer appears to be attributable in great part to the proportionately higher number of lip cancers that occur in men. The preponderance of cases in men may also be partly accounted for by outdoor occupations and recreational activities, as well as histories of heavier daily tobacco and alcohol consumption by male patients. Varying frequencies of lip cancer do occur in metropolitan centers, but explanations usually are not evident. Again, the decreasing frequency of lip cancer may reflect public education about the dangers of sunlight exposure and preventive measures.

Table 1–3. CHARACTERISTICS OF ORAL CARCINOMAS IN 595 PATIENTS: ASSOCIATION OF SITE, STAGE, AND DIAGNOSTIC PATTERNS

Site	Localized Stage at Diagnosis (%)	Mean Delay Time (mo)*	Pain as First Complaint (%)	First Consultation with a Dentist (%)
Tongue	51	4.2	66	36
Oropharynx	43	3.0	56	16
Mouth floor	64	3.4	59	44
Gingiva	56	3.5	64	52
Buccal	79	3.4	52	50
Lip	88	5.0	27	46
Hard palate	75	4.5	50	57

Adapted from the Oral Medicine Clinic, University of California at San Francisco.
*Time from patient's recognition of first sign/symptom to diagnosis.

STAGE AT DIAGNOSIS AND SURVIVAL

Approximately half of all patients with oral and pharyngeal cancers will survive their disease 5 years following treatment (see Chapter 5, "Spread of Tumor, Staging, and Survival"). The outcomes are more favorable for whites than for blacks (58% versus 34% 5-year survival rates). Although genetics must play some critical role, socioeconomic status, education, and access to the health care system also have an influence. However, the primary explanation is based on the poor survival rates for advanced tumors compared with early, localized cancers (Table 1–4). If all diagnosed and treated oral cancer cases were early, localized tumors, almost 4 of 5 patients would survive 5 years. Unfortunately, unsatisfactory progress has been made during the last three decades in regard to early diagnosis (Table 1–5). Additionally, based on more than 25,000 SEER Program oral/pharyngeal cases for which there was adequate information, localized/early oral cancers were outnumbered by advanced tumors 59 to 41%. The lip was the only major site where local-

Table 1–4. ORAL CANCER: RELATIVE 5-YEAR SURVIVAL RATES BY STAGE AT DIAGNOSIS, 1992–1997

Stage	Distribution (%)	Alive at 5 Yr (%)
Localized	41	82
Regional	48	46
Distant	11	21
All stages	100	56

Adapted from the National Cancer Institute's SEER (Surveillance, Epidemiology, and End Results) Program, 1973–1998.
Localized = tumor confined to the oral cavity; Regional = tumor spread to cervical lymph node(s); Distant = tumor spread to other organ(s).

ized cancers were more frequently found than cancers that were advanced. Because advances in treatment approaches have not led to significantly improved survival, earlier diagnosis is obviously a key factor in improving oral cancer control and reducing morbidity and mortality.

RACE AND GENETICS

Ethnic background is known to influence many types of cancer. For example, cancer in blacks is increasing at a faster rate than in whites. Oral and pharyngeal cancer is the fourth leading cancer site in black men and the seventh leading site of cancer in non-Hispanic white men. Oral cancers in men and women occur less frequently in Asians and Hispanics compared to whites and blacks. Although this finding suggests genetic factors, differences in habits and lifestyle are strongly implicated (see Chapter 2, "Etiology and Predisposing Factors"). As another example, cancer of the nasopharynx is 20 to 30 times more prevalent in Chinese than in whites. The rate of nasopharyngeal carcinoma is highest in Chinese who have remained in Asia, for example, those in Southeast Asia, where it is one of the most common cancers (see Chapter 11, "Other Malignancies and Oral Oncology").

Studies of human cancer of specific types have shown aggregation in some families, implying a genetic influence.[8] Examples of these types include rare cancers with mendelian inheritance, such as retinoblastoma in childhood; more common cancers, such as breast, prostate, or colon; and familial cancer syndromes, which can include leukemias, sarcomas, and brain tumors. No such evidence of familial grouping has been presented for oral cancer. As the genetic code becomes further unraveled, inherited risks undoubtedly will be clarified.

Most human tumors show chromosome aberrations that are usually proportional to the degree of malignancy and vary with each tumor and patient (Figure 1–1). It is not known whether the chromosomal abnormalities are the cause or the result of malignancy. However, identification of chromosomal deletions and gene mutations will surely help our understanding of causes, prevention, treatments, and prognosis of malignancies.

MULTIPLE CANCERS

The data unequivocally show that persons with oral and pharyngeal cancers are at an increased risk for developing subsequent additional malignancies.[9–13] In one study of 153 patients with carcinoma of the mouth floor who were treated and observed between 1957 and 1973 at the University of California at San Francisco (UCSF), 36% of the patients had at least one second primary cancer. Twenty-three patients (15%) had a second primary oral cancer. In a similar follow-up study at UCSF involving 204 patients with carcinoma of the oral tongue who were observed between 1940 and 1971, 19% had second primary cancers, and 61% of these were second oral primary malignancies (12% of the total group). A 1981 report of 377 patients treated for cancer in the floor of the

Table 1–5. ORAL CANCER: COMPARING SITES AND STAGE AT DIAGNOSIS, UNITED STATES, 1973–1996

	1973–1984		1985–1996	
Site	*n*	L (%)	*n*	L (%)
Tongue	4,794	44	5,993	45
Lip	4,014	86	3,402	94
Mouth floor	3,042	43	2,804	44
Other sites	4,135	41	4,701	43

Adapted from the National Cancer Institute's SEER (Surveillance, Epidemiology, and End Results) Program.
L = localized tumor (cancer stages 1 and 2); *n* = number of cases.

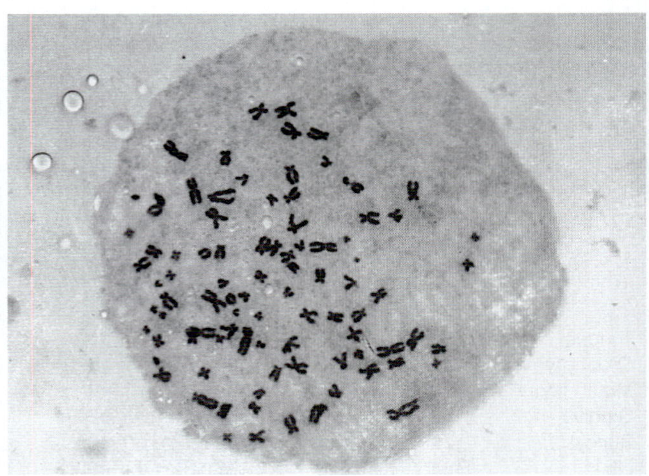

Figure 1–1. Chromosome preparation from a malignant cell; note aneuploidy. Karyotyping is used to characterize aberrations of cancer cells.

mouth found that 18% developed new cancers of the respiratory and upper digestive tracts and 9% had second primary cancers occurring in the mouth. Studies reported in 1992, 1994, and 1995 from three different centers further support the previous findings. Second primary tumors were common in those patients who already had oral and pharyngeal carcinomas, with occurrences ranging as follows: 9.1% in a median time of 36 months in 3,436 patients; a yearly rate of 3.7% among 21,371 patients from data collected between 1973 and 1987; and 19% of 851 patients followed from 1978 to 1990. In all three reports, tobacco increased the risks, and most second primaries were in oral and oropharyngeal sites. Second primary tumors occurred more often than expected.

A report from our clinic in 1994 showed that 72% of 403 patients with oral and pharyngeal cancers smoked.[14] Of those who continued to smoke after diagnosis and treatment, 36% developed second primary oral/oropharyngeal cancer, compared with 14% in those patients who never smoked, stopped smoking, or greatly reduced their smoking. In a recent Japanese study reported in 2002,[15] among 1,609 early-stage oral and pharyngeal squamous cell carcinoma patients, 333 second primary cancers were documented in 258 patients; 235 (71%) of the second primary carcinomas occurred in respiratory and upper digestive anatomic sites.

MORTALITY

Worldwide, cancer of various forms accounts for more than 2 million deaths each year. In the United States, cancer is a leading killer, second only to cardiovascular disease (Table 1–6). In women over 50, cancer is the leading cause of death. Cancer is responsible for about 1 of every 4 American deaths—more than 550,000 deaths each year (more than 10,000 deaths every week!). Someone in the United States dies of cancer almost every minute.

The number of cancer deaths has risen almost without interruption in the United States. Oral and pharyngeal cancers cause nearly 10,000 deaths yearly, accounting for about 0.4% of all deaths (see Table 1–6). The relative survival rate of black patients is lower than that of white patients and, in recent years, these figures have apparently not improved (Table 1–7). This observation may be attributable to socioeconomic disadvantages in the health care system, as well as to the known greater prevalence of smoking and alcohol consumption in that population. Oral and pharyngeal cancer occurrence and mortality rates are lower in Asians and Hispanics than in whites and blacks. For a comparison with some other cancer sites, see Table 1–8. Death rates from around the world (Table 1–9) suggest marked differences in the occurrence of oral cancer, variations that probably reflect different combinations of ethnic, cultural, and environmental factors.

Table 1–6. SELECTED CAUSES OF DEATH, UNITED STATES, 2001 (2,337,256)

Rank	Disease	*n*	Rate	% of Deaths
1	Heart disease	724,860	189.0	31.0
2	Cancer	541,530	162.0	23.2
3	Stroke	158,450	39.0	6.8
6	Pneumonia	91,870	21.9	3.9
7	Diabetes	64,750	18.5	2.8
10	Cirrhosis	25,190	8.1	1.1
15	AIDS	13,430	4.0	0.6

Adapted from the National Center for Health Statistics, Centers for Disease Control and Prevention.
n = number of cases.

ACQUIRED IMMUNE DEFICIENCY SYNDROME

The current epidemic of the acquired immune deficiency syndrome (AIDS) continues unabated, with more than 36 million persons throughout the world now infected with the human immunodeficiency virus (HIV). As the virus multiplies and mutates, producing immune deficiency, the now immunocompromised host is at risk of developing malignancies as well as opportunistic infections. The malignancies associated with HIV infection can occur in the head and neck and involve the oral cavity and pharynx. These primarily

Table 1–7. ORAL CANCER: 5-YEAR RELATIVE SURVIVAL RATES (%), UNITED STATES

Race	1974–1976	1983–1985	1992–1997
White	55	55	58
Black	36	35	34
All races	53	53	56

Adapted from CA Cancer J Clin 2001;51:35.

Table 1–8. CANCER IN THE UNITED STATES, 2002: ESTIMATES FOR SELECTED SITES			
Site	New Cases	M:F*	Deaths
All sites	1,284,900	1.00	555,500
Breast	202,000	—	39,600
Prostate	189,000	—	30,200
Lung	169,400	1.10	154,900
Colorectal	148,000	0.96	56,600
Urinary bladder	56,500	2.80	12,600
Kidney	31,800	1.50	11,600
Pancreas	30,300	0.94	29,700

Adapted from the American Cancer Society, Cancer Facts and Figures, 2002. Oral and pharyngeal cancers account for about 30,100 new cases.
*Male-to-female ratio.

include Kaposi's sarcoma, non-Hodgkin's lymphoma, and squamous cell carcinoma. Therefore, establishing the diagnosis, infection control, and treatment are all-important considerations for health professionals (see Chapter 12, "Human Immunodeficiency Virus–Associated Oral Malignancies").

Table 1–9. AGE-ADJUSTED DEATH RATES FOR ORAL CANCER PER 100,000 POPULATION*		
Country	Men (Rank)	Women (Rank)
Hungary	20.0 (1)	2.4 (1)
Slovakia	16.8 (2)	1.2 (15)
France	11.3 (5)	1.3 (9)
Russian Federation	9.1 (8)	1.1 (26)
Spain	7.0 (14)	0.9 (36)
Germany	6.5 (15)	1.2 (14)
Cuba	5.5 (20)	1.5 (4)
Denmark	4.5 (23)	1.6 (3)
Canada	3.8 (27)	1.2 (17)
United States	3.2 (29)	1.1 (23)
Japan	3.1 (31)	0.8 (37)
United Kingdom	2.9 (32)	1.1 (22)
Netherlands	2.8 (33)	1.0 (32)
China	2.6 (36)	1.1 (24)
Venezuela	2.5 (37)	1.2 (11)
Sweden	2.2 (40)	0.9 (35)
Chile	2.1 (42)	0.6 (43)
Mexico	1.9 (43)	0.7 (41)
Israel	1.5 (45)	0.7 (40)

Adapted from CA Cancer J Clin 2000;50:32–3.
*Selected from 45 nations studied by the World Health Organization, 1994–1997.

REFERENCES

1. Mahboubi E. The epidemiology of oral cavity, pharyngeal and esophageal cancer outside of North America and Western Europe. Cancer 1977;40:1879–86.
2. Myers JN, Elkins T, Roberts D, Byers RM. Squamous cell carcinoma of the tongue in young adults: increasing incidence and factors that predict treatment outcomes. Otolaryngol Head Neck Surg 2000;122:44–51.
3. Pitman KT, Johnson JT, Wagner RL, Myers EN. Cancer of the tongue in patients less than forty. Head Neck 2000;22: 297–302.
4. Schantz SP, Yu G-P. Head and neck cancer incidence trends in young Americans, 1973-1997, with a special analysis for tongue cancer. Arch Otolaryngol Head Neck Surg 2002;128:268–74.
5. Edwards BK, Howe HL, Ries LA, et al. Annual report to the nation on the status of cancer, 1973–1999, featuring implications of age and aging on U.S. cancer burden. Cancer 2002;94:2766–92.
6. Shiboski CH, Shiboski SC, Silverman S Jr. Trends in oral cancer rates in the United States, 1973-1996. Community Dent Oral Epidemiol 2000;28:249–56.
7. Silverman S Jr. Demographics and occurrence of oral and pharyngeal cancers: the outcomes, the trends, the challenge. J Am Dent Assoc 2001;132:7S–11S.
8. Albert S, Child M. Familial cancer in the general population. Cancer 1977;40:1674–9.
9. Day GL, Blot WJ. Second primary tumors in patients with oral cancer. Cancer 1992;70:14–9.
10. Jones AS, Morar P, Phillips DE, et al. Second primary tumors in patients with head and neck squamous cell carcinoma. Cancer 1995;75:1343–53.
11. Schwartz LH, Ozahin M, Zhang GN, et al. Synchronous and metachronous head and neck carcinomas. Cancer 1994;74:1933–8.
12. Tepperman BS, Fitzpatrick PJ. Second respiratory and upper digestive tract cancers after oral cancer. Lancet 1981; 2:547–9.
13. Wynder EL, Mushinski MH, Spivak JC. Tobacco and alcohol consumption in relation to the development of multiple primary cancers. Cancer 1977;40:1872–8.
14. Gorsky M, Silverman S Jr. Tobacco use in patients with head and neck carcinomas: habit changes and second primary oral/pharyngeal cancers in patients from San Francisco. Cancer J 1994;7:78–80.
15. Yamamoto E, Shibuya H, Yoshimura R, Miura M. Site specific dependency of second primary cancer in early stage head and neck squamous cell carcinoma. Cancer 2002; 94:2007–14.

2

Etiology and Predisposing Factors

SOL SILVERMAN JR., MA, DDS
CRAIG S. MILLER, DMD, MS (Viruses)
JOAN S. THOMPSON, PhD, RD, CD (Nutrition)

The exact cause of oral cancer is unknown and may remain a mystery because of the multifactorial nature of carcinogenesis. Evidence indicates that although inherited genes do influence cancer risk, heredity alone explains only a fraction of all cancers. Mutations of genes and the proteins they produce can alter cell biochemistry and function, causing disease. On the other hand, alterations of genes (gene therapy) may prevent mutations, control cell growth and apoptosis (cell death), and become an important approach in cancer treatment.

Because time is needed for the cellular events involved in the development of neoplasia to take place, the most prominent associated factor determining susceptibility to cancer is age (see Chapter 1, "Epidemiology"). Variations in incidence rates among different groups or populations may be influenced by differences in exposure to carcinogenic initiators or promotors. For example, the use of tobacco or alcohol significantly increases the risk of cancer, indicating an etiologic role. The role of other factors in promoting human cancer remains important but unclear. For example, immunologic susceptibility, gene mutations, epithelial cell growth, suppressor proteins, and enzyme action all influence cell stability and health. At a certain time, a cell or group of cells may undergo uncontrolled growth. This capacity for disorderly division continues in daughter cells, and if dysregulation remains uncontrolled, a cancer may develop through the production or inactivation of proteins, causing local destruction of tissues and organs, extensions, and metastasis. In 20 generations, 1 cell, with progeny that maintain the ability to duplicate themselves, becomes the source of more than 1 million cells. However, because some of the cells comprising a malignant tumor do not maintain the ability to divide, and the number of generations varies considerably, growth patterns of tumors are highly irregular and unpredictable.

Humans are exposed continually and simultaneously to a broad spectrum of biologic agents, chemical substances, and physical forces. To complicate matters even more, each individual reacts somewhat differently to these events. As indicated above and from the occurrence and demographics of oral and pharyngeal cancer described in Chapter 1, individual reactions differ, conditioned by heredity, age, gender, and a multitude of other modifiers, including lifestyles and behavior. Current evidence suggests one conclusion more strongly than any other: there are probably multiple causes for every type of cancer.

MOLECULAR PROGRESSION

Neoplasms arise clonally from transformed cells that have undergone specific genetic alterations in proto-oncogenes or tumor suppressor genes.[1] As just one example, loss of chromosomal region 9p21 is a common genetic change that occurs early in tumor progression. This leads to an inhibition of cyclin-dependent kinase that is important in cell-cycle regulation. Additionally, a large number of malignant cells express a mutation of the suppressor *p53* gene, which, in turn, diminishes cell senescence and indirectly promotes growth. Molecular genetics is gradually enabling us to unravel some of the critical events associated with the development of head and neck cancer and precancer.[1a] Unfortunately, early genetic alterations do not necessarily correlate with gross or microscopic changes, which obviously can complicate clinical observations and judgments.

As already stated, activation of proto-oncogenes and/or loss of tumor suppressor genes can result in the stimulation of cell division. As another phenomenon, telomeres, composed of repeating sequences of six nucleotides, are situated at the end of chromosomes. They influence the longevity of cells and regulate their biologic clock by progressive shortening. When activated by telomerase, telomere growth may prevent cell senescence by maintaining chromosomal integrity. Thus, telomeres may be a potentially important target in controlling cancer. The complexity and multifactorial aspects of explaining neoplasia are evident.

IMMUNE SYSTEM

Immune competence and immune cell surveillance diminish with age. These facts undoubtedly contribute to the association between age and malignancy. Furthermore, studies have shown that the risks of cancer increase in individuals whose immune systems are either congenitally defective or have been suppressed or altered by disease and/or medications. For persons in the general population who develop oral cancers and who are not otherwise known to have or be at risk of immunodeficiency, it is not clear whether differences found in some immunologic variables cause or result from the malignancy. As our understanding and control of the immune system progress, a role in prevention and treatment (immunotherapy) will attain increasing importance.

TOBACCO

Smoking may be viewed as a worldwide epidemic, causing serious diseases and immense health problems.[2] Apart from its effect on mortality, smoking results in a considerably increased morbidity rate with consequent losses in working days and productivity, excessive demand on medical services, and increased health expenditures.[3]

Tobacco was first introduced to western civilization by the Spanish explorers of America in the early sixteenth century. At first, it was simply smoked in pipes, but, as it became more popular, it was also chewed and snuffed. Cigarettes were first made in Spain in the mid-seventeenth century, and, in the twentieth century, they became the most popular form of the tobacco habit.

Suspicion of an association between the use of tobacco and oral cancer dates back to the early eighteenth century, when cancer of the lip was noted among tobacco users. Several other serious diseases, among them lung cancer, emphysema, bronchitis, laryngeal cancer, and heart disease, affect smokers more often than nonsmokers. For the heaviest smokers, the risks are greatest.

Tobacco Components

More than 4,000 compounds have been identified in tobacco smoke. In the combustion mainstream of one cigarette, there are approximately 500 mg of gas (92%) and particulate matter (8%). Eighty-five percent of the gaseous phase is composed of carbon dioxide, oxygen, and nitrogen. Even though the percentage of carbon monoxide is low, it raises blood levels of this gas significantly, in turn influencing the hemoglobin exchange system. "Tars" (aromatic hydrocarbons) range from < 1 mg to 35 mg and contain the most potent carcinogens. Nicotine ranges from < 1 mg to 3 mg and contributes to habituation, platelet adhesion associated with cardiovascular disease, ulcer susceptibility from decreased pancreatic bicarbonate, and hypertension. Effective filtering can reduce these substances. However, reductions in nicotine (the habituation factor) and tars (the basis for tobacco's "taste") often lead to increased smoking, negating the potential advantage.[4] In addition, many filters do not filter effectively. Tobacco substitutes (ie, vegetable and wood products) and "smokeless" cigarettes have not been popular and have therefore been financial as well as therapeutic failures.

Tobacco Use and Health

Globally, the consequences of tobacco use are staggering. By the year 2020, it is estimated that 8.4 million people will die annually from tobacco-related diseases, more than two-thirds occurring in developing countries. If current trends continue, more people will perish annually from tobacco-related illness than from any single disease.

Reports from the US surgeon general and others conclude that cigarette smoking is the main single cause of cancer mortality in the United States, contributing to an estimated 30% of all cancer deaths and substantially to cancers of the head and neck. A federal law requires that health warnings be printed on all cigarette packages sold in the United States.

Despite intensified warnings about the health hazards of smoking, American consumption continues at substantial rates, exceeding 600 billion cigarettes annually. About 23% of adult Americans smoke regularly (Table 2–1). The level of schooling has an important influence because the prevalence of smoking is inversely proportional to years of education. Smoking habits tend to decrease after middle age, most likely owing to medical reasons requiring cessation. There is no question that high taxes have also been a deterrent.

A recent federal report describing smoking trends among American high school students indicated that in 2001, almost 29% of students in grades 9 through 12 were current smokers and 14% were everyday smokers.[4a] However, this is a significant decline from the 36% rate found in 1997. Smoking frequency was about equal between males and females, with only a very slight predominance in boys. There was a marked increase in smoking from ninth graders (24%) to twelfth graders (35%). There were also racial differences noted, with the greatest use being in whites and declining in order from Hispanics, to Asians, to blacks. Whereas the smoking rate in black adolescents is the lowest among all racial and ethnic groups in the United States (except American Indians), in adulthood, they have the highest rate. The most popular form of tobacco use was smoking cigarettes, followed by cigars, pipes, and bidis. About 6% of the students had tried a tobacco product by age 11.

Although over 45 million Americans have quit smoking, the exact magnitude of their lowered risk for oral cancer is unclear. The percentage of dentists and physicians who smoke has dropped from more than 30% to less than 20% during the past two decades.

Table 2–1. ADULT SMOKING, UNITED STATES, 2000

Region	Men Range % (avr)	Women Range % (avr)	Total Average (%)
Northeast	16–26 (21.7)	16–27 (21.0)	20.8
Midwest	17–35 (26.4)	17–28 (22.0)	23.7
South	17–32 (25.2)	15–29 (21.0)	23.2
West	14–33 (22.4)	12–31 (19.4)	20.6
	14–35 (24.0)	12–31 (21.4)	22.7

Adapted from MMWR Morb Mortal Wkly Rep, December 2001.

Oral Cancer Risk and Smoking

The association between cigarette use and oral carcinoma has been firmly established from epidemiologic studies, revealing that there are more than twice as many smokers among oral cancer patients as among control populations. A study of 403 oral and pharyngeal cancer patients followed for a mean of 5.1 years at the University of California at San Francisco (UCSF) found that 72% were smokers and 58% smoked more than one pack daily (Table 2–2), demonstrating the very high risk for tobacco users. As discussed in Chapter 1, smoking increases the already high risk for developing second primary oral and pharyngeal cancers.

Table 2–3 shows, in a follow-up study, that almost one of five patients (17.7%) developed second primary oral/oropharyngeal cancers in a mean time of 5 years. Those who did not change their original tobacco habits incurred the greatest risk as a second primary oropharyngeal cancer developed in 25.6% of that group. Discontinuing smoking led to the same rate of second primary oropharyngeal cancer as in nonsmokers. There was also an increased risk for multiple cancers in males, probably because they smoked more per day than women and for a greater number of years.

A similar degree of correlation between smoking and second primaries has been reported in other studies. One study concerned a group of 203 oral and laryngopharyngeal cancer patients in whom the disease had been eradicated for more than 3 years. Of 120 patients who continued to smoke, 37% developed second primary cancers, whereas only 6% of 81 ex-smokers developed second primaries.

Table 2–2. TOBACCO USE IN 403 PATIENTS WITH ORAL/PHARYNGEAL CARCINOMAS

		Sex (%)		Age (yr)			
Cancer Site	*n*	M	F	Mean	Range	Tobacco Users (%)	More Than 1 Pack/Day (%)
Floor of the mouth	70	59	41	57	(29–76)	94	81
Larynx	33	48	52	59	(40–82)	94	79
Lip	7	71	29	61	(25–87)	86	43
Oropharynx	52	48	52	59	(25–81)	83	63
Tongue	142	64	36	55	(25–81)	69	56
Buccal mucosa	16	44	56	66	(29–84)	56	50
Hard palate	4	25	75	61	(48–77)	50	25
Gingiva	34	47	53	55	(43–81)	44	38
Nasopharynx	45	71	29	44	(24–71)	42	29
Total	403	58	42	56	(24–87)	72	58

Source: University of California at San Francisco.

The combined effects of tobacco and alcohol were illustrated in another study of 351 patients treated for tongue cancer. Forty-three patients abstained from both tobacco and alcohol, and 308 were users of one or both. The abstainers had a mortality of 14% in 5 years, whereas the users had a mortality rate of 31%. A second primary cancer occurred in 11% of the abstainers compared with 20% of the users. Obviously, cofactors are critically important.

Numerous laboratory studies have shown that some hydrocarbons isolated from tobacco products have induced buccal carcinomas in animals under certain experimental conditions. Benzo[*a*]pyrene, the most potent of these carcinogens, binds to nucleoproteins and is mutagenic as well as carcinogenic. The association between tobacco use and oral malignancies also appears to include cigars, pipes, and smokeless preparations.

Pipes, Cigars, Snuff, and Smokeless Tobacco

Carcinogenic agents have been isolated from pipe, cigar, and smokeless tobaccos. Although studies of these forms of tobacco use have not been as extensive as those of cigarettes, the data show a strong association between noncigarette forms of tobacco and mouth cancer. The surgeon general's report of 1964 concluded that "the causal relationship of the smoking of pipes to the development of cancer of the lip appears to be established" (Figures 2–1 and 2–2). Fortunately, the incidence of lip cancer has been declining slowly (see Chapter 1).

Whereas the production and consumption of pipe tobacco have decreased slightly over the years, there has been a recent increase in cigars and cigarillos. Regarding cigar smoking in the United States, approximately 5 million cigars are smoked each year, and the use has increased 50% during the past 5 years; women now account for about 5% of all cigar smokers.[5] Twenty-seven percent of teenagers between 14 and 19 years of age have smoked cigars. There are no government regulations on labels, which further complicates control. Studies have shown an increased risk for heart and lung diseases, as well as cancers of the mouth, larynx, esophagus, and lungs, in cigar users. An explanation in part is because, in general, cigars have 7 times greater tar content, contain 4 times greater amounts of nicotine, and produce 11 times greater amounts of carbon monoxide than do cigarettes. Furthermore, cigar wrappings using tobacco leaf further increase the amounts and dangers of

Table 2–3. SMOKING HABITS AMONG 277 ORAL CANCER PATIENTS

	Smoking Status (*n*)		Cancer Status (*n*)
Tobacco Use	At Time of Cancer Diagnosis (%)	1-Year Post-treatment (%)	Second Primary Oropharyngeal Cancer (%)*
Yes	187 (67.5)	90 (48)	23 (25.6)
Discontinued	97 (52)	13 (13.4)	
No†	90 (32.5)	90 (100)	13 (14.4)

Source: Oral Medicine Clinic, University of California at San Francisco, 1989.
*Follow-up mean = 5 years.
†Never smoked or stopped > 1 year.

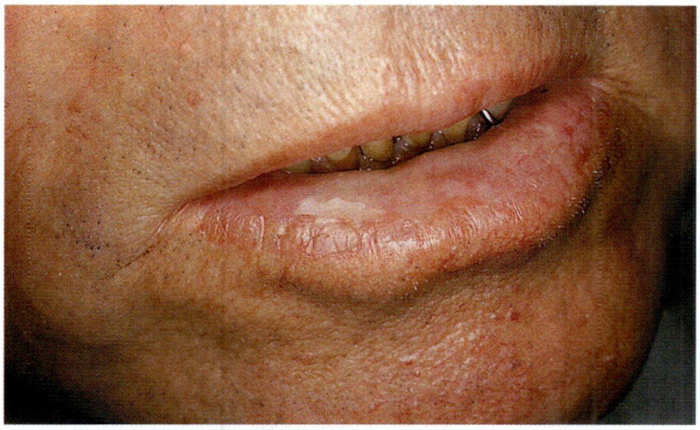

Figures 2–1, 2–2. Relationship between pipe smoking and lip cancer.
Figure 2–1. Precancerous leukoplakic lesion at site of chronic contact with pipe stem.

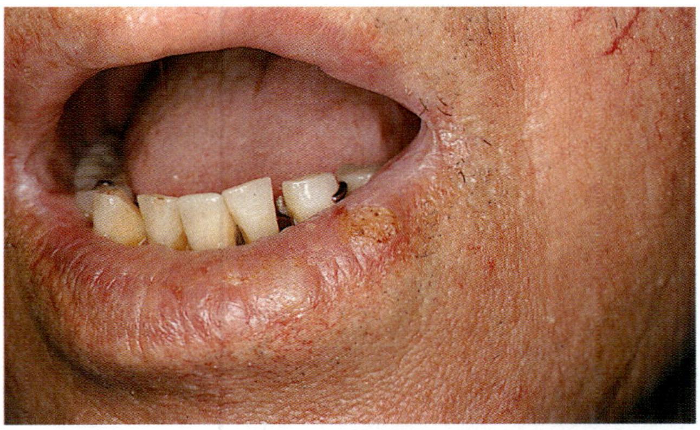

Figure 2–2. Early squamous cell carcinoma at site where pipe stem was habitually held for more than 10 years.

these substances. Obviously, the levels of toxic substances vary between brands and with patient smoking profiles. Given these variations, some comparisons between cigarettes and cigars have shown that the amount of nicotine and tars in one cigar is equivalent to those contained in as much as half a pack to a full pack of cigarettes.

The carcinogenic hazard of snuff dipping and tobacco chewing causes special concern because of the marked upswing of smokeless tobacco consumption in the United States (Figures 2–3 to 2–8). It has been estimated that over 12 million Americans (3 million under age 21) use smokeless tobacco.[6] Its use among teenagers is increasing and poses a danger for increased oral cancer in the future (see Table 2–2). In the southeastern United States, where women frequently use snuff or chewing tobacco, there is a higher than expected incidence of oral cancer in women, together with a higher mortality. A case-control study in North Carolina of 255 women with oral and oropharyngeal cancer showed an up to 50-fold risk for cancers of the gingiva and buccal mucosa in long-term habitual snuff dippers. A report on 201 oral cancer patients at M. D. Anderson Cancer Center in Texas showed that 46 (23%) used snuff or chewing tobacco. Twenty of these patients reported that, for an average of 44 years, they had consistently held the tobacco at the site where the cancer developed. Smokeless tobacco's influence on carcinogenesis appears to be associated with long-term use, information that should encourage people in cessation programs, particularly young athletes. It must be pointed out that there are different risks with different brands, obviously depending on the ingredients. Reflecting geographic differences, in a recent report regarding Swedish snuff users, there was no association with oral cancer. In summary, though, smokeless ("spit") tobacco is not a safe substitute for combustible tobacco products.

Nitrosamines (*N*-nitrosonornicotine being the most potent) have been identified as noncombustible products in snuff and chewing tobacco that possess carcinogenic activity.[7] Other carcinogens are found in smaller quantities (hydrocarbons and polonium). Interestingly, tobacco products are not regulated by the US Food and Drug Administration (FDA), and the nitrosamine levels far exceed those permitted in foods (as preservatives). Both sugar and fluoride contents are higher in chewing tobacco than in other forms of tobacco.[8] However, a firm relationship between different tobacco forms and dental caries has not been established. On the other hand, many studies have shown an association between smoking and periodontal disease.[9]

Nicotine levels are high and serve as a potent factor in habituation, addiction, and hypertension. The salt contained in smokeless tobaccos also contributes to high blood pressure. The most common conditions found with the use of smokeless tobacco are gingival recession, hyperkeratosis, and staining. Once again, the risk of oral epithelial dysplasia or carcinoma increases with long-term use of smokeless tobacco products.

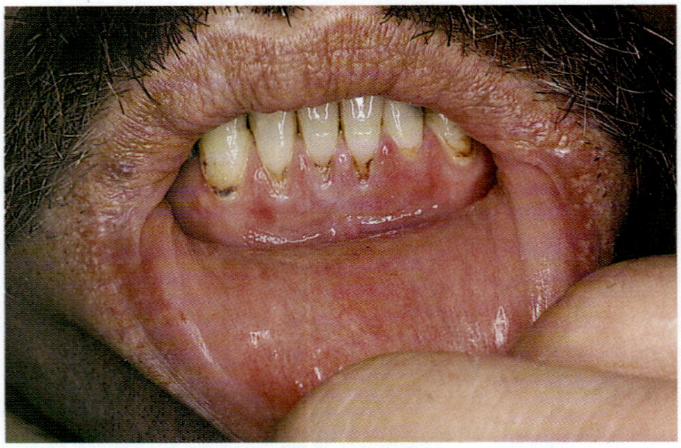

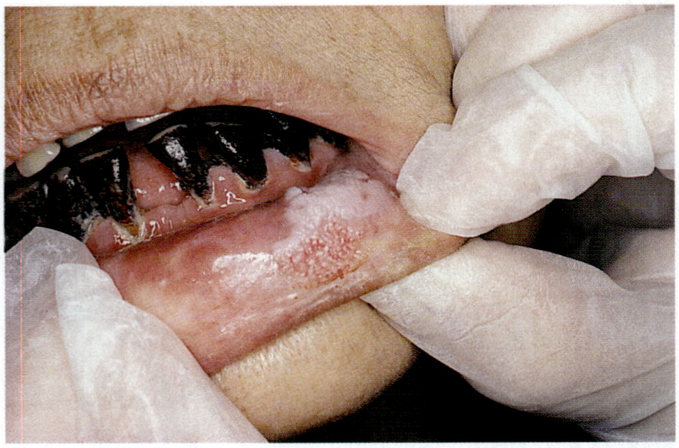

Figures 2–3 to 2–8. Tissue changes caused by prolonged contact with tobacco.

Figure 2–3. Gingival recession and loss of attachment are common early changes at sites where smokeless tobacco is held.

Figure 2–6. Leukoplakia of the lower labial mucosa at site where patient held tobacco during a 27-year habit. Microscopic epithelial dysplasia and intense dental staining occurred.

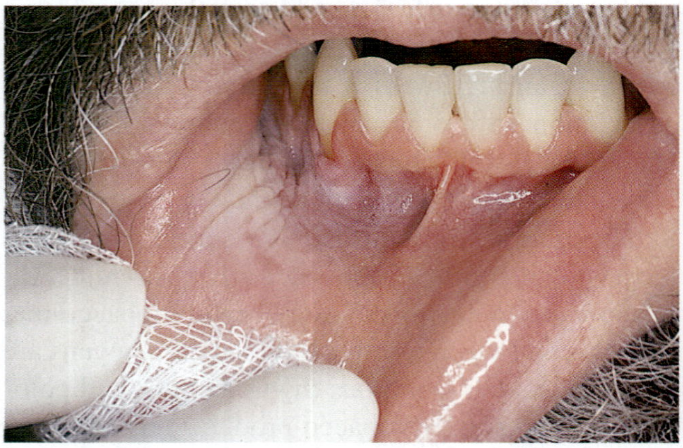

Figure 2–4. Patient habitually held tobacco at this site for more than 5 years.

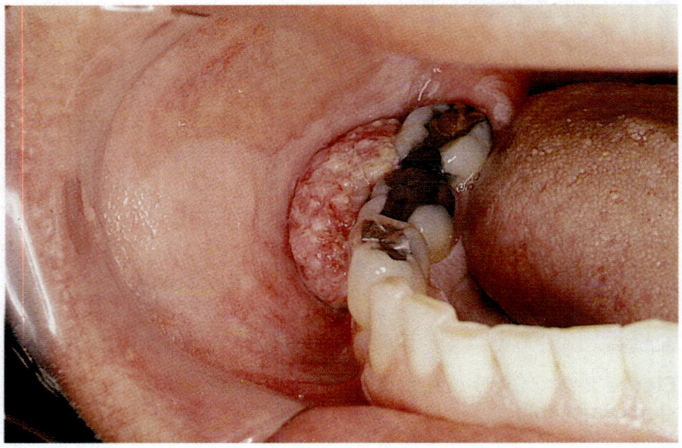

Figure 2–7. Snuff was held daily buccal to lower right molars for 20 years. A biopsy showed verrucous carcinoma.

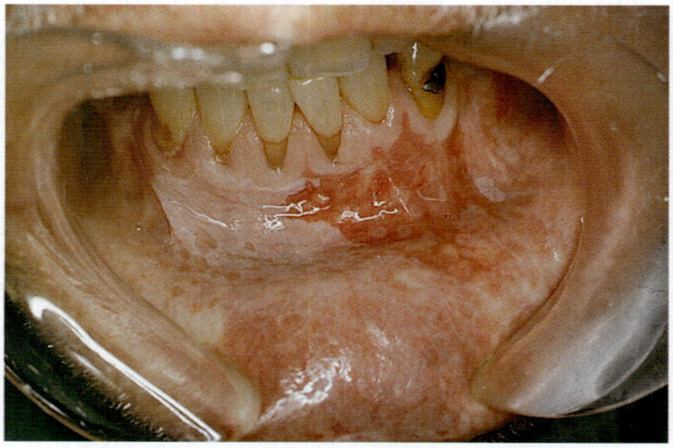

Figure 2–5. Patient held tobacco between lower lip and gingiva for more than 5 years, inducing this erythroleukoplakic mucosal lesion.

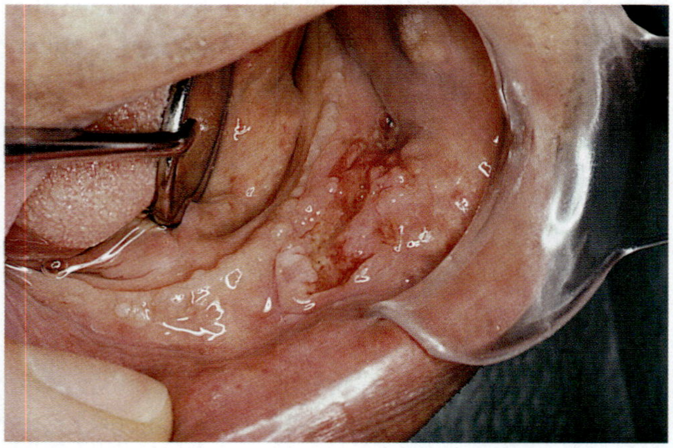

Figure 2–8. Squamous cell carcinoma at site where snuff was habitually held for more than 30 years.

Smoking and Survival

The hazards of smoking can also be demonstrated by the survival time of oral cancer patients after diagnosis and treatment. In a UCSF report of 874 patients with intraoral squamous cell carcinoma, the 5-year survival rate for nonsmokers was 43%, compared with 27% for smokers. In a group of 203 oral and laryngopharyngeal cancer patients studied at another center, 65% of the nonsmokers were alive at the end of 13 years, whereas only 30% of the smokers survived the same period.

Smoking Cessation

Because tobacco plays such an important role in oral carcinogenesis, stopping the habit is a fundamental part of prevention and treatment.[10,11] Many approaches have been used, with varying degrees of success.

Fear

Although fear motivates some people to stop smoking, in others it may backfire and even increase tobacco use by promoting fear as well as inducing other psychological problems.

Filters

Apparently, as filters become more effective in reducing tar and nicotine, their effectiveness in breaking the tobacco habit decreases. This finding points out the importance of taste and habituation, which are related to tar and nicotine content.

Aversive Conditioning

Methods to make tobacco smoking or taste objectionable, such as chemical additives, electric shock, and hypnosis, have not been reproducibly effective. Clinics, organized groups, self-help methods, and manuals have helped some persons and are promoted widely. Studies have not yet convincingly documented their long-term value.

"Cold Turkey"

Stopping abruptly rather than gradually has been successful for some patients who are well motivated and can effectively assign priorities to their lifestyle and goals.

Advertising Regulations and Legislation

These approaches have been ineffective in stemming the increasing consumption of tobacco and habituation at an early age. However, taxation and the increased cost of smoking seem to have some influence in reducing tobacco use.

Counseling

Counseling can be accomplished in brief or intense sessions with individuals or in groups. Leadership can involve a variety of professionals with special training in tobacco cessation.

Pharmacotherapy

Nicotine replacement. Because of nicotine habituation and/or addiction, "breaking the habit" may be accomplished by substituting other sources for nicotine needs. Probably the most popular have been the transdermal patches, which yield a stable, fixed dose in decreasing amounts. These patches can be obtained over the counter without prescription. Gum (Nicorette, 2 or 4 mg of nicotine per stick), a nasal spray, and vapor inhalers are other alternatives for nicotine replacement. Amounts needed vary from patient to patient, and, of course, a patient's physician should be notified. The nicotine from these sources can irritate oral and pharyngeal mucosae as well as cause other side effects, such as nausea and dizziness. Also, they lead to rapid peak blood levels followed by irregular and varying concentrations in amount and duration.

Drugs. Some antidepressant medications have been useful. The most widely used has been bupropion (Zyban) in doses up to 300 mg per day. Bupropion has dopaminergic and noradrenergenic properties. There can be many adverse side effects, including xerostomia, irritability, insomnia, and behavior changes.

Clinical trials involving pharmacotherapy have demonstrated some limited efficacy—usually a 40 to 60% smoking cessation by individuals at the end of treatment but only 25 to 30% at 1-year follow-up

(Table 2–4). The best results are seen when pharmacotherapy and counseling are combined.

Other Carcinogenic Habit Forms

Social customs that can lead to cancer are complex and far-reaching. Some customs, such as betel and tobacco dipping, are widespread and seem to satisfy important human cravings. In the areas of the world where these habits are practiced, the incidence of oropharyngeal tumors is comparatively high. Prevalence varies considerably in different countries, depending on the manner in which the ingredients are prepared for chewing.

Reports from India reveal that oral carcinoma accounts for a high percentage of total cancers, ranging from 15 to 65%, with the largest prevalence in the south. A relationship appears to exist between this extremely high occurrence of oral malignancy and the use of various forms and combinations of tobacco, slaked lime, areca nuts, and spices (Figures 2–9 to 2–11). In Taiwan, betel (areca nut prepared with lime) is widely used, resulting in an unusually high rate of oral cancer, with the main site being buccal mucosa (Figure 2–12).

In many areas throughout the world, members of low socioeconomic groups smoke rolled tobacco leaves or small cigars with the lit end placed in the mouth, termed "reverse smoking" (Figures 2–13 to 2–15). In some of these areas, the incidence of palatal carcinoma is high.

Precancerous Lesions

Tobacco may clearly induce benign clinical changes of the oral mucosa in the form of red and/or white lesions (leukoplakia, erythroplakia, erythroleukoplakia). These changes are considered premalignant because

Table 2–4. SMOKING CESSATION: GENERAL RESPONSE AFTER 1 YEAR

	Counseling (%)		
Pharmacotherapy	None	Brief	Full
None	5	10	15
Drug/nicotine*	10	20	30

*Bupropion and/or nicotine replacement.

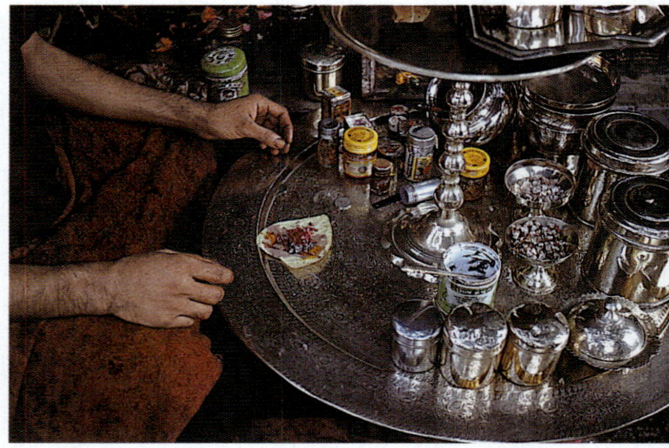

Figures 2–9 to 2–11. Pan habit in India.
Figure 2–9. Varying ingredients, including tobacco, areca (betel) nut, lime, and spices, are placed in the betel leaf, which is then folded and held in the mouth for prolonged periods of time.

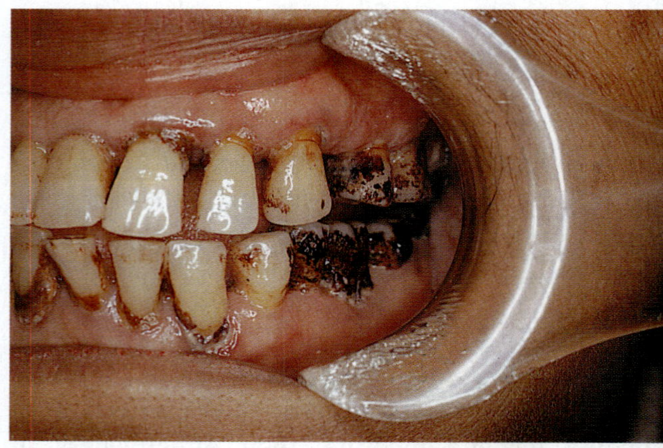

Figure 2–10. Note usual tooth staining resulting from the use of pan.

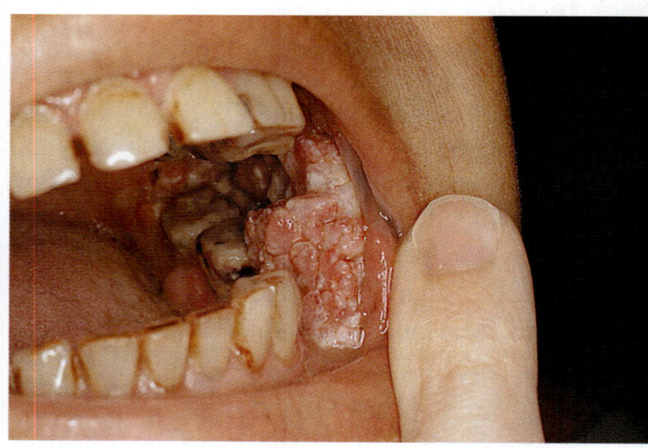

Figure 2–11. After prolonged pan usage, the risk of squamous cell carcinoma at the habit site increases.

some may transform into malignancies. Those with certain clinical features or degrees of epithelial cell dysplasia are at greater risk (see Chapter 3, "Leukoplakia and Erythroplakia"). However, not all oral cancers are preceded by clinical, precancerous lesions.

Summary

The use of tobacco in all forms—cigarettes, cigars, pipes, chewing preparations, and snuff—increases the risk of eventually developing oral carcinoma, which appears to be causally related to this use. This association is based on the following facts:

1. Carcinogenic agents have been isolated from tobacco condensates.
2. Tobacco can induce cellular change and tissue atypia.
3. Patients with oral carcinoma use tobacco more than persons in control groups do.
4. Tobacco used in various forms has been associated with an unusually high prevalence of carcinoma of specific oral sites.
5. Continued smoking is a factor in the development of multiple oral carcinomas.
6. The mortality ratio from oral carcinoma for smokers is greater than for nonsmokers.

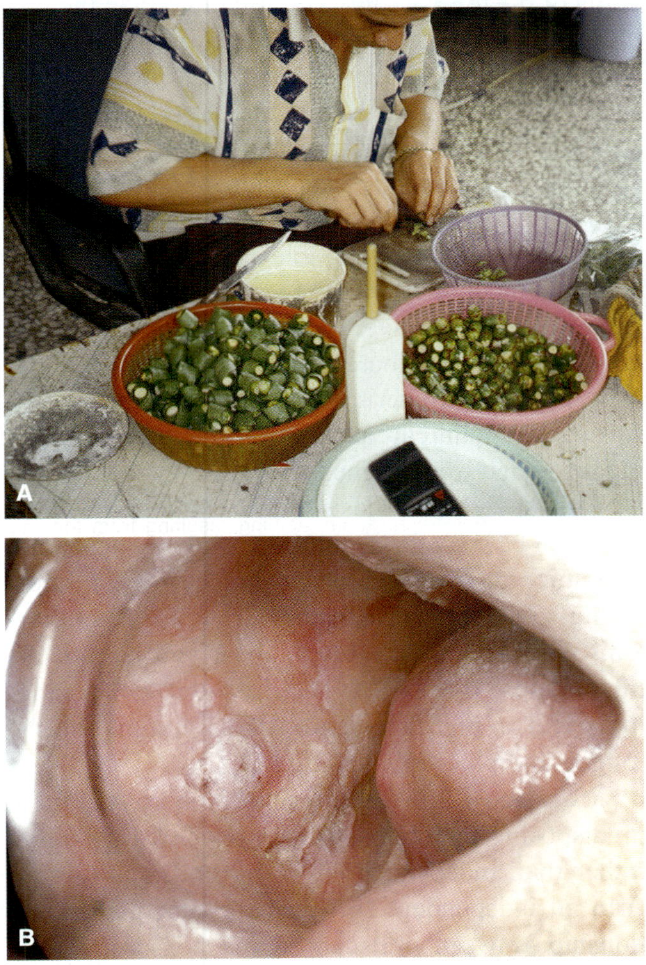

Figure 2–12. Areca nut–chewing habit in Taiwan. *A*, Areca nut prepared with lime (calcium hydroxide). The lime increases mucosal absorption of arecoline (a parasympathomimetic agent that has some carcinogenic properties). *B*, Long-standing leukoplakia at the site of holding the nut.

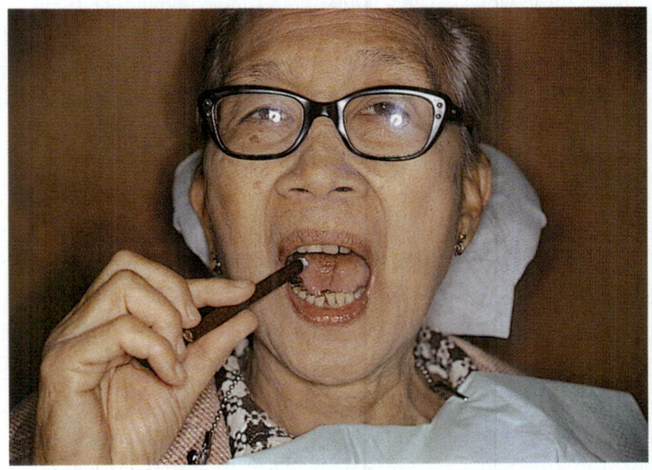

Figures 2–13, 2–14. Reverse smoking habit of many decades' duration.

Figure 2–13. Lit end of the cigarillo is held inside the mouth.

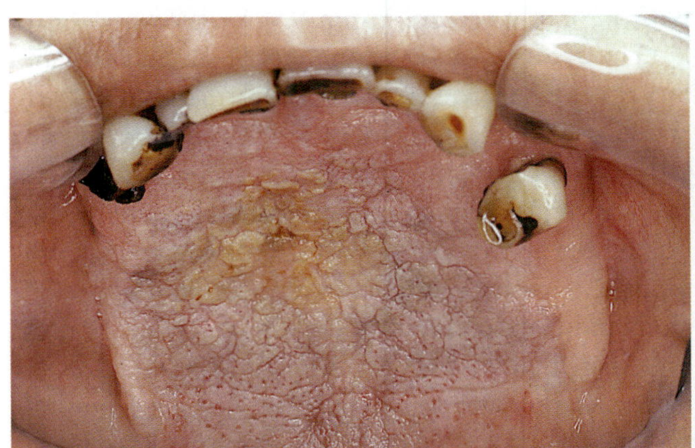

Figure 2–14. The palatal leukoplakia is mildly symptomatic. The risk of dysplastic and malignant changes is moderately high.

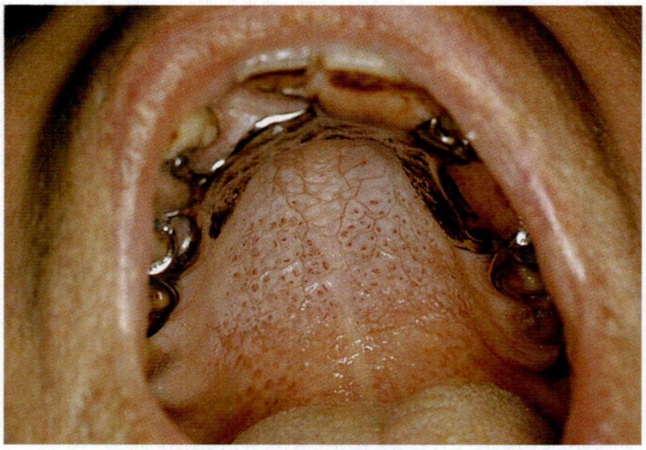

Figure 2–15. Smoker's palate (nicotinic stomatitis), primarily seen in pipe smokers. Typical clinical picture includes hyperkeratosis and swollen minor salivary glands with dilated and reddened orifices (giving the speckled appearance). Malignant transformation is very rare.

ALCOHOL, CIRRHOSIS, AND CANCER

Death from cirrhosis (primarily owing to alcohol intake) is the eighth leading disease cause of death in the United States. This high incidence of alcoholism is relevant because alcohol intake has been related to an increased risk of developing oral cancer and a higher than expected mortality.[12,13]

More than 35 years ago, a study determined that heavy alcohol consumption was a significant factor in the development of mouth cancer. In that study, one-third of the 543 male oral cancer patients drank more than 7 ounces of whiskey per day compared with 12% of a control group.

The association between alcoholism and oral and laryngeal cancer was further affirmed in a study showing a large excess mortality (observed-expected ratio more than 3:1) in a group of alcoholics with oropharyngeal carcinoma. In Utah, a state with a population approximately two-thirds Mormon, a religious group abstaining from alcohol and tobacco, a study indicated an incidence of oropharyngeal cancer less than that of the western United States or the nation as a whole.

One group of investigators found that 44% of 108 patients with cancer of the tongue and 59% of 68 patients with cancer of the floor of the mouth, palate, or tonsillar fossa had unequivocal evidence of alcoholic cirrhosis. Approximately 75% drank alcohol excessively. In a 1977 study of 408 oral cancer patients with age-matched controls, Keller confirmed a previously observed correlation between cirrhosis of the liver and cancer of the floor of the mouth. He found clinically diagnosed cirrhosis in 20% of the cases of floor of the mouth carcinoma in contrast to 9% of controls. He concluded that cirrhosis, heavy drinking, and smoking were associated with cancer of the floor of the mouth.

Of 213 evaluable patients studied at the University of California, 41 (19%) had laboratory-diagnosed cirrhosis and an additional 26 (12%) demonstrated clinical cirrhotic changes. In the 41 patients with diagnosed cirrhosis, 40% had carcinoma of the tongue (only slightly more than the distribution of tongue cancer in the entire group), but 46% had floor of the mouth carcinoma (significantly higher than the rate in the entire group).

The underlying mechanisms for this association are poorly understood.[14] The cause might be related to (1) the dehydrating effects of alcohol, rendering the mucosa more susceptible to carcinogens contained in alcoholic beverages (nitrosamines, hydrocarbons), or (2) to liver-induced cellular changes in target tissues (eg, increased cytoplasmic acetaldehyde content). Experiments in animals have confirmed the clinical association between alcohol ingestion and tumorigenesis.

Patients with cirrhosis often demonstrate what appear to be smooth, erythematous, glossy-appearing oral mucosae (atrophic mucous membranes). Interestingly, in the past, patients with Plummer-Vinson syndrome (atrophic-appearing oral mucous membranes, dysphagia, and iron deficiency anemia) had a high incidence of carcinoma of the tongue and pharynx.

Most heavy drinkers are also smokers, and these predisposing factors probably work in combination rather than independently.[15,16] Several studies confirm an independent as well as a synergistic relationship between oral cancer and consumption of tobacco and alcohol.

Risk associations between alcohol-containing mouthrinses and the development of oral cancer have not been established. This was confirmed by a panel convened by the FDA in 1996.

SYPHILIS

The rate of syphilis in the United States is decreasing, with currently (2002) slightly over 100 new cases of primary syphilis reported each week to the Centers for Disease Control and Prevention. This rate is lower than any previous year but about the same as 2001 and almost 30% lower than the occurrence reported in 1998. Past reports of patients with oral cancer have indicated positive histories and/or serologic tests varying between 6 and 19%. However, little evidence currently supports an association between syphilis and oral cancer. Oral syphilitic lesions (chancres and gummas) may clinically resemble carcinoma. When any doubt exists in these cases, appropriate serologic and microscopic examinations must be performed.

ORAL LICHEN PLANUS

Oral lichen planus (OLP) is a complex, chronic, inflammatory disease. Mucosa and skin may both be affected, microscopic features vary, and the oral lesions appear in different forms (Figures 2–16 to 2–19). The prevalence of OLP is unknown, but it may be present in as much as 1% of the adult population.

The etiology of OLP is unknown, but it is thought to be an immunopathologic disease. There is no definitive curative treatment, although corticosteroids are beneficial for control. The oral lesions are frequently symptomatic and chronic, persisting indefinitely in most patients. OLP is primarily a disease of adults, with the average age of onset about 50 years. It is rarely found in persons less than

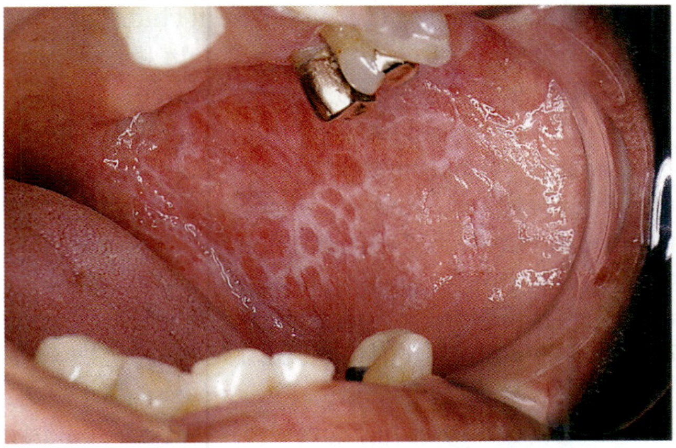

Figures 2–16 to 2–21. Forms of lichen planus (LP) and associated carcinoma.
Figure 2–16. Reticular LP, buccal.

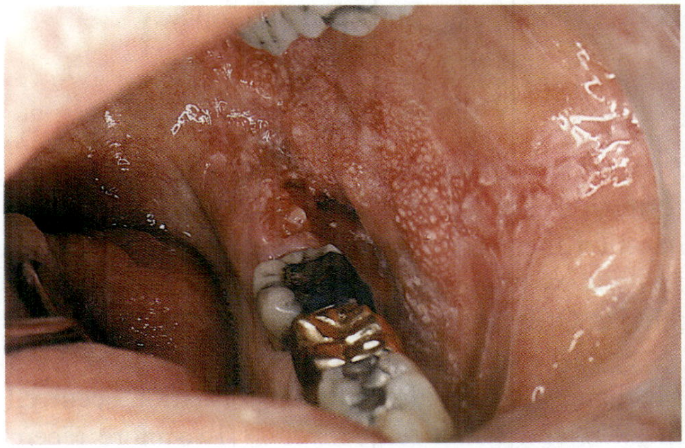

Figure 2–18. Atrophic LP, buccal, transforming to carcinoma in posterior buccal after 13 years.

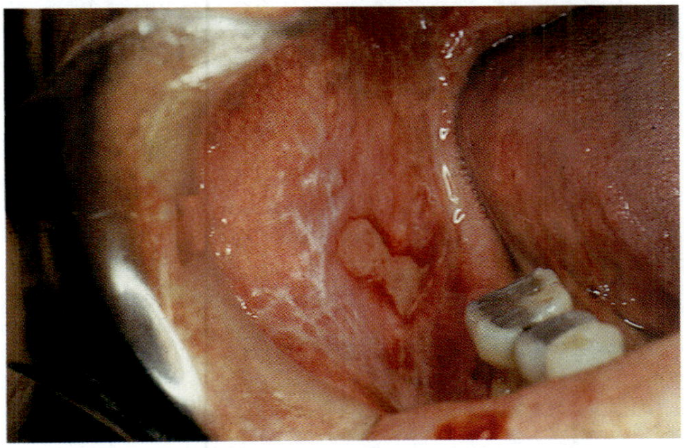

Figure 2–17. Erosive LP, buccal.

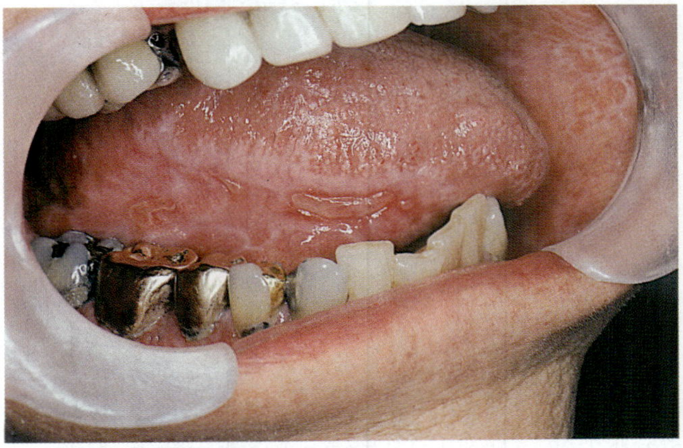

Figure 2–19. Erosive LP, tongue.

30 years old. Women predominate, in a ratio of about 2 to 1. OLP can be found in all ethnic groups, with little evidence of familial clustering. Although OLP can occur in any oral site, the buccal mucosa is by far the most common location.

Diagnosis

OLP can usually be recognized by the unique clinical features of reticular, annular, or punctate keratotic (white) patterns on the mucosal surface.[17] The diagnosis, however, can be confusing because these keratotic changes may be associated with pseudomembrane-covered ulcerations and marked erythema. Because many OLP patients are asymptomatic, signs are sometimes recognized unexpectedly during routine oral examination or by chance observation. The majority of OLP patients do not have skin involvement. Diagnosis is confirmed by biopsy.

Malignant Association

Reports have associated OLP with malignant transformation (see Figures 2–18, 2–20, and 2–21). The question therefore centers around the magnitude of risk and whether it justifies attaching a precancerous label to OLP. In two prospective and follow-up studies of 214 and 570 OLP patients at the UCSF Oral Medicine Clinic, malignant transformation occurred in 2.5% and 1.2%, respectively.[18] Two more recent and independent follow-up studies of an additional 95 and 229 OLP patients in the UCSF Oral Medicine Clinic reconfirmed a malignant association.[19] The rates of malignant transformation were 3.2% and 1.7%, respectively. The mean age of both cohorts was 54, and the mean duration in time after the diagnosis of OLP to transformation of carcinoma approximated 6 years. The prevalence of oral cancer in both groups exceeded that expected in a comparable sample of the general population. All of the UCSF studies failed to reveal associations between the development of carcinoma and gender, smoking, systemic disease, medications, or site of OLP.

A 1993 report from the United Kingdom, a review of 241 OLP patients with associated squamous cell carcinoma, found that 3.7% developed a carcinoma with a transformation time varying up to 12 years.[20] In this review of studies performed since 1981, the authors reported OLP-associated malignancies varying from 0.4 to 5.6% in seven different countries.

It is of interest to compare OLP with leukoplakia (see Chapter 3). The similarities between patients with OLP and those with leukoplakia include a comparable age of onset and a hyperkeratotic propensity of the epithelium. Red areas seem to increase the risk for dysplasia and carcinoma in both lesions. The two diseases differ in that OLP seems to be more common in women, is primarily inflammatory, and bears no relationship to tobacco use.

In summary, the findings indicate a risk of associated malignancy in patients with OLP, particularly in the erosive form and in erythematous areas.

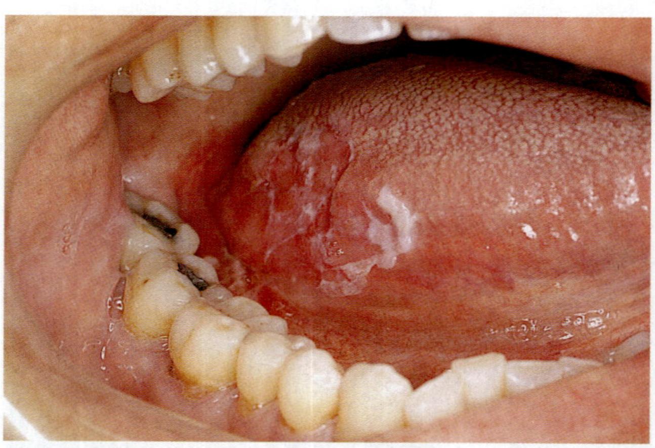

Figure 2–20. Atrophic LP, tongue, transforming to carcinoma after 3 years.

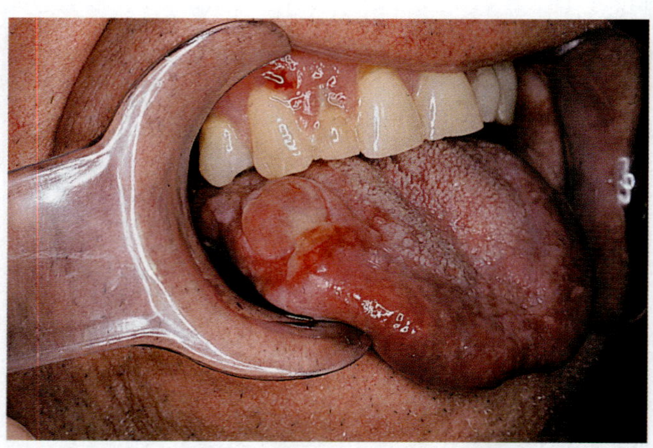

Figure 2–21. Erosive LP of gingiva, buccal mucosa, and tongue, with development of carcinoma of right lateral tongue after 15 years.

However, a formal classification as a precancerous lesion is reserved until transformation rates can be more reproducibly established. Therefore, all patients with OLP should be carefully evaluated and observed periodically.

DENTURES

Although some carcinomas develop in areas covered by or adjacent to a prosthetic appliance (Figures 2–22 to 2–25), adequate studies have not been designed to demonstrate conclusively whether this is a coincidental or a cause-and-effect relationship. More than 35 million Americans over 30 years of age wear complete upper and/or lower dentures, yet carcinomas of the palate and alveolar mucosa together account for less than 14% of all oral cancers (less than 0.4% of all cancers). However, in some patients, even though the risk is low, irritation in addition to other unidentified factors may possibly promote neoplastic activity.

In the UCSF Oral Medicine Clinic, we studied 400 patients with oral cancer to evaluate the risk of wearing dentures.[21] Forty-three percent of the group wore dentures. The study found no correlation between the wearing of dentures and any specific cancer site (Table 2–5). Furthermore, denture wearers and other patients did not differ in age, gender, time from first signs or symptoms to diagnosis, tumor stage, or tobacco use. Other studies have also shown no difference between denture wearers and control groups in the occurrence of oral cancer.

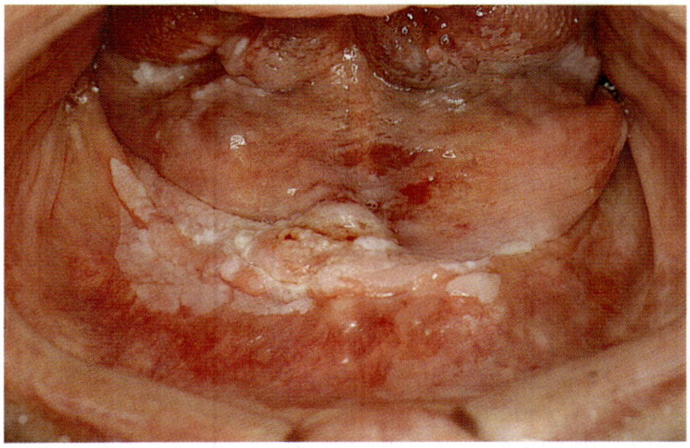

Figure 2–22. Carcinoma developed under a lower denture in anterior alveolar mucosa after a 15-year history of leukoplakia.

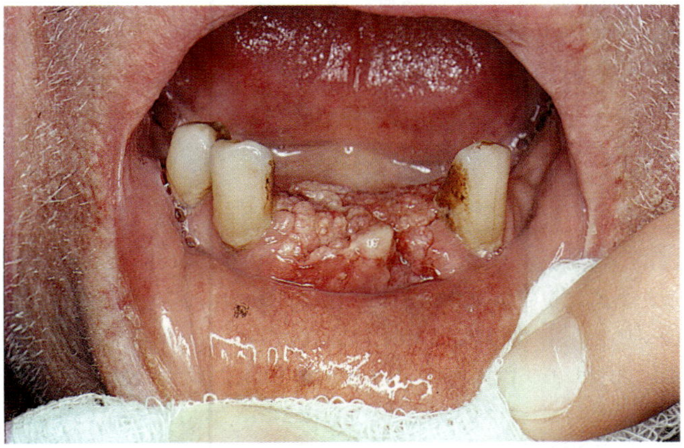

Figure 2–23. Verrucous carcinoma developed under the saddle of a lower partial denture.

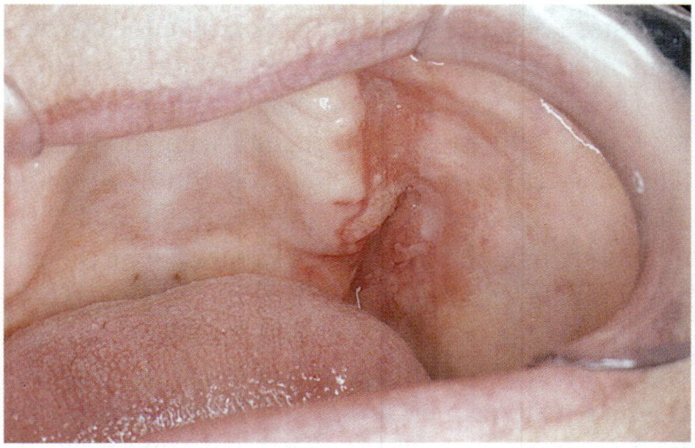

Figure 2–24. A carcinoma, at first thought to be an epulis, at the denture flange of a full upper denture.

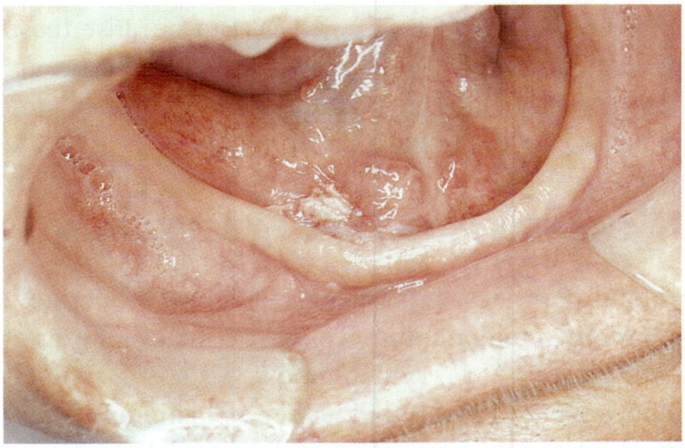

Figure 2–25. A carcinoma, at first thought to be a benign keratotic change stemming from chronic lower-denture flange irritation, involving the anterior floor of mouth and lingual alveolar mucosa.

Table 2–5. COMPARISON OF CANCER SITE AND USE OF DENTURES IN 400 ORAL CANCER PATIENTS

Cancer Site	Cancers (%)	Denture Wearers (%)	Complete Upper and Lower (%)	Complete Upper or Lower (%)	Other Combinations (%)
Tongue	34	42	60	30	10
Floor of the mouth	23	49	56	27*	17
Oropharynx	20	35	54	36	10
Gingiva†	10	43	61	28	11
Buccal mucosa	6	54	62	23	15
Palate	3	43	0	67	33
Lip	4	29	75	0	25
Total	100	43	56	30	14

Source: University of California at San Francisco.
*All upper dentures.
†Seven in maxilla.

Therefore, at this time, denture irritation does not appear to promote carcinogenesis. However, because chronic denture irritation and oral cancer have been associated, care should be taken by patients, as well as dentists, to minimize local irritation and to examine any changes with utmost care.

The same principle may apply to patients who have poor oral hygiene or jagged teeth or fillings that may act as irritants. However, little controlled evidence supports this supposition, although it is frequently mentioned in articles dealing with the etiologic factors of oral cancer. In a few animal experiments testing various carcinogenic agents, oral tumor induction has been facilitated by trauma. Denture material per se has not been shown to be carcinogenic.

Placement of jawbone implants with various materials and techniques is increasing at a rapid pace. However, there has been no indication of a carcinogenic factor (see Chapter 8). But because these patients are generally in the higher-risk age group, careful examinations and follow-up, at least, are indicated for coincidental oral tumors.

PALATAL PAPILLARY HYPERPLASIA

Palatal papillary hyperplasia, which is moderately common among denture wearers, consists of grapelike clusters of erythematous tissue on palatal mucosa that is covered by either a plastic or a metal prosthetic appliance (Figure 2–26).[22] It is found mainly in patients who do not have good adaptation. Paradoxically, poor adaptation does not necessarily indicate that a subsequent tissue hyperplasia will develop. Candidiasis can complicate the diagnosis by producing palatal erythema and symptoms of burning or pain (Figure 2–27). The microscopic picture of palatal papillary hyperplasia may sometimes be confusing because the chronic tissue irritation can cause a reactive-type hyperplasia with resultant cellular atypia. Therefore, lack of familiarity with this lesion may lead to an erroneous interpretation of a neoplastic process. Numerous years of observing patients, plus a lack of reports in the literature correlating this lesion with carcinoma, lead to the conclusion that palatal papillary hyperplasia is not a premalignant change.

Management demands careful follow-up and elimination of irritation. In case of doubt, biopsy is advised. Removal of the lesion is elective. However, when indicated for denture adaptation, hygiene purposes, or discomfort, many surgical techniques and prosthodontic approaches have been useful to modify the hyperplastic tissue.

NUTRITION

Dietary factors, such as high fat and low fiber, may play a role in carcinogenesis in some sites. However, no dietary characteristics have been recognized that distinguish patients with cancer of the oral cavity. In addition, no body of evidence links oral cancer with deficiencies or excesses of dietary proteins, fats, or carbohydrates. Some have suggested that poor dental health and denture status might be related to oral cancer risk by causing chewing difficulties that

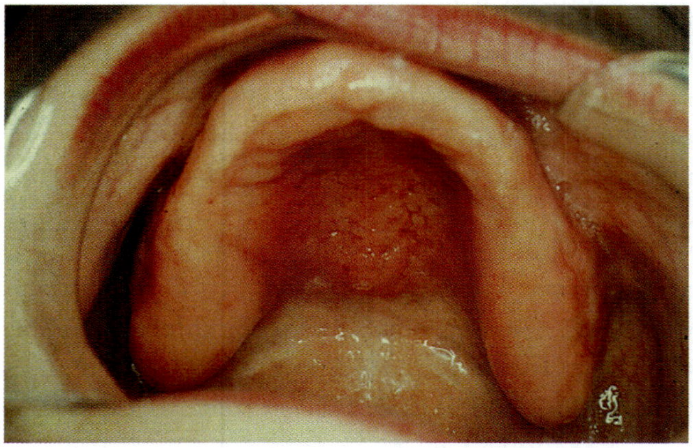

Figure 2–26. Palatal papillary hyperplasia. This usually asymptomatic lesion is attributable to a nonspecific tissue reaction to dentures and is not considered precancerous.

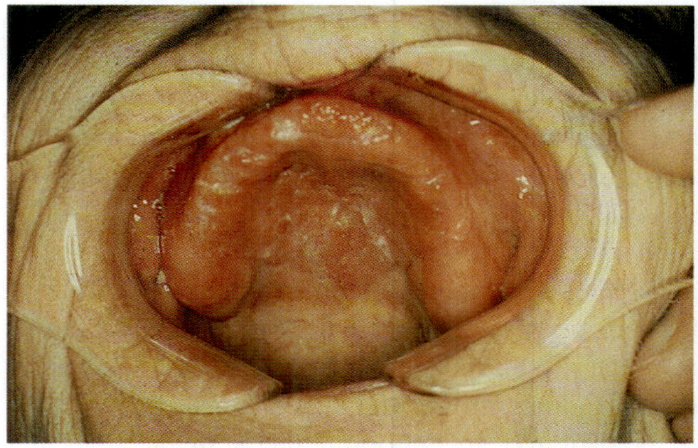

Figure 2–27. Denture stomatitis owing to chronic candidiasis. There is little evidence to link candidiasis with carcinoma (see Chapter 3).

could adversely affect nutrition. However, no studies have confirmed this indirect relationship.

Antioxidant Vitamins and Minerals

Deficiencies of antioxidant vitamins and nutrients have been postulated as cofactors in carcinogenesis. There have been reports of an inverse relationship between ingestion of carotenoids (carotene-rich vegetables) and cancer risk. More specifically, cancers of the mouth, larynx, and esophagus have been related to low intake of fruits and vegetables. Additionally, active ingredients in fruits and vegetables that may act as suppressor agents to control cell growth include indoles, flavonoids, isothiocyanates, terpenes, rutin, and phenolic antioxidants. Vegetables are also a source of fiber, which has been associated with a reduced risk of oral cancer.

Low dietary and/or serum levels of vitamin A have been associated with oral precancerous lesions and subsequent cancer (see Chapter 3). This association has been based on the correlation between vitamin A deficiencies and hyperkeratosis, as well as on demographic studies showing high rates of oral cancer in countries where vitamin A intake is low. Beta-carotene, a weak precursor to vitamin A, is abundant in some fruits and vegetables. Although it is a potent antioxidant (free radical scavenging), beta carotene has not been effective in the control of premalignant or cancerous oral lesions. However, it must be remembered that there are more than 400 carotenoids that may act as effective antioxidants in the control of cell free radicals. For example, lycopene, found in tomatoes, has shown effective antioxidant activity in some experimental systems. Recall that free radicals are molecules that contain an unpaired set of electrons. These highly unstable molecules are capable of causing mutagenesis and carcinogenesis.[23]

As for vitamin C, it appears to help block the conversion of nitrites to nitrosamines (potent carcinogens).[24] However, no data indicate that vitamin C deficiencies occur in oral cancer patients or that vitamin C supplements are helpful in preventing oral malignancies.

Vitamin E is an antioxidant vitamin that has aroused much interest. However, no studies have confirmed that either a deficiency state increases the risk of oral cancer and precancer or that vitamin E supplementation reduces the risk.

Minerals have also been studied. Iron deficiency anemia is part of the Plummer-Vinson syndrome, which has been associated with an increased risk of developing carcinoma of the tongue. Iron deficiency has not been shown to be a common finding in patients presenting with oral cancer, although high iron storage has been indicated as a possible marker or factor in cancer.[25] Zinc and copper also have been implicated in head and neck cancer, but one study of zinc and copper in oropharyngeal cancer patients found that serum levels of these elements were not different from those of control subjects and were not useful as markers.[26] Although hypercalcemia indicates a poor prognosis in patients with head and neck cancer (usually reflecting bone involvement), alterations in calcium metabolism have no cause-and-effect relationship. Some studies have indicated a risk for developing cancer in individuals with low serum levels of selenium. The role of selenium in head and neck cancer is unknown.[27] Selenium is considered an antioxidant mineral that works in conjunction with vitamin E. Selenium is mainly found in meats, fish, and grains and to lesser degrees in dairy products, fruits, and vegetables.

Nutrition is an important factor in the management of patients during treatment and rehabilitation (see Chapter 7, "Complications of Treatment," and Chapter 8). Poor nutrition and abnormal weight loss are usually associated with cachexia, intercurrent infections, and a poor prognosis.[28] On the other hand, obesity appears to be equally associated with poor survival. Obviously, then, factors that encourage adequate food intake and a nutritious diet are important to survival in conjunction with tumor control.[29]

To reduce the risk factors for oral cancer, a diet high in fruits and vegetables appears to be prudent and in order.[30,31] Dietary Reference Intakes (DRIs) are directed for general health and not targeted for cancer prevention or treatment. Use of large, excessive amounts of vitamin supplements may cause imbalances in absorption and function and, therefore, is not necessarily prudent. For example, large amounts could stimulate epithelial growth by diminishing the activity of cell suppressor proteins (eg, in vitro studies of excess beta carotene serving as a pro-oxidant and altering the function of *p53*). In general, prevention of vitamin and mineral deficiencies is achieved through nutritional intake of fruits, vegetables, whole grains, dairy products, meats, poultry, and fish. When there are difficulties in appetite, mastication, and swallowing, nutritional supplements, including calorie-dense foods, are necessary. Nasogastric tubes and gastrostomies may be required in patients with severe undernutrition (see Chapter 7).

Complementary Medicine

The usefulness of complementary or adjunctive medicines ("alternative medicine") is primarily based on non–evidence-based reports. Although there may be merit in many nutritional approaches in control of wellness, some nutritionals (eg, herbs) may have some adverse side effects and may even be dangerous (eg, liver damage as reported in the use of *kava,* an herb taken to alleviate anxiety and insomnia; *ginseng*, an herb that affects clotting by interaction with warfarin; and *yellow jessamine*, an herb that causes xerostomia). Alternative medicine approaches are often used in cancer quackery, which often delays the diagnosis and offers improper and inappropriate treatment to control malignant disease.

The National Cancer Institute has reported that a large number of cancer patients use herbal medicines and nutritional supplements to improve their quality of life. Unfortunately, many patients believe that they are safe and may even prevent or cure cancer. As stated above, many of these supplements have adverse side effects and should be used with caution and not as substitutes for proven therapies. Often patients do not volunteer that they are using these agents, which obviously complicates management.

Nutritional Biochemistry

Current areas of nutrition-related research include the following: (1) enzymatic activity of glutathione S-transferase and (2) low folic acid status associated with elevated homocysteine levels and carcinogenesis.[32] Glutathione S-transferase enzymes are essential for a multitude of chemical detoxification reactions, including tobacco carcinogenesis. Genetic mutations that alter these enzymes have shown some association with oral squamous cell carcinoma in some studies.

Adequate folic acid levels may be chemopreventive. The mechanism appears to involve the inverse relationship between blood folate levels and homocysteine, the latter showing an increase in some cancer patients. Smokers appear to have lower folate and higher homocysteine levels. Homocysteine is an inflammatory agent to mucosal cells and accumulates in the blood when folic acid and vitamins B_6 and B_{12} are below normal. The most common sources of folate include fruits, vegetables, and whole grains. Most multiple vitamin preparations provide 400 μg of folic acid (100% of the DRI), which minimizes the circulating levels of homocysteine.

DENTAL RADIATION

There is no evidence to indicate that exposure to radiation from periodic, routine, diagnostic dental radiographic examination is mutagenic or carcinogenic.[33–35] However, to minimize any potential risk to patients, all procedures that reduce radiation exposure (consistent with patients' diagnostic requirements) should be used. Years ago, some dentists carelessly exposed themselves to radiation over a period of years, leading to carcinomas of their fingers.

FLUORIDATED WATER

In 1977, Dr. Arthur Upton, director of the National Cancer Institute, made the following statement to the House Committee on Government Operations of the US Congress: "No trends in cancer rates can be ascribed to the consumption of water that is artificially or naturally fluoridated." Numerous studies and comprehensive reviews that compare mortality data between communities with fluoridated and nonfluoridated water document this statement.[36,37] Evidence-based studies have not shown that fluoridation poses any hazard to health or an increased risk of cancer.

VIRUSES

The role of viruses in development of oral cancer has been a matter of speculation for a long time. Although viruses are not known to cause oral squamous cell carcinoma, other head and neck cancers have a defined relationship with viruses (Table 2–6). Of the viruses that infect oral tissues, those having oncogenic potential are from two groups: the herpesviruses and the papillomaviruses.

Herpesviruses

Herpesviruses are enveloped viruses containing double-stranded deoxyribonucleic acid (DNA) within an icosahedral capsid of 110 to 150 nm in diameter. They cause two types of infections, lytic and latent infection, with periodic reactivation from the latent state to cause recurrent and chronic disease. There are eight herpesviruses that infect human tissues: herpes simplex virus 1 (HSV-1), herpes simplex virus 2 (HSV-2), varicella-zoster virus (VZV; human herpesvirus 3 [HHV-3]), Epstein-Barr virus (EBV; HHV-4), human cytomegalovirus (CMV; HHV-5), and human herpesviruses 6, 7, and 8 (HHV-6, HHV-7, HHV-8). Some of these do not require consideration in the discussion of oral cancer. For example, HSV-2 does not normally infect oral tissues, and neither has VZV, CMV, or HHV-7 been implicated in oral cancer. The remaining herpes virus may play some role in oral oncogenesis.

Herpes Simplex Virus 1

HSV-1 is a well-known cause of primary herpetic stomatitis and recurrent herpes labialis (cold sores). More than 90% of the population has been infected. Following the primary infection, the virus remains latent in the trigeminal or other sensory ganglion for the remainder of the person's life and can be reacti-

Table 2–6. VIRUS ASSOCIATIONS WITH HEAD AND NECK CANCER

Virus	Genotype	Association with Head and Neck Cancer	Type of Cancer Association
Human herpesvirus	HHV-1 (HSV-1)	?	—
	HHV-2 (HSV-2)	No	—
	HHV-3 (VZV)	No	—
	HHV-4 (EBV)	Yes	Hodgkin's and non-Hodgkin's lymphomas, nasopharyngeal carcinoma
	HHV-5 (CMV)	No	—
	HHV-6	Cofactor?	Lymphoma
	HHV-7	No	—
	HHV-8 (KSHV)	Yes	Kaposi's sarcoma
Human papillomavirus	HPV-16, HPV-18	Yes	Oral squamous cell carcinoma

CMV = cytomegalovirus; EBV = Epstein-Barr virus; HHV = human herpesvirus; HSV = herpes simplex virus; KSHV = Kaposi's sarcoma herpesvirus; VZV = varicella-zoster virus.

vated either to produce recurrent lesions or be shed asymptomatically from infected epithelium into the saliva. Although the virus is highly cytolytic and destroys infected cells efficiently, it has the ability to transform cells to a malignant phenotype under certain circumstances.[38] This could be important as HSV-1 infection of oral epithelium could, in theory, increase the odds for malignant changes to occur.

If HSV-1 is partially inactivated by exposure to ultraviolet light, then it does not kill the cells it infects. In this experimental situation, the infected cells can transform to a malignant phenotype. They become immortal in cell culture and will invade and metastasize if they are injected into an experimental animal. The mechanism by which HSV-1 causes malignant transformation is not known but probably involves mutagenesis. The virus expresses at least one protein that raises the mutation frequency in cells, although the types of mutations, and their location in the chromosomes, appear to be random.

Presumably, an occasional random mutation will occur in an oncogene, a tumor suppressor gene, or at some other important site, and the cell that contains that mutation develops a growth advantage over adjacent cells and will produce a malignant clone. Similarly, a viral infection can cause a cellular mutation or up-regulation of a growth protein. Subsequently, the viral DNA can be lost from the tumor cells (hit and run), yet the cell continues becoming malignant. Because mutagenesis can also result from environmental or tobacco carcinogens, and many at-risk patients both smoke tobacco and shed HSV-1 in the oral cavity, it is difficult to show convincingly that a particular tumor arose because of exposure to HSV-1. However, in vivo experiments have shown that HSV-1 can interact with potential oral carcinogens to produce tumors. In the well-known hamster cheek pouch model, HSV-1 is co-oncogenic with the tobacco carcinogen benzo*[a]*-pyrene for the production of oral tumors.[39]

Epstein-Barr Virus

EBV infects most humans and is best known for causing infectious mononucleosis. It resides latently in lymphocytes and is found frequently in the saliva of healthy persons. Experimentally, EBV infection of human lymphocytes can show features of malignancy. Malignant transformation requires alterations of the apoptotic and growth pathways by the up-regulation of EBV latency membrane protein 1 (LMP1) and the nuclear factor-κB pathway. EBV is associated with a number of head and neck cancers, including endemic Burkitt's lymphoma, certain Hodgkin's lymphomas, and undifferentiated nasopharyngeal carcinoma that occurs primarily in Asian countries. EBV can infect oral epithelial cells and is present in hairy leukoplakia, a benign proliferative condition of the tongue (see Chapter 3). The virus is seldom found in oral cancers. Because oral cancer does not appear to arise in hairy leukoplakia, it seems doubtful that EBV plays any role in the development of oral cancer.

Human Herpesvirus 6

HHV-6 was originally discovered in patients with acquired immune deficiency syndrome (AIDS) and might play a role in the progression of that disease because it can increase expression of several functions of the human immunodeficiency virus (HIV). Like other herpesviruses, it is known to be widespread in the human population. It causes the mild childhood infection roseola (exanthema subitum) and febrile seizures. It is harbored latently in peripheral blood mononuclear cells, salivary glands, mucosa, and tonsils and can be reactivated in persons who are immunosuppressed. HHV-6 DNA has been detected in biopsies from lymphoma tissue. However, its role in malignant transformation remains to be defined. HHV-6 proteins have been detected in oral cancer cells, and these proteins can transactivate other viruses (eg, HIV, HDV) associated with malignant disease.

Human Herpesvirus 8 (Kaposi's Sarcoma Herpesvirus)

This most recently discovered human herpesvirus is found in lesions of AIDS-associated Kaposi's sarcoma (KS) (see Chapter 12, "Human Immunodeficiency Virus–Associated Malignancies"). The fact that HHV-8 DNA is present in KS lesions, a majority of persons with KS have antibodies to HHV-8, and the virus can produce lesions similar to KS in experimental animals provides strong evidence that HHV-8 is the etiologic agent of KS. Recently, the virus has been identified to infect endothelial cells, and this infection, under certain circumstances, results in the recruitment of inflammatory cells.[40] The inflammatory cells locally produce interleukins and other chemokines that contribute to the hyperplastic, angiogenic tumor response. KS lesions present commonly on the face and intraorally (gingival and palate). HHV-8 is not unique to patients with AIDS or KS but is widespread in the healthy population. Immune factors that regulate the recruitment of inflammatory cells may dictate which infected patients develop KS.

Papillomaviruses

Human papillomaviruses (HPVs) are a large group of related viruses. Over 90 HPVs have been identified. They infect mucosa and skin, causing a variety of conditions, including warts, condyloma, papilloma, and cervical and anogenital cancers. HPVs can either alter epithelial cell growth and replication or dysregulate the cell cycle, resulting in malignant changes.[41,42] Infection outcomes are dependent on the infecting HPV genotype, anatomic site, and immune response. Benign or low-risk HPVs (types 6, 11, 44, 55) replicate in the lower epidermis and differentiated cells (keratinocytes), producing increased numbers of epithelial cells and koliocytosis. The principal high-risk genotypes (HPV-16, -18, -31, -33, -35) are associated with premalignant and malignant epithelial disease, especially cervical cancer.

Two HPV genes, E6 and E7, are expressed continuously in infected tumor cells. The function of these genes is known and involves blocking the effects of tumor suppressor proteins p53 and Rb. In vitro, cells that are transfected with DNA that encodes E6 and E7 of HPV-16 or -18 can become malignant.

Cell lines derived from cervical cancer usually contain HPV DNA in an episomal or extrachromosomal form in early passages, but the virus becomes integrated into the cellular DNA quickly. In oral cancer, on the other hand, the DNA of HPV is usually lost after cells have been in culture for a short time. Whether these observations indicate an important difference between the role of HPV in the two types of cancer is unknown. However, a small number of oral cancer cell lines retain HPV DNA sequences, such as the 1483 line. Normal oral keratinocytes can be transformed to an immortal phenotype by the high-risk HPVs, but the cells are not tumorigenic in nude mice. They do, however, become tumorigenic if they are exposed to low doses of chemical carcinogens, a fact that seems to indicate the potential role of HPV in the development of oral cancer, along with other necessary factors.

HPV has been detected in oral cancer, but the importance of this finding is not clear. Not all oral cancers contain HPVs. However, HPV is often present in proliferative verrucous leukoplakia (a premalignant oral lesion), and meta-analysis has shown that the probability of detecting HPV increases with increasing dysplastic changes of oral mucosa. The use of the most sensitive testing methods has shown that up to two-thirds of oral cancer cases harbor HPV DNA in their tumor cells. Although the virus is present in these cancers, at present, the function of HPV DNA in oral cancers has not been fully examined. Many people harbor HPV DNA in oral mucosa, and only a small percentage of these persons develop oral cancer. HPV-16 and -18 may play a role in the neoplastic transformation of oral precancerous lesions to malignancy and are considered by the scientific community as risk factors for oral cancer. Still undetermined are important questions regarding the need for screening of patients who may harbor latent high-risk HPV in oral mucosa and whether HPV-associated premalignant and malignant lesions should be managed differently from uninfected lesions. Interestingly, patients who have HPV-positive head and neck squamous cell carcinomas have improved survival compared with patients who have HPV-negative head and neck squamous cell carcinomas.

There are few drugs that will inhibit the growth of HPVs, either in vitro or in vivo. However, if HPVs could be confirmed to be important in the growth of some oral cancers, then several therapeutic methods could be useful for the prevention and treatment of these oral cancers. Immunomodulating drugs (eg, imiquimod) applied topically might help reduce HPV-induced epithelial proliferation. The ribonucleic acid (RNA) transcript from the transforming genes of the virus could be used as a target for therapy. By inactivating the E6 and/or E7 RNA, E6 and E7 proteins would not be synthesized, and the cellular tumor suppressor machinery could remain intact. Studies in the 1483 oral cancer cell line have shown that antisense RNA can be directed against these transcripts and will slow tumor cell growth. An alternative method of inhibition is to use ribozymes—antisense RNA with enzymatic activity—to cut HPV RNA molecules. This technique has been shown to be effective in cervical cancer cells and on the *bcl2* oncogene of oral cancer cells.

Another way to exploit active papillomavirus infections is to use the genetic promoter from the high-risk HPVs. If this promoter was used to drive expression of toxic genes, the construct would kill cells in which HPVs are active but not kill other cells. However, these various methods of antipapillomavirus therapy remain to be tested in vitro and validated in human trials.

VIRUSES IN GENE THERAPY

Although viruses have long been suspected of a role in the cause of oral cancer, recent research suggests that they might be adapted to a role in treatment.[43] Gene therapy for cancer is a new research area that shows much promise and offers several new approaches to managing cancer.[44,45]

The thymidine kinase gene of HSV-1 has been explored in many laboratories for possible use in cancer therapy. This gene sensitizes cells to the effects of antiviral drugs such as acyclovir and ganciclovir, which are phosphorylated and made biologically active by the gene product. Therefore, when the thymidine kinase gene is introduced to cancer cells, without the rest of the virus, the cancer cells are altered or killed by exposure to specific antiviral drugs, such as ganciclovir (Figure 2–28). This approach has been shown to be effective in animal tumors, human oral cancer cells in vitro, and human oral cancers that are transplanted to nude mice. Preliminary studies in human oral cancer have begun.

Another possible use for HSV-1 in cancer therapy is to use the virus as a vector so that it carries new fragments of DNA into a cell and, thus, replaces a missing gene or counters the effects of a defective one. Unfortunately, the nonspecific toxic effects of HSV-1 have limited its use in this way. Several laboratories have tried to reduce the cellular toxicity of the virus by stripping away the virulence genes. A theoretical, alternative approach would be to modify the genome of HSV-1 so that it would grow only in oral cancer cells and not in nonmalignant cells. Such a virus would kill cancers but not spread to surrounding or distant tissues.

Other adenovirus, adeno-associated virus vectors and retrovirus vectors that can transfer specific frag-

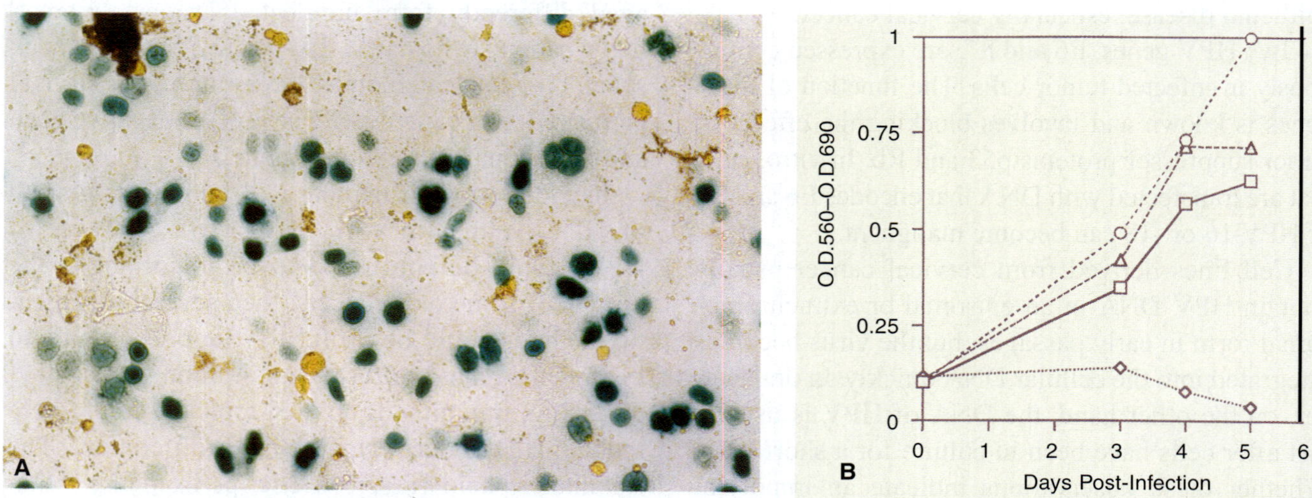

Figure 2–28. Potential use of viruses in gene therapy of oral cancer. The 686-LN oral cancer cell line was exposed to an adenovirus vector, which carries the genes for beta-galactosidase and the herpes simplex gene for thymidine kinase. *A,* The cells that acquired the genes are stained blue. *B,* The growth curves show that the thymidine kinase gene sensitizes the cells to the toxic effects of ganciclovir at the low dose of 5 μg/mL (◇). The cells are relatively unaffected by either ganciclovir without the virus (△) or the virus without ganciclovir (□), when compared with untreated cancer cells (○). This suggests that viruses can be modified to provide new forms of gene therapy for oral cancer.

ments of DNA to oral cancer tissues have been developed over the last decade.[46–48] These vectors have less nonspecific toxicity than herpes-based vectors and can transfer marker genes, toxic genes, or tumor suppressor genes to oral cancer cells. Human trials for some of these approaches have begun, and data should be available soon.

REFERENCES

1. Forastiere A, Koch W, Trotti A, Sidransky D. Head and neck cancer. N Engl J Med 2001;345:1890–900.

1a. Ziober BL, Silverman S Jr, Kramer RH. Adhesive mechanisms regulating invasion and metastasis in oral cancer. Crit Rev Oral Biol Med 2001;12:499–510.

2. Waxman H. The future of the global tobacco treaty negotiations. N Engl J Med 2002;346:936–8.
3. Jones RB. Tobacco or oral health: past progress, impending challenge. J Am Dent Assoc 2000;131:1130–45.
4. National Cancer Institute. Risks associated with smoking cigarettes with low machine-measured yields of tar and nicotine. Smoking and tobacco control monograph no. 13. Bethesda, MD; 2001.

4a. National Cancer Institute. Changing adolescent smoking prevalence. Where it is and why. Smoking and tobacco control monograph no. 14. Bethesda, MD; 2001.

5. Baker F, Ainsworth SR, Dye JT, et al. Health risks associated with cigar smoking. JAMA 2000;284:735–40.
6. Robertson PB, Derouen TA, Ernster V, et al. Smokeless tobacco use: how it affects the performance of major league baseball players. J Am Dent Assoc 1995;126:1115–24.
7. Hoffman D, Djordjevic MV, Fan J, et al. Five leading U.S. commercial brands of moist snuff in 1994: assessment of carcinogenic N-nitrosamines. J Natl Cancer Inst 1995;87: 1862–9.
8. Going RE, Hsu SC, Pollack RL, et al. Sugar and fluoride content of various forms of tobacco. J Am Dent Assoc 1980;100:27–33.
9. Gonzalez YM, de Nardin A, Grossi SG, et al. Serum cotinine levels, smoking and periodontal attachment loss. J Dent Res 1996;75:796–802.
10. Christen AG. Tobacco cessation, the dental profession, and the role of dental education. J Dent Educ 2001;65:368–74.
11. Rigotti NA. Clinical practice. Treatment of tobacco use and dependence. N Engl J Med 2002;346:506–12.
12. Mashberg A, Garfinkel L, Harris S. Alcohol as a primary risk factor in oral squamous cell carcinoma. CA Cancer J Clin 1981;31:146–55.
13. Thun MJ, Peto R, Lopez AD, et al. Alcohol consumption and mortality among middle-aged and elderly U.S. adults. N Engl J Med 1997;337:1705–14.
14. Harty LC, Caporaso NE, Hayes RB, et al. Alcohol dehydrogenase 3 genotype and risk of oral cavity and pharyngeal cancers. J Natl Cancer Inst 1997;89:1698–705.
15. Keller AZ. Alcohol, tobacco and age factors in the relative frequency of cancer among males with and without liver cirrhosis. Am J Epidemiol 1977;106:194–202.
16. Lewin F, Norell SE, Johansson H, et al. Smoking tobacco, oral snuff, and alcohol in the etiology of squamous cell carcinoma of the head and neck. Cancer 1998;82:1367–75.
17. Vincent SD, Fotos PG, Baker KA, Williams TP. Oral lichen planus: the clinical, historical and therapeutic features of 100 cases. Oral Surg Oral Med Oral Pathol 1990;70:165–71.
18. Silverman S Jr, Gorsky M, Lozada-Nur F, Giannotti K. A prospective study of findings and management in 214 patients with oral lichen planus. Oral Surg Oral Med Oral Pathol 1991;72:665–70.
19. Chainani-Wu N, Silverman S Jr, Lozada-Nur F, et al. Oral lichen planus: patient profile, disease progression and treatment responses. J Am Dent Assoc 2001;132:901–9.
20. Barnard NA, Scully C, Everson JAW. Oral cancer development in patients with oral lichen planus. J Oral Pathol Med 1993;22:421–4.
21. Gorsky M, Silverman S Jr. Denture wearing and oral cancer. J Prosthet Dent 1984;52:164–6.
22. Bhaskar SN, Beasley JD III, Cutright DE. Inflammatory papillary hyperplasia of the oral mucosa: report of 341 cases. J Am Dent Assoc 1970;81:949–52.
23. Miller EC, Miller JA. Carcinogens and mutagens that may occur in foods. Cancer 1986;58:1795–803.
24. Mirvish SS. Effects of vitamins C and E on N-nitroso compound formation, carcinogenesis and cancer. Cancer 1986;58:1842–50.
25. Stevens RG, Jones DY, Micozzi MS, et al. Body iron stores and the risk of cancer. N Engl J Med 1988;319:1047–52.
26. Silverman S Jr, Thompson JS. Serum zinc and copper in oral/oropharyngeal carcinoma. A study of seventy-five patients. Oral Surg Oral Med Oral Pathol 1984;57:34–6.
27. Petridou E, Zavras AI, Lefatzis D, et al. The role of diet and specific micronutrients in the etiology of oral carcinoma. Cancer 2002;94:2981–8.
28. Heber D, Byerly LO, Chi J, et al. Pathophysiology of malnutrition in the adult cancer patient. Cancer 1986;58:1867–73.
29. Lupulescu AP. Hormones, vitamins, and growth factors in cancer treatment and prevention. Cancer 1996;78:2264–80.
30. American Cancer Society. Guidelines on diet, nutrition, and cancer prevention: reducing the risk of cancer with healthy food choices and physical activity. CA Cancer J Clin 1996;46:325–41.
31. Calle EE, Rodriquez C, Jacobs EJ, et al. The American Cancer Society cancer prevention study II nutrition cohort. Cancer 2002;94:2490–501.
32. Almadori G, Bussu F, Galli J, et al. Serum folate and homocysteine levels in head and neck squamous cell carcinoma. Cancer 2002;94:1006–11.
33. Campbell JA. Where does dentistry stand on radiation? J Calif Dent Assoc 1986;14:17–20.
34. Underhill TE, Kimura K, Chilvarguer I, et al. Radiobiologic risk estimation from dental radiology. Part II. Cancer incidence and fatality. Oral Surg Oral Med Oral Pathol 1988;66:261–7.
35. White SC, Frey NW. An estimation of somatic hazards to the United States population from dental radiology. Oral Surg Oral Med Oral Pathol 1977;43:152–9.
36. Clemmesen J. The alleged association between artificial fluoridation of water supplies and cancer: a review. Bull World Health Organ 1983;61:871–3.

37. Newbrun E. Water fluoridation and fluoride supplements in caries prevention. J Calif Dent Assoc 1980;8:38–47.
38. Das C, Schantz SP, Shillitoe EJ. Antibody to a mutagenic peptide of herpes simplex virus in young adult patients with cancer of the head and neck. Oral Surg Oral Med Oral Pathol 1993;75:610–4.
39. Park K, Cherrick HM, Min BM, Park NH. Active HSV-1 immunization prevents the cocarcinogenic activity of HSV-1 in the oral cavity of hamsters. Oral Surg Oral Med Oral Pathol 1990;70:186–91.
40. Shillitoe EJ, Hwang CBC, Silverman S Jr, Greenspan JS. Examination of oral cancer tissue for the presence of the proteins ICP4, ICP5, ICP6, ICP8 and gB of herpes simplex virus type-1. J Natl Cancer Inst 1986;76:371–4.
41. Gillison ML, Koch WM, Capone RB, et al. Evidence for a causal association between human papillomavirus and a subset of head and neck cancers. J Natl Cancer Inst 2000; 92:709–20.
42. Miller CS, Johnstone BM. Human papillomavirus as a risk factor for oral squamous cell carcinoma: a meta-analysis, 1982-1997. Oral Surg Oral Med Oral Pathol Oral Radiol Endod 2001;91:622–35.
43. Shillitoe EJ, Greenspan D, Greenspan JS, Silverman S Jr. Five-year survival of patients with oral cancer and its association with antibody to herpes simplex virus. Cancer 1986;58:2256–9.
44. Shillitoe EJ, Lapeyre J-N, Adler-Storthz K. Gene therapy—its potential in management of oral cancer. Eur J Cancer 1994;30B:143–54.
45. Shillitoe EJ, Gilchrist E, Pellenz C, Murrah V. Effects of herpes simplex virus on human oral cancer cells, and potential use of mutant viruses in therapy of oral cancer. Oral Oncol 1999;35:326–332.
46. Clayman GL, Frank DK, Bruso PA, Goepfert H. Adenovirus-mediated wild-type p53 gene transfer as a surgical adjuvant in advanced head and neck cancers. Clin Cancer Res 1999;5:1715–22.
47. Gibson SA, Pellenz C, Hutchinson RE, et al. Induction of apoptosis in oral cancer cells by an anti-bcl-2 ribozyme delivered by an adenovirus vector. Clin Cancer Res 2000;6:213–22.
48. Nakashima T, Sun SY, Lotan R, et al. All-trans-retinoic acid enhances the effect of adenovirus-mediated wild-type p53 gene transfer in head and neck squamous cell carcinoma. Laryngoscope 2001;111:1459–64.

3

Leukoplakia and Erythroplasia

SOL SILVERMAN JR., MA, DDS

Decreasing morbidity and mortality from oral carcinoma in part depends on improved understanding of precancerous lesions. The risk for malignant transformation is multifactorial, depending on the type of leukoplakia, the presence of epithelial dysplasia, lifestyle and habits, microbial agents, genomics, duration, and other undefined factors. White and red lesions of the oral mucosa are the most common precancerous clinical lesions. Although not all oral cancers are preceded by clinically evident premalignant mucosal changes, such changes give a warning of risk and present an opportunity for preventive measures. Additionally, early cancer can also appear as an innocuous white and/or red lesion. Although white changes (leukoplakia) are the most common premalignant lesion, red changes (erythroplasia, erythroplakia) or white changes with a red component (speckled leukoplakia, erythroleukoplakia) carry a greater risk.

LEUKOPLAKIA

The term leukoplakia is used to designate a clinical white patch or plaque on the oral mucous membranes that cannot be removed by scraping and cannot be classified clinically or microscopically as another disease entity.[1] Most of these lesions, which can occur in all areas of the oral cavity, are reflections of benign hyperkeratosis (Figures 3–1 to 3–6). Although tobacco or acute/chronic irritation may induce hyperkeratosis, the causes of many leukoplakias are unknown.

EPIDEMIOLOGY OF LEUKOPLAKIA

The age range and the tobacco habits of patients with oral leukoplakia are similar to those of patients with oral carcinoma. These facts indicate possible biologic similarities and comparable risks. The rela-

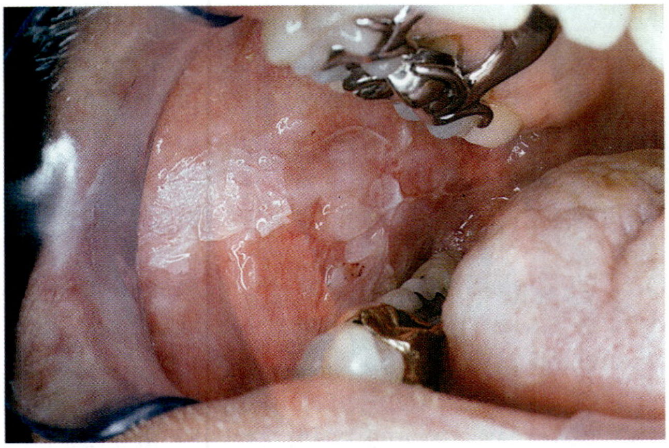

Figure 3–1. Leukoplakia, buccal mucosa.

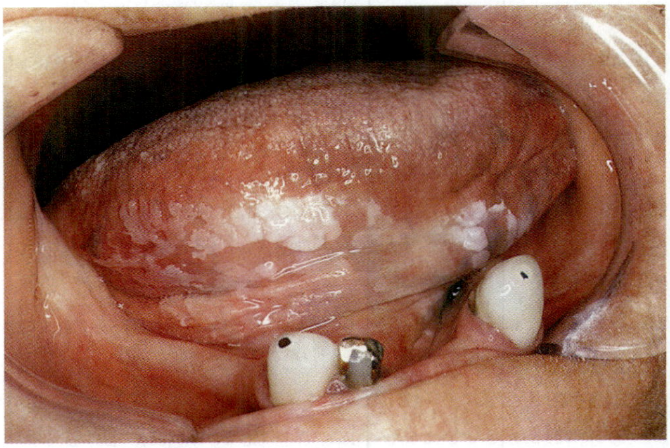

Figure 3–2. Leukoplakia, tongue.

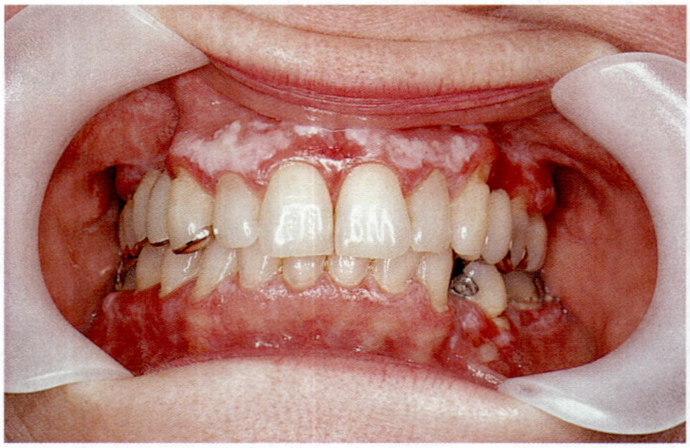

Figure 3–3. Leukoplakia, gingiva.

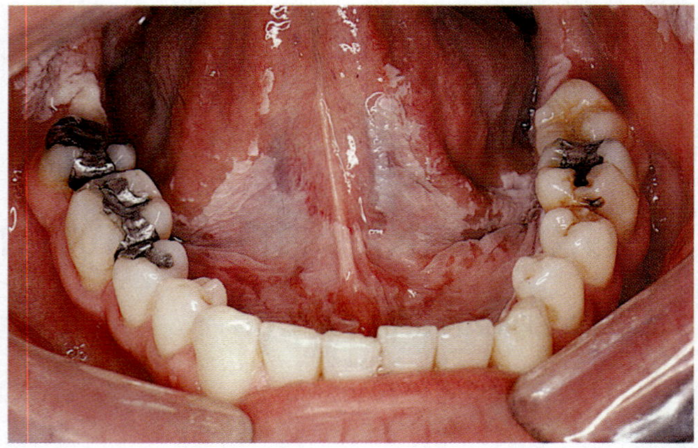

Figure 3–5. Leukoplakia, ventral tongue, floor of the mouth.

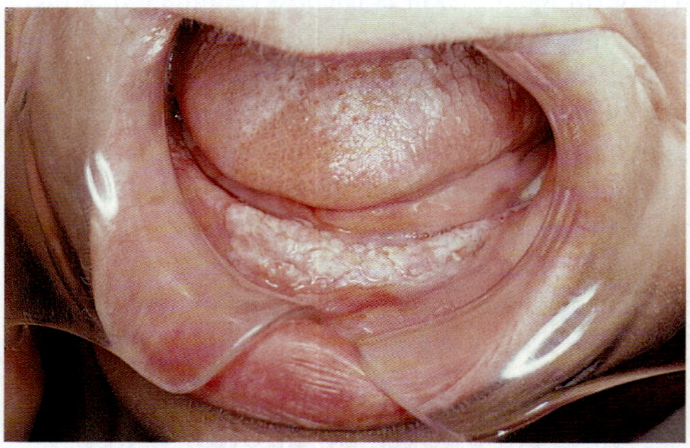

Figure 3–4. Leukoplakia, alveolar mucosa, tongue.

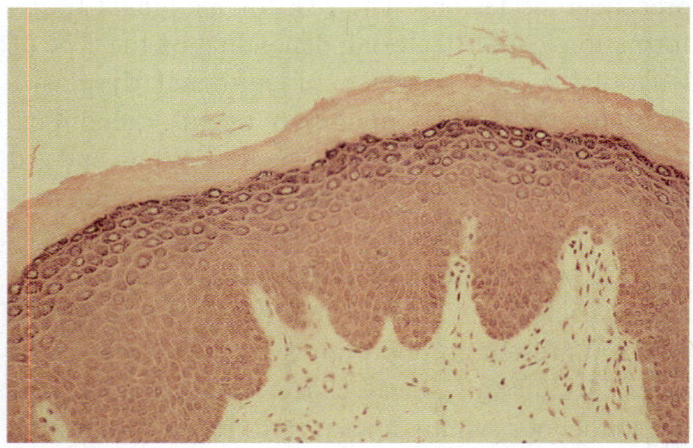

Figure 3–6. Hyperkeratosis, stratified squamous epithelium.

tionship between smoking and leukoplakia is not always clear because abstinence from tobacco may not lead to remission of the lesion, and some patients with leukoplakia have never smoked. However, if associated with the use of smokeless tobacco, an induced leukoplakic change almost always reverses when the use of snuff or chewing tobacco stops (Figures 3–7 and 3–8).

The prevalence of oral leukoplakia in the general population is unknown. Prevalence studies have been attempted in certain parts of the world, but the results are variable and do not support any generalizations as to rates. Variability in both classifications and etiologic factors add to the difficulty of carrying out such a study. In a Minnesota study of 27,443 adults, the occurrence of leukoplakia was found to be 0.1%, yet in a study of more than 180,000 army recruits ranging in age from 17 to 26 years, 1.5% had oral leukoplakia.[2] A study of 51,000 villagers in southern India found that the prevalence rates in four states ranged from 0.2 to 5%. On the other hand, a study from Ahmedabad, in northwest India, indicated that the occurrence of leukoplakia was close to 12%. However, this study examined a selected population of 57,518 textile mill workers over 35 years of age who belonged to a lower socioeconomic class.

PRECANCEROUS CLASSIFICATION

Oral leukoplakia is a premalignant lesion, that is, there exists a risk of transforming to carcinoma. This conclusion is based on the following: (1) a large number of oral carcinomas have been associated with leukoplakic changes (Tables 3–1 and 3–2), and (2) in prospective studies, occurrences of malignant transformations in oral leukoplakias exceed the

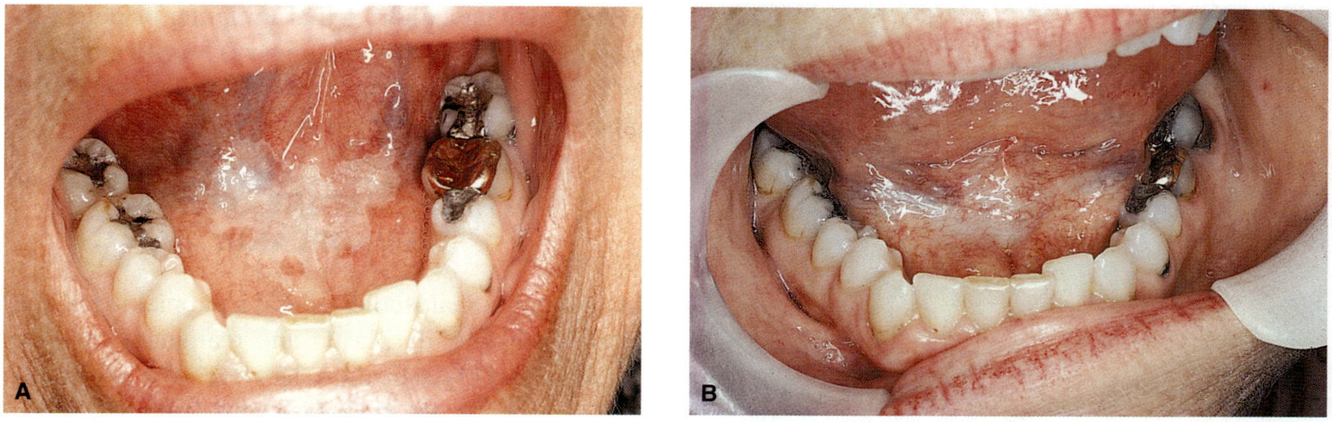

Figure 3–7. Leukoplakia and smoking cessation. *A,* Leukoplakia, floor of the mouth, associated with years of smoking one pack of cigarettes daily. *B,* Four months after discontinuation of smoking, the leukoplakia is regressing, with complete disappearance in 6 months.

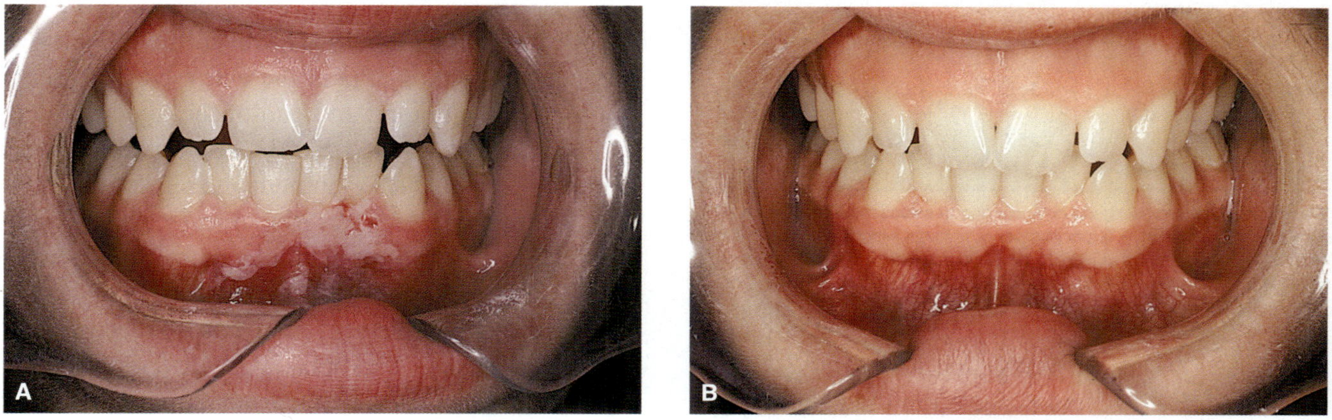

Figure 3–8. A 16-year-old athlete who held snuff between his lower lip and anterior teeth for almost 4 years. *A,* Asymptomatic gingival leukoplakia. *B,* Complete disappearance 1 month after discontinuing the use of snuff.

Table 3–1. MALIGNANCIES AND PREMALIGNANT CHANGES FOUND IN BIOPSY SPECIMENS CLINICALLY DIAGNOSED AS LEUKOPLAKIA

Source (Country)	Year	No. of Patients	Frequency of Malignancy or Premalignant Changes
Pindborg (Denmark)	1963	185	3% carcinoma 12% dysplasia
Silverman (United States)	1968	117	10% carcinoma
Waldron (United States)	1975	3,256	3% carcinoma 17% dysplasia
Banoczy (Hungary)	1976	500	10% carcinoma 24% dysplasia

Table 3–2. PROGRESSION OF DYSPLASIA TO CANCER IN PATIENTS WITH ORAL LEUKOPLAKIA

Source (Country), Year	No. of Patients	Follow-up: Years	Follow-up: Cancers (%)
Mincer (United States), 1972	45*	1–8	5 (11.1)
Banoczy (Hungary), 1976	68†	1–20	9 (13.2)
Pindborg (India), 1977	21	7	3 (14.3)
Silverman et al (United States), 1984	22‡	1–39	8 (35.4)
Lumerman et al (United States), 1995	44	1–7	7 (15.9)
Cowan (Ireland), 2001	165	1–11	14 (8.5)
Sudbo et al (Norway), 2001	150§	1–14	36 (24.0)

*22 persisted, 3 resolved, and 20 were excised (7 recurred).
†45 of 68 were excised; 8 cancers in untreated lesions.
‡20 of 22 lesions were erythroleukoplakia.
§All initially treated by excisional biopsies.

Table 3–3. MALIGNANT TRANSFORMATION IN ORAL LEUKOPLAKIAS

Source (Country), Year	*n*	Malignant Transformation (%)*	Observation Period Years (Mean)
Silverman (Gujarat, India), 1976	4,762	0.13	2 (2)
Gupta (Bhavnagar, India), 1980	360	0.3	1–10 (7)
Gupta (Ernakulan, India), 1980	410	2.2	1–10 (7)
Roed-Petersen (Denmark), 1971	331	3.6	> 1
Einhorn (Sweden), 1967	782	4.0	1–20
Pindborg (Denmark), 1968	248	4.4	1–9
Kramer (England), 1969	187	4.8	1–16
Banoczy (Hungary), 1977	670	5.9	1–30 (9.8)
Silverman (United States), 1968	117	6.0	1–11 (3.5)
Schepman (Netherlands), 1998	166	12.0	5–17 (2.7)
Silverman et al (United States), 1984†	257	17.5	1–39 (7.2)

*Number of transformations varied according to selection of patients and duration of observation. A larger number of patients with leukoplakic lesions, selected at random and followed up over a longer period of time, would be necessary to determine a transformation rate in a given population.
†See Tables 3–4 through 3–6.

number of oral cancers expected in the general population (Tables 3–3 to 3–6, Figures 3–9 to 3–14). A biochemical and pathophysiologic explanation for the potential association between hyperkeratosis and malignant transformation is not forthcoming.

TOBACCO-INDUCED RISKS

Tobacco use increases the risk for developing oral cancer. Paradoxically, in patients with oral leukoplakia, nonsmokers are at higher risk. This finding was shown in a study of patients from the University of California at San Francisco (UCSF) Oral Medicine Clinic (Table 3–7) and has also been reported by others. Einhorn (Sweden) cited an eightfold risk, and Roed-Petersen (Denmark) cited a fivefold risk of developing a carcinoma for nonsmoking leukoplakic patients. Although no one has proposed a clear explanation for this finding, it might be speculated that patients without tobacco as a causative irritant may have more lethal initiating or potentiating factors. Banoczy (Hungary) confirmed this increased risk in nonsmokers in her long-term reports on leukoplakic patients.[3]

DYNAMIC NATURE OF ORAL LEUKOPLAKIA

Most longitudinal studies of oral leukoplakia patients focus on habits, dysplastic and malignant transformations, and classification. However, the possibility of spontaneous regression of oral leukoplakia has been confirmed in several reports. In a 2-year follow-up study of 4,762 persons with oral leukoplakia in Gujarat, India, although essentially none of the cohorts reported changed habits during the 2-year interval, almost one-third experienced complete regression of their lesions. However, the prevalence rates for oral leukoplakia in the entire Gujarat study group at the beginning and end of the 2-year period were similar, 11.7% and 12.0%, respectively. These results indicate that development and regression rates were comparable, so that the occurrence of oral leukoplakia in this population was relatively constant. The incidence was 2.6% per year.

Because others have found cases of complete regression in oral leukoplakia in different Indian populations, at rates ranging from 26 to 45% in 5-year intervals, this remission phenomenon appears to be real. Similarly, a Danish study found that 37% of 214 leukoplakic lesions were totally or partially reversed without any intervention during a follow-up period that ranged up to 15 years, and a study of 520 Hungarian patients with oral leukoplakia observed from 1 to 25 years found regressive changes in 9%.

Table 3–4. TRANSFORMATION RATES OF LEUKOPLAKIC FORMS

Leukoplakia	No. of Patients	Subsequent Carcinoma	Transformation Rate (%)
Homogeneous*	107	7	6.5
Erythroleukoplakia†	128	30	23.4
Dysplasia‡	22	8	36.4
Total	257	45	17.5

Adapted from Silverman S et al.[6]
*All-white appearance.
†Red component.
‡20 of 22 appeared clinically as erythroleukoplakia.

Table 3–5. OCCURRENCES OF CARCINOMAS RELATED TO FOLLOW-UP PERIODS IN 257 PATIENTS WITH LEUKOPLAKIA

Follow-up Years	Occurrences of Carcinoma in 45 Patients (%)	Patients Followed for Each Period (%)	Rate of Carcinoma in Patients Followed (%)	Rate of Carcinoma per Year (%)
0.5–1	9	100	2	4
1–2	24	84	5	5
2–5	20	70	5	1.6
5–10	22	46	8	1.6
10–20	16	27	10	1
20–39	9	8	19	1

Adapted from Silverman S et al.[6]

Over the years, we have also observed a spontaneous disappearance and/or regression unexpectedly in some patients.

DYSPLASIA AND MALIGNANT TRANSFORMATION

The risk of subsequent malignant transformation increases when a biopsy specimen reveals an associated epithelial dysplasia (see Table 3–2). However, specific data regarding the correlation among degrees of oral epithelial dysplasia, time-related progression, and the influences of a variety of cofactors remain uncertain.[4,5] Well-designed studies to collect and evaluate this type of information have not been conducted.

In a retrospective review from a large New York City biopsy service, Lumerman and colleagues reported a follow-up study of oral epithelial dysplasia in 44 patients for whom they were able to obtain adequate follow-up material.[5a] These patients represented 14% of a pool of 308 recorded epithelial dysplasia cases in their service. Obviously, the question arises as to whether this small group of evaluable cases is representative of all of their cases or even of similar patients at other centers. Thirty-nine patients (89%) presented with white and/or red lesions, indicating the probable clinical diagnosis of leukoplakia and/or erythroplakia. The mean age was 61 years, and 55% were women. Although most reports indicate a similar age grouping, this preponderance of women was unusual. After the biopsy diagnosis and management, 7 (16%) developed oral carcinomas 7 to 78 months later (mean, 34 months); the average age was 63, and 4 were men. Two of the 7 had microscopic descriptions consistent with the high-risk type of leukoplakia termed "proliferative verrucous leukoplakia" (see below).

From a prospective study of 257 oral leukoplakia patients followed up for a mean time of 8.1 years in the author's clinic in San Francisco, 22 of these patients with oral leukoplakia also had microscopic dysplasia.[6] In the time frame of this study, 37 of 235 patients (15.7%) without biopsy evidence of epithelial dysplasia developed oral carcinomas; however, 8 of the 22 patients (36.4%) with existing epithelial dysplasia found in their initial biopsies developed oral carcinomas (see Tables 3–4 and 3–6). No evident factors distinguished these 8 patients and the 14 who had epithelial dysplasia but did not develop oral carcinomas. A

Table 3–6. PROFILE OF 45 PATIENTS WITH TRANSFORMATION OF LEUKOPLAKIA TO CARCINOMA

Transformation Site	F	M	% of Lesions	Age at Onset of Leukoplakia (yr) Range	Mean	Transformation Time (yr) Range	Mean	Preexisting Dysplasia	Tobacco Use* Cigarette	Pipe	Cigar
Tongue	9	4	28.9	37–79	55	1–18	6.4	1	2		1
Gingiva	6	5	24.4	46–84	66	1–21	8.6	3	2	1	
Floor	2	5	15.6	30–69	50	1–30	10.2	2	6	1	
Buccal	3	2	11.1	48–71	60	1–16	8.8	1	1	1	
Palate	4	1	11.1	38–76	54	2–39	9.3	1	2		1
Lip	2	2	8.9	45–65	54	3–11	6.6	0	3		
Total	26	19	100.0	30–84	57	1-39	7.2	8	16	3	2

Adapted from Silverman S et al.[6]

*Of the 24 nonsmokers, 18 had never smoked and 6 stopped smoking when diagnosed.

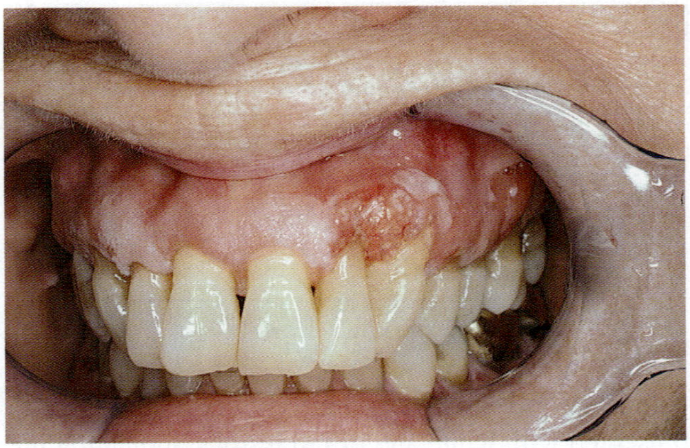

Figures 3–9 to 3–12. Some varying appearances of squamous cell carcinomas associated with preexisting areas of long-standing leukoplakia.

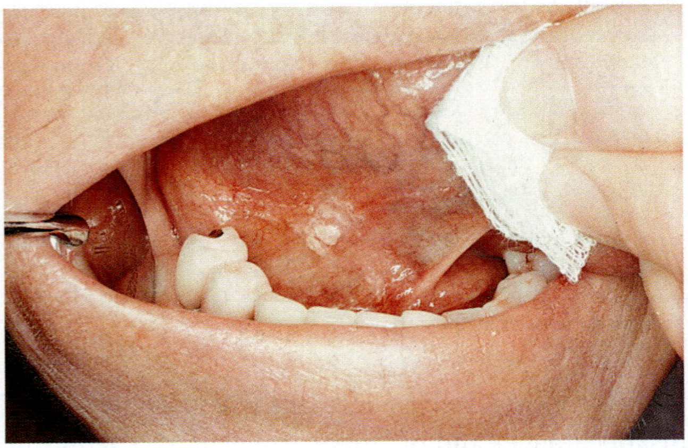

Figure 3–11.

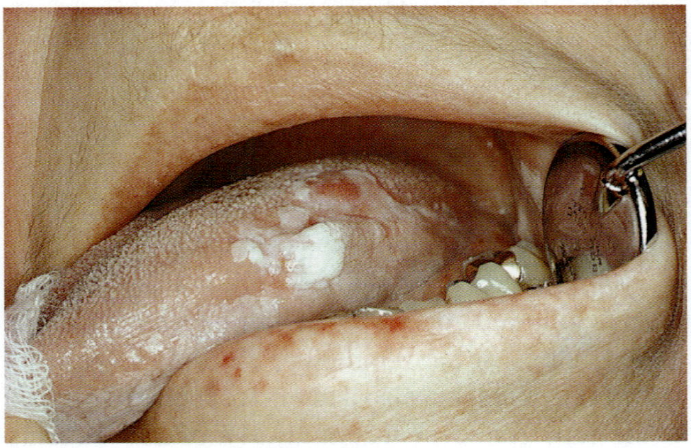

Figure 3–10.

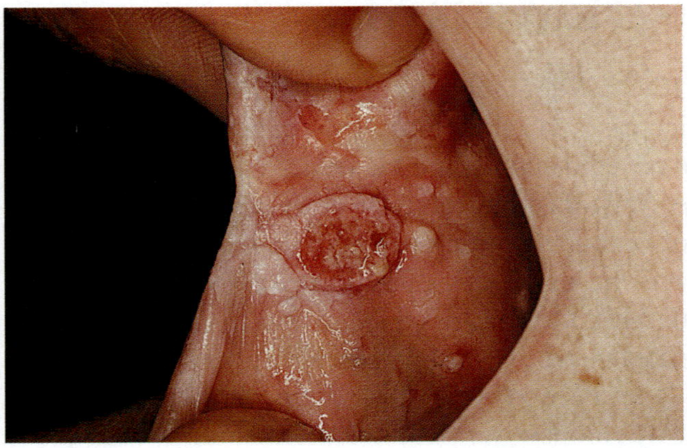

Figure 3–12.

longer follow-up may well have shown more malignant transformations. The mean age of the 8 patients was 59 years (range 30–77), and 5 were women. Four of the patients smoked, 91% had a red component in their leukoplakic lesion, and microscopic candidiasis was found in 44%. Although oral leukoplakia is generally asymptomatic, half of the patients had complaints of discomfort. The overall follow-up time from when the 8 patients first noticed their clinical leukoplakia was 9.5 years (range 1–29). Obviously, no one knows when the dysplastic changes actually occurred.

The above findings prompt the following conclusions regarding the clinical recognition and diagnosis of oral leukoplakia, the development of epithelial dysplasia, and subsequent malignant transformation:

1. In oral leukoplakia, the occurrence and time of dysplastic changes are uncertain. De novo transformation from hyperkeratosis to carcinoma may occur without recognizable dysplasia.
2. An erythematous component and discomfort should raise suspicion of dysplastic or malignant transformation.[7]
3. Because epithelial dysplasia increases the risk of the development of a malignant tumor, surgical removal of dysplastic lesions is indicated. This limits prospective follow-up studies.
4. Proliferative verrucous forms of leukoplakia have a high risk of dysplasia and malignant transformation and should be treated aggressively.
5. Although the severity of the degrees of dysplasia has clinical significance regarding neoplasia, patients with mild dysplasia, or even without evidence of dysplasia, are at risk of transformation. Therefore, all patients with chronic white and/or red lesions, whether treated or not, should

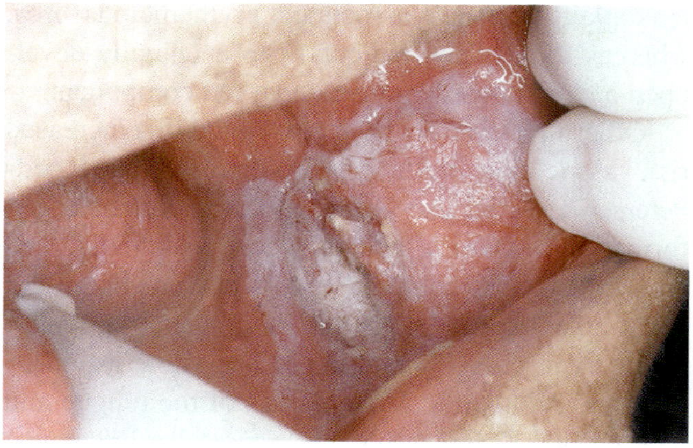

Figure 3–13. Asymptomatic leukoplakia of the left buccal mucosa, present for more than 10 years, became painful and indurated in the posterior portion of the lesion. A biopsy showed well-differentiated squamous cell carcinoma.

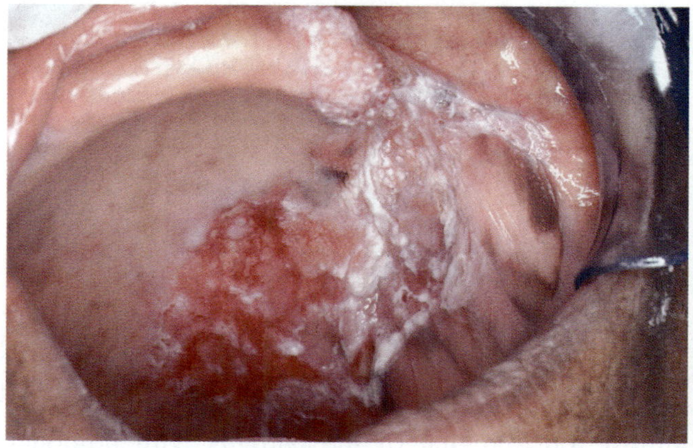

Figure 3–14. After being present for more than a decade, a large area of asymptomatic leukoplakia became erythematous and painful in the palatal portion. A biopsy showed squamous cell carcinoma.

be followed carefully. This advice holds true even after surgical intervention because recurrences are common.

6. Reproducible interexaminer agreements in diagnosing oral epithelial dysplasia are difficult to achieve, adding to the confusion regarding treatment approaches and aggressiveness.[8] Therefore, the development of biologic markers (eg, monoclonal antibodies, deoxyribonucleic acid (DNA)/ribonucleic acid (RNA) probes, special stains) emerges as extremely important, and even critical, in producing fundamental advancements in the diagnosis, prognosis, and treatment parameters of precancerous lesions (see section in Chapter 5, "Advanced Molecular Analysis").

GENOMICS

As studies continue regarding the role of chromosomes and genes in influencing the development and progression of oral leukoplakia to malignancy, risks and prognoses will undoubtedly be clarified to some degree. In a recent follow-up study by Sudbo and colleagues of nuclear DNA content (ploidy) in 150 Norwegian patients with dysplastic leukoplakia, there was a direct risk association between chromosome ploidy and progression to malignancy (Table 3–8).[9]

ERYTHROLEUKOPLAKIA AND ERYTHROPLASIA

Leukoplakia that clinically has an erythematous or red component (erythroleukoplakia) is far more likely to undergo dysplastic or malignant epithelial changes than other forms of leukoplakia (Figures 3–15 to 3–20). Because red lesions without a white component may also represent either dysplasia or carcinoma, such lesions must be carefully evaluated (see Chapter 4, "Diagnosis"). In our oral medicine clinic, the risk of malignant transformation in the

Table 3–7. ASSOCIATION BETWEEN TOBACCO HABITS AND FOLLOW-UP CHANGES IN LEUKOPLAKIA IN 257 UNTREATED PATIENTS

	Tobacco Use		Leukoplakia		
No. of Patients	At Diagnosis	After Diagnosis*	Unchanged or Extended (%)	Improved or Disappeared (%)	Transformed to Carcinoma (%)
74	–	–	73	3	24
133	+	+	47	37	16
50	+	–	44	44	12

Adapted from Silverman S et al.[6]
*More than 1 year.
+ = current tobacco users; – = never smoked or stopped permanently at time of diagnosis.

Table 3–8. ORAL LEUKOPLAKIA WITH DYSPLASIA: PROGRESSION TO CARCINOMA		
Chromosome Ploidy	Nuclear DNA *n* (%)	Squamous Carcinoma *n* (%)
Diploid	105 (70)	3 (3)
Tetraploid	20 (13)	12 (60)
Aneuploid	25 (17)	21 (84)

Adapted from Sudbo J et al.[9]
Mean follow-up: 103 months (range 4–65).

patients with erythroleukoplakia was shown to be almost fourfold that of the patients with homogeneous leukoplakia (see Table 3–4). With this in mind, clinicians should take biopsy specimens that include erythematous areas because of the increased risk of representing dysplasia or neoplasia. In our study group of 257 patients, 58% of the patients with leukoplakia had an associated erythematous area, whereas 84% of the patients who eventually developed a carcinoma demonstrated a red component.

Other investigators have also found this increased risk associated with erythroleukoplakia. Roed-Petersen reported a sevenfold risk of malignant transformation in Danish patients whose leukoplakia had an erythematous component. His patients showed a 1.3% transformation rate in homogeneous leukoplakia versus a 9.1% rate in red and white lesions.[10] In a study limited to leukoplakias of the tongue and mouth floor, Kramer (England) reported a 15% transformation rate in an average period of 4.3 years.[11] The risk of formation of carcinoma in the red and white lesions was five times that of the homogeneous leukoplakias. Banoczy (Hungary) described an erosive form of leukoplakia with an erythematous com-

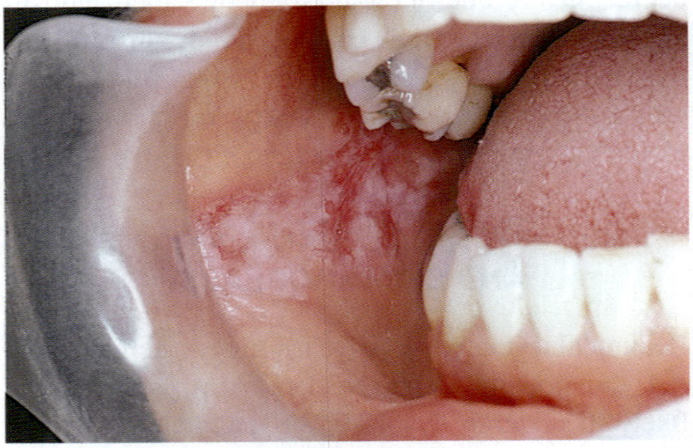

Figures 3–15 to 3–18. Erythroleukoplakias associated with transformations to dysplasia and carcinoma.
Figure 3–15. Dysplasia, buccal mucosa.

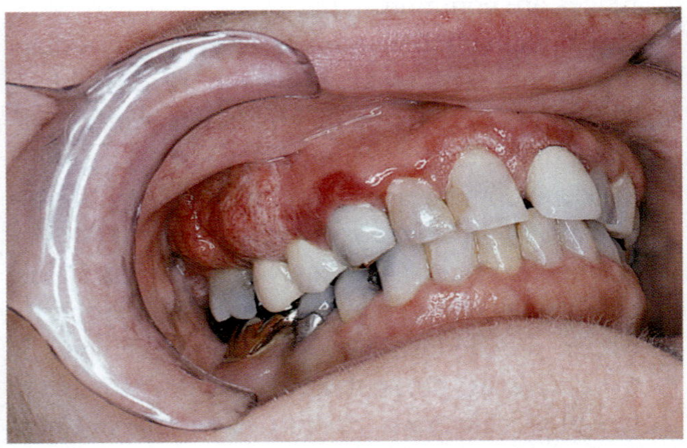

Figure 3–17. Gingival dysplasia (areas 6–9) and carcinoma (areas 3–5).

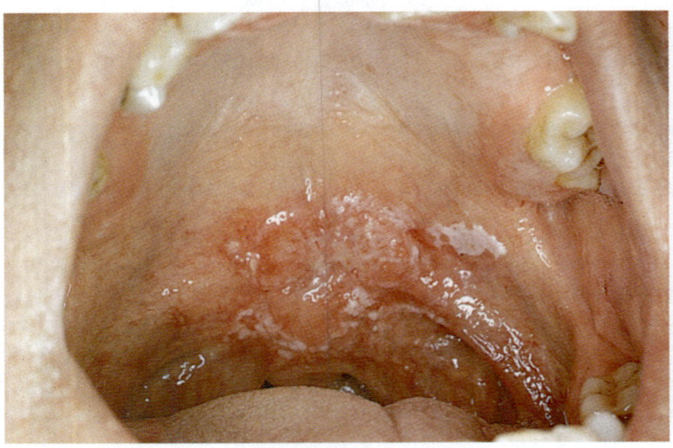

Figure 3–16. Carcinoma, oropharynx.

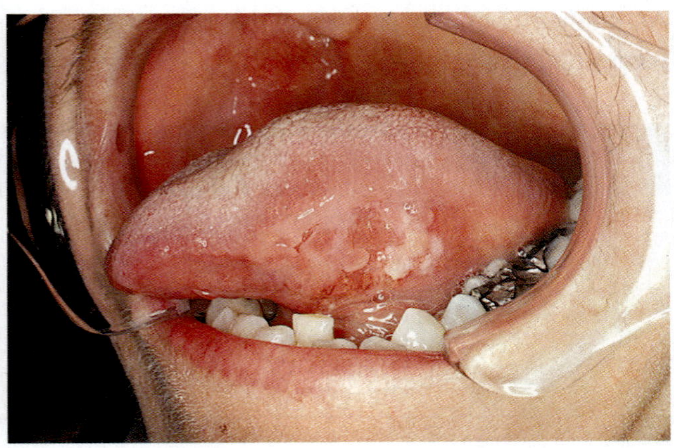

Figure 3–18. Carcinoma, tongue.

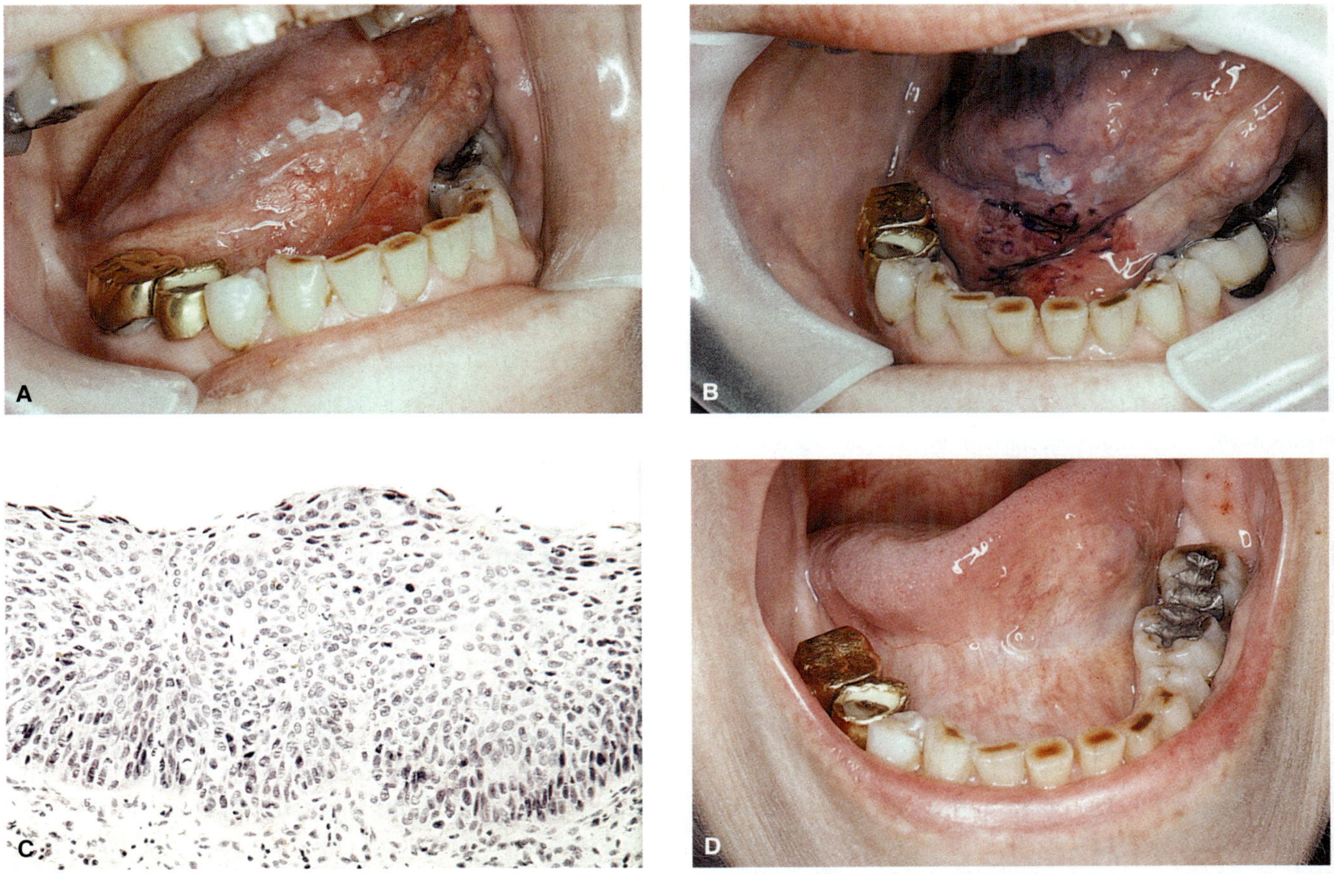

Figure 3–19. *A,* Patient complained of floor of the mouth irritation of 1 month duration. *B,* The red and white lesion was painted with 1% toluidine blue and decolorized with 1% acetic acid. Note retention in red area. *C,* A biopsy from the red area showed carcinoma in situ. *D,* Two months after carbon-dioxide laser excision. The lesion had not recurred at 5 years, and the patient was asymptomatic.

ponent that had a fivefold greater risk of malignant transformation than other leukoplakias.

In the United States, the high risk of malignancy in erythroplasia was reaffirmed further by Waldron and Shafer in a microscopic review of more than 3,000 leukoplakias.[12] Fifty-eight were described as clinically red lesions, of which 91% were found to be either invasive carcinoma, carcinoma in situ, or severe dysplasia. Mashberg and Samit directed another series of studies of high-risk patients (older men, high tobacco and alcohol consumption) in a New Jersey Veterans Administration Hospital. These studies showed that persistent erythroplasia, rather than leukoplakia, in high-risk sites is the earliest and predominant sign of oral carcinoma.[7] In Mashberg and Samit's prospective study of 222 asymptomatic oral carcinomas, 28% were red only; 62% were red and white; 97% occurred in the mouth floor, oral tongue, and oropharynx; and 84% were less than 2 cm at their largest diameter.

ERYTHROPLASIA WITH ULCERATION

Another rare but high-risk premalignant lesion is the chronic erythematous change associated with constantly recurring erosive changes. These lesions are often mistaken for "recurrent aphthous stomatitis of the herpetiform variety" or "nonspecific inflammatory immunopathologic vesiculoerosive disease" (Figure 3–21). A biopsy of the early lesion may show only hyperkeratosis and inflammation not suggestive of any specific disease. Clinical responses to empirical corticosteroid therapy may help rule out a premalignant status by indicating a benign inflammatory response associated with a vesiculoerosive disease. However, even a nondysplastic pattern in this type of

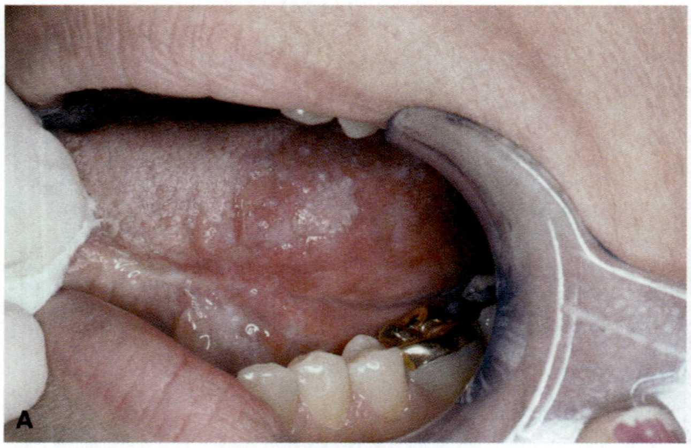

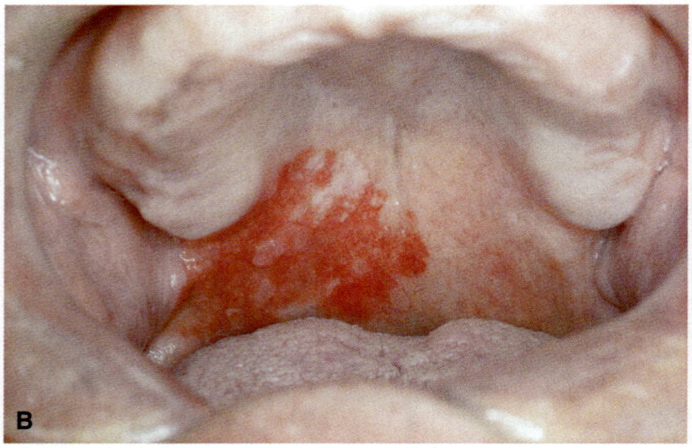

Figure 3–20. *A,* Erythroleukoplakia of the tongue microscopically showing severe dysplasia. *B,* Erythroleukoplakia of the palate, at first thought to represent a chronic infection, on biopsy was shown to be a squamous cell carcinoma.

lesion that cannot be classified deserves close follow-up, or even attempted removal, because of the risk that it may eventually develop into a carcinoma.

PROLIFERATIVE VERRUCOUS LEUKOPLAKIA

In 1985, we first described a unique form of leukoplakia found in 30 patients.[13] This group of lesions had a high risk of malignant transformation. Because of the characteristic appearance—an expanding, exophytic/fissured white lesion—we coined the name "proliferative verrucous leukoplakia" (PVL) (Figures 3–22 and 3–23).

To complicate matters, these growths displayed variable histologic appearances even within the same patient specimen, variations that could range from a benign hyperkeratosis through degrees of epithelial dysplasia to verrucous or squamous carcinoma (Figure 3–24). The inflammatory infiltrate also appeared quite variable, ranging from a mild, diffuse, white cell appearance to a dense, subepithelial clustering.

Subsequently, our follow-up study in 1997 of 54 PVL patients confirmed our initial findings as follows: (1) PVL is a very high-risk precancerous lesion with high transformation and mortality rates, (2) women outnumber men, (3) less than one-third of PVL patients smoke, and (4) there is usually multisite oral involvement (see Table 3–9).[14]

Therapeutic approaches have been only moderately encouraging. In our clinic at UCSF, the best results have been obtained with surgical removal using the carbon-dioxide laser. Often the procedure requires serial removal because of the large size and extensions of the lesion, enabling us to observe step-by-step control in an orderly fashion and to assess the high potential for recurrences because of possible inadequate margins and/or "field" involvement. The surgical failures appear to be related to early changes in subcellular elements that are not as yet clinically or microscopically evident, thereby leading to recurrences because of "inadequate margins."

Another laser-type procedure involves "photodynamic therapy," using cell-sensitizing compounds (ie, porfimer sodium or 5-aminolevulinic acid), followed by applications of laser energy of specific wavelengths that is directed to the sensitized cells.[15,16] This permits a more exacting target for dysplastic and/or cancer cell destruction. The side effects of the sensi-

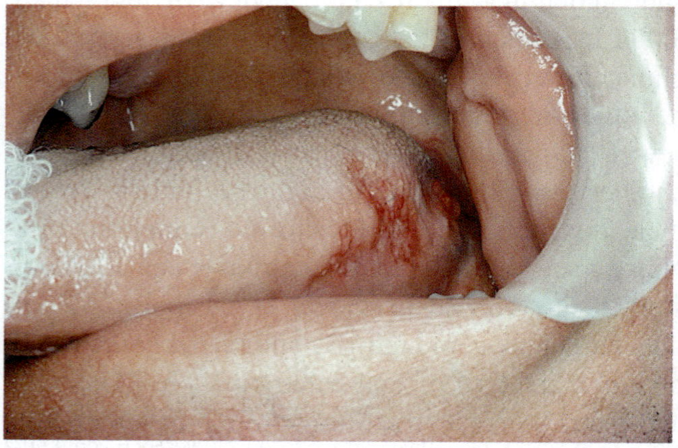

Figure 3–21. Squamous cell carcinoma presenting as a symptomatic erosive erythematous lesion of 3 months duration.

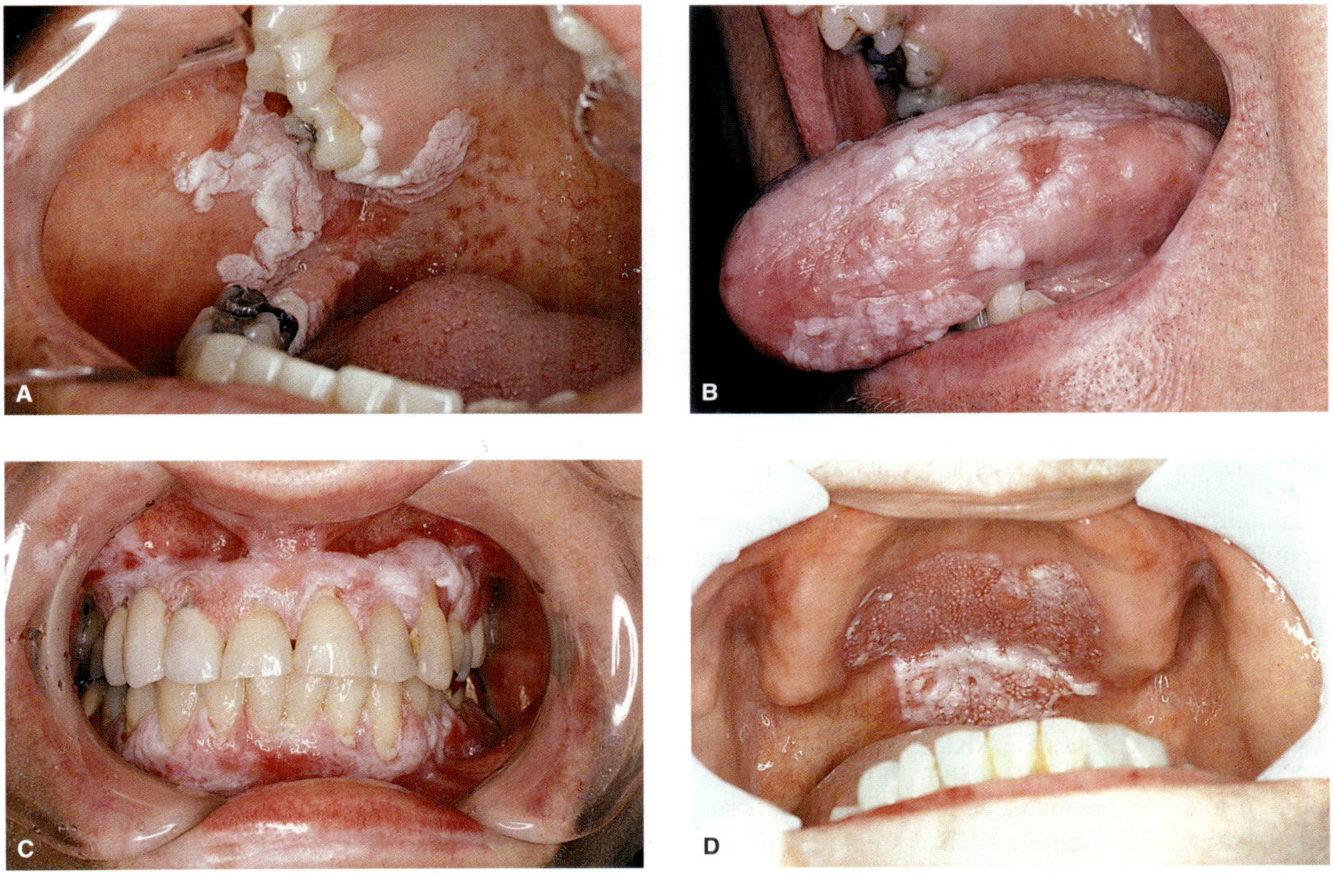

Figure 3–22. *A–D,* Proliferative verrucous leukoplakia.

tizing drugs, few long-term studies, and erratic results limit the practical and accepted use of this technique at present. Radiation and chemotherapeutic agents do not appear to be effective in controlling PVL.

Diagnostic and prognostic biomarkers for PVL have not as yet been identified. Human papillomaviruses (HPVs) have been isolated from some PVL lesions, but their role in the occurrence and/or

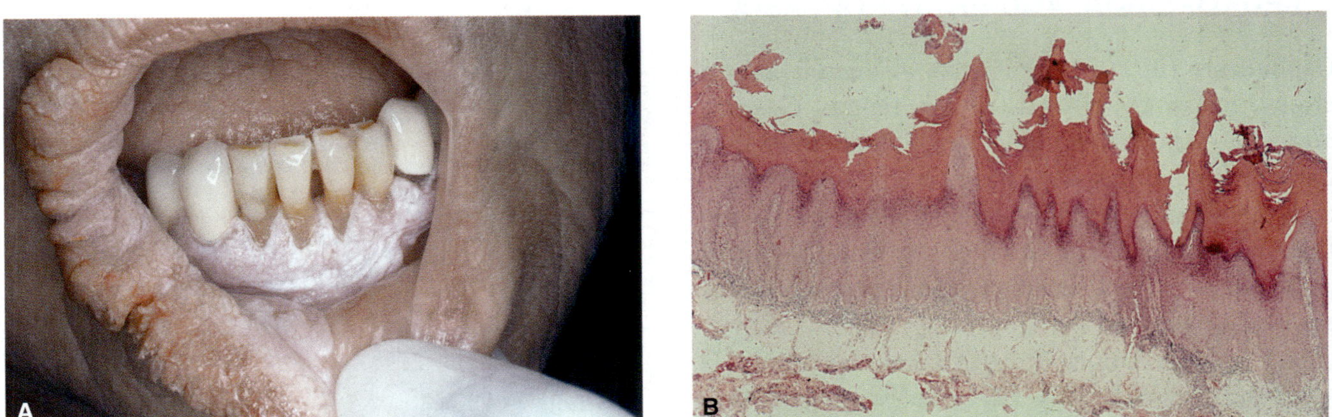

Figure 3–23. *A,* Proliferative verrucous leukoplakia of 5 years duration in a nonsmoking 78-year-old woman. *B,* A biopsy revealed characteristic changes of hyperorthokeratosis, surface papillary projection, epithelial hyperplasia, and an inflammatory infiltrate. There was a malignant transformation during the sixth year.

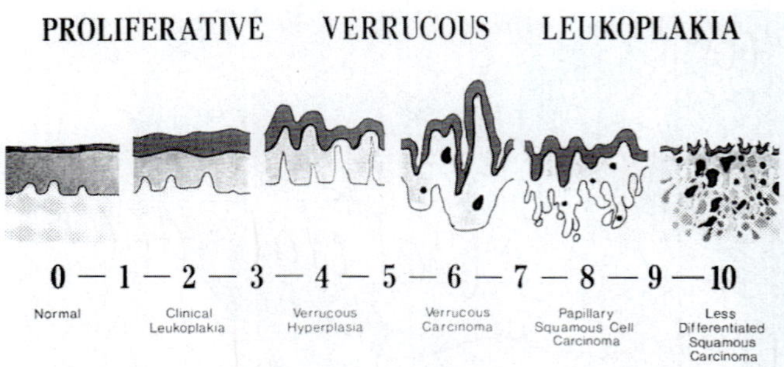

Figure 3–24. Varying histologic findings in proliferative verrucous leukoplakia specimens.

progression of PVL remains speculative.[17,18] However, the known effects of HPV E6 protein, which is capable of inactivating p53 suppressor protein, may account for ineffective control of epithelial growth factors and subsequent neoplasia. A recent study of HPV-associated PVL found that excision plus adjunctive use of an antiviral agent led to improved results compared with surgery alone.[19]

Because of the extreme variations in PVL appearance, natural history, histopathology, and outcome, it logically seems to be a multifactorial condition. Additionally, factors such as smoking and the presence of *Candida* have not demonstrated any influence on either occurrence or progression. At the present time, then, careful clinical and microscopic assessment combined with surgical techniques, clinical judgment, and close follow-up offer the best approaches to management.

CANDIDIASIS (CANDIDOSIS), LEUKOPLAKIA, AND ERYTHROPLASIA

Candidiasis (thrush, moniliasis) is caused almost always by an overgrowth of the fungus *Candida albicans*. Although this fungus is found in more than one-third of normal-appearing mouths, overgrowth does not occur unless the normal balance of the oral flora is disturbed, for example, by debilitating or acute illness, immune suppression, xerostomia, or antibiotic therapy. The following factors support clinical manifestations of candidal colonization: (1) adherence mechanisms between fungi and oral epithelial cells; (2) yeast overgrowth (which is probably dependent on and reflective of proteins expressed by *Candida*), host cell and extracellular matrix proteins, host cation influence on adhesion, and possible coaggregation between fungi and bacteria; and (3) host immune incompetence. The diagnosis of candidiasis is suspected with the observation of creamy-white and/or erythematous mucosal changes (Figure 3–25). Candidiasis can be confirmed by smear, culture, biopsy, or response to antifungal therapy.

Our studies indicate that candidiasis may add a potential risk factor for malignant transformation of leukoplakia (Figure 3–26). Although cultures showed that 31% of our leukoplakia patients fostered *Candida* as part of their oral flora, a rate similar to the occurrence in normal populations, 53% of the leukoplakia patients who developed carcinomas were *Candida* positive prior to tumor formation. However, mutagenicity and carcinogenicity of *C. albicans* have not been shown. Formation of nitrosamines (potential carcinogens) by *Candida* species in vitro has been implicated.

Other reports have demonstrated a higher prevalence of *Candida* in speckled leukoplakia compared with homogeneous (all-white) leukoplakia. In one study of 235 Danish patients with leukoplakia, 23.4% were *Candida* positive. However, whereas in the homogeneous group, 4 of 152 (2.6%) were *Candida* positive, in the speckled leukoplakia group, 51 of 83 (61.4%) were *Candida* positive. Our experience confirms the greater risk of fungal infection in the red and white lesion. It seems that the *Candida* organisms in these situations are secondary residents because treatment will most often convert erythroleukoplakia only into the homogeneous form. It

Table 3–9. SITES OF SQUAMOUS CARCINOMA IN 38 OF 54 PATIENTS WITH PROLIFERATIVE VERRUCOUS LEUKOPLAKIA

	No. of Carcinomas			
Site	Both Sexes (%)	Women (n = 43)	Men (n = 11)	Smokers
Gingiva	11 (29%)	9	2	1
Tongue	10 (26%)	8	2	5
Buccal	6 (16%)	5	1	3
Mouth floor	5 (13%)	5	0	1
Palate	5 (13%)	4	1	2
Lip	1 (3%)	1	0	0
Total	38 (100%)	32 (74.4%)	6 (54.5%)	12 (31.6%)

Adapted from Silverman S et al.[12]

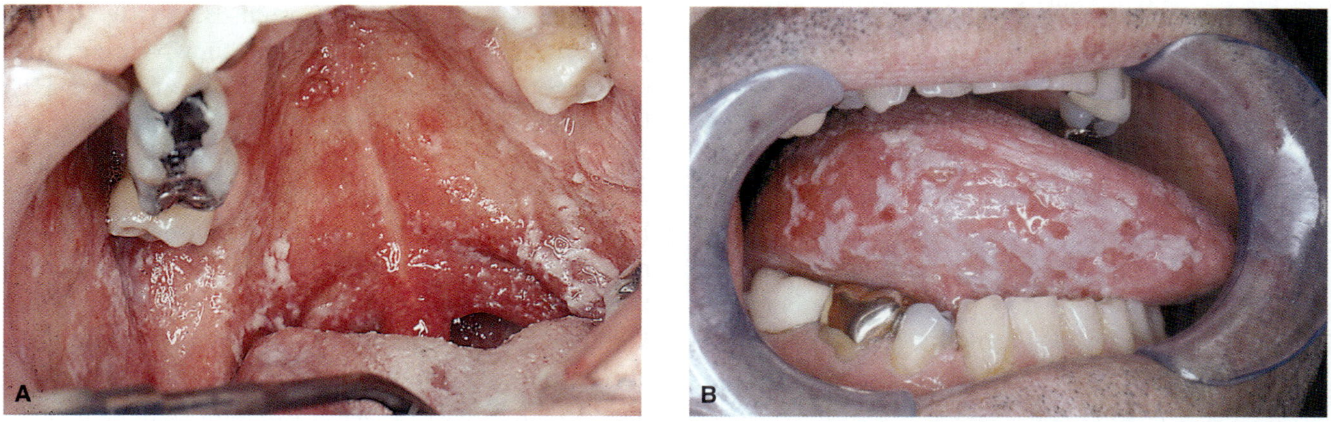

Figure 3–25. *A*, Candidiasis presenting as a red and white lesion. *B*, Plaque-form candidiasis mimicking leukoplakia. The lesion could not be scraped off but disappeared following antifungal therapy. A biopsy showed fungal hyphae in the epithelial surface layers.

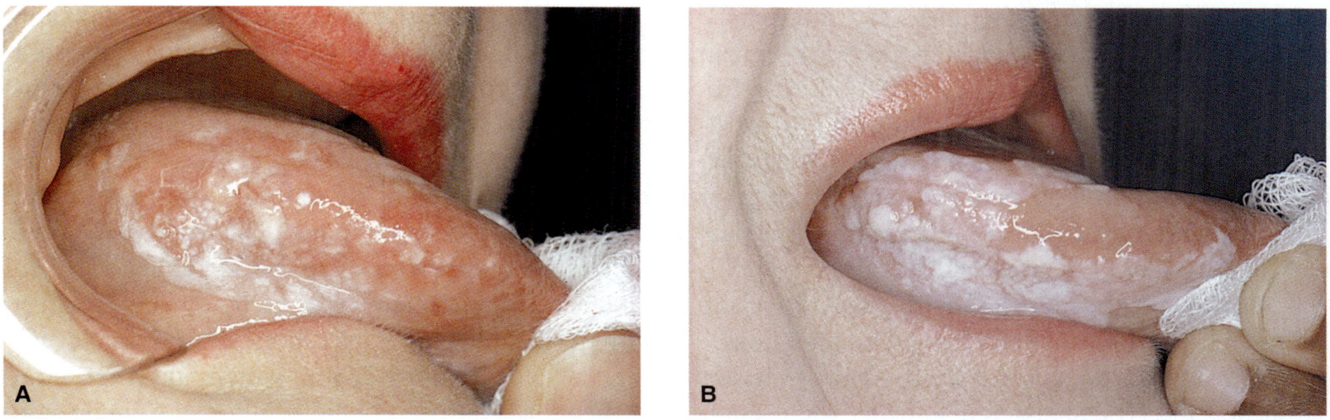

Figure 3–26. *Candida*-associated leukoplakia. *A*, Uncomfortable lesion of 6 months duration. Biopsy showed hyperkeratosis, inflammation, and *Candida* hyphae in the surface cell layers. *B*, Antifungal medication transposed the lesion to an asymptomatic homogeneous leukoplakia. The patient suffered recurrent bouts of candidiasis, and, after almost 2 years, the lesion transformed into a squamous cell carcinoma.

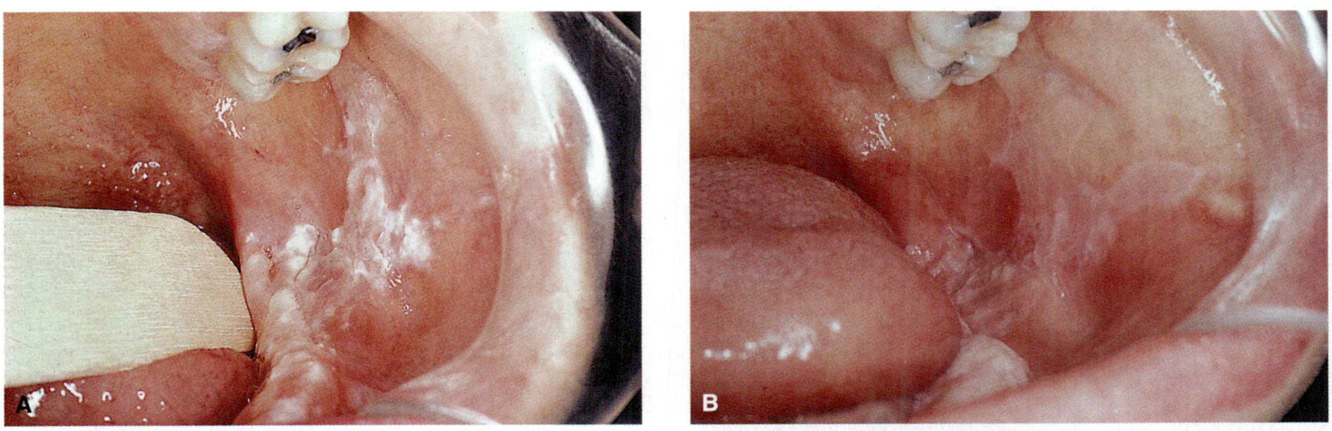

Figure 3–27. *Candida*-associated leukoplakia. *A*, Biopsy of this painful, long-standing leukoplakia showed hyperkeratosis, inflammation, and surface *Candida* organisms. *B*, Antifungal treatment led to control of symptoms and a marked reduction in the leukoplakia. Years later, this 60-year-old nonsmoking woman developed a squamous cell carcinoma in this area.

is possible, but infrequent, that *Candida* organisms stimulate hyperkeratosis leading to hyperplastic candidiasis because adequate antifungal treatment of the *Candida* infection may lead to disappearance of the clinical lesion (Figure 3–27).

The above reports show that candidiasis may complicate the observation and management of oral leukoplakia, but no studies have definitively documented a cause-and-effect relationship between *Candida*-associated leukoplakia and malignant transformation.

HAIRY LEUKOPLAKIA

Oral hairy leukoplakia (HL) describes white-appearing lesions that almost always occur unilaterally or bilaterally on the borders of the tongue. The significance of HL is that it serves as a marker for human immunodeficiency virus (HIV) infection. HL frequently appears as hairlike projections and/or corrugations, but it may also have a plaque-like appearance (Figure 3–28). It appears occasionally on other oral sites such as the buccal mucosa, oropharynx, and mouth floor. No evidence suggests that HL shares biologic similarities with hyperkeratotic leukoplakia, which has premalignant connotations.

The diagnosis is confirmed by biopsy and/or serology if the HIV status is unknown. Microscopically, HL appears as an epithelial hyperplasia with a parakeratotic surface and vacuolated cells often referred to as koilocytes (cells suggestive of viral infection). The presence of Epstein-Barr virus (EBV) in these vacuolated cells has been shown by electron microscopy and DNA probes. Because non-HL lesions can sometimes have a similar clinical or even microscopic appearance as HL, ultimate confirmation may depend on the demonstration of EBV or HIV-positive serology. Connective tissue inflammation may vary from moderate white cell infiltrates to the appearance of a noninflammatory lesion. The keratotic surface appears to comprise immature keratin because it is not preceded by keratohyaline granules. In about half of cases, *Candida* organisms can be demonstrated on the epithelial surface; however, antifungal treatment does not appreciably alter HL.

Whether EBV is a cause or result is as yet not clear. HL can occur in all HIV-infected groups, although far more often in homosexual men than in heterosexual men or women. This finding suggests a cofactor or cofactors that possibly may be transmitted more readily by oral and anal sexual practices.

Treatment is elective because these lesions are usually asymptomatic but chronic. They are treated only if they bother the patient in some way (mild irritation or appearance) or by coincidence when another disease is the target of treatment. HL may disappear following high doses of antiviral drugs (eg, acyclovir, zidovudine), which interrupt viral replication; topical tretinoin solution or retinoic acid solution; sulfa-type antibiotics given for controlling *Pneumocystis carinii* pneumonia; or topical applications of a podophyllum solution (a keratinolytic

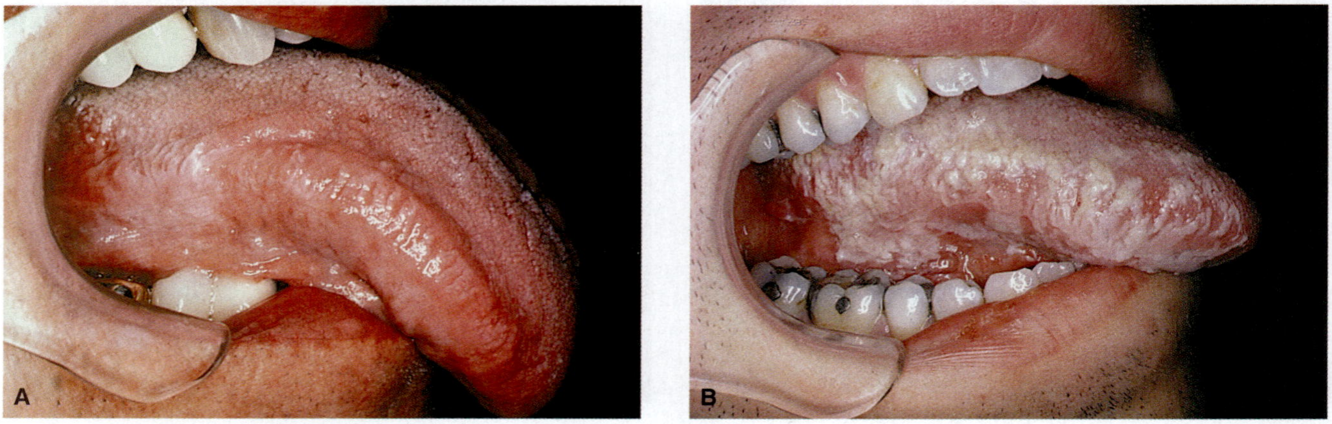

Figure 3–28. Hairy leukoplakia (HL). HL is not related to dysplasia or carcinoma. *A,* Mild, asymptomatic lesion in a 38-year-old HIV-positive homosexual male. *B,* Marked, asymptomatic lesion in a 32-year-old HIV-positive male.

agent). HL usually recurs when treatment is modified or discontinued. In any event, HL augurs a poor prognosis and is most definitely a marker for the acquired immune deficiency syndrome (AIDS). Since the institution of aggressive combination antiretroviral therapy for HIV-positive patients, HL is less frequently seen. It must be remembered that the only association between HL and leukoplakia is the white appearance; there is no other biologic similarity and most certainly not a precancerous risk.

DIAGNOSIS AND MANAGEMENT

Patients with leukoplakia are usually asymptomatic. The lesion is usually discovered by a clinician during a routine examination or by patients themselves because of a feeling of roughness in their mouths. No consistent or reliable clinical signs and symptoms associated with oral leukoplakia allow differentiation between or accurate prediction of a premalignant or early malignant change. However, even mild symptoms are often suggestive of a dysplastic epithelial change or even an early invasive tumor. Because the clinical appearance of oral leukoplakia—thick or scant, large or small—does not reliably indicate its biologic potential, clinicians should be suspicious of all white lesions and should carefully evaluate and observe these patients.

The first step in management of leukoplakia is the removal of all irritants. If the leukoplakia is not reversible, excision is the most effective treatment. However, because these lesions may spread over a large area, they cannot always be surgically excised. In addition, recurrence after excision is common, possibly owing to continuation of an irritant or the biologic potential in adjacent tissue that appears normal morphologically (field cancerization).

The use of the carbon-dioxide laser has proved extremely useful and effective (Figures 3–29 to 3–31).[20,21] Preceding the laser procedure, a diagnostic biopsy in part determines the biology of the lesion, the extent of the lesion, and a guide for the aggressiveness of removal. Removal, then, is usually accomplished by vaporization under local anesthesia in single or serial operations (depending on the extent of the leukoplakia). Healing occurs without suturing by secondary intention. Recurrences may occur, but they are almost always well localized, contained, and highly controllable with limited follow-up laser procedures. Complications are minimal, bleeding and infections are rare, and pain is variable and manageable with analgesic agents.

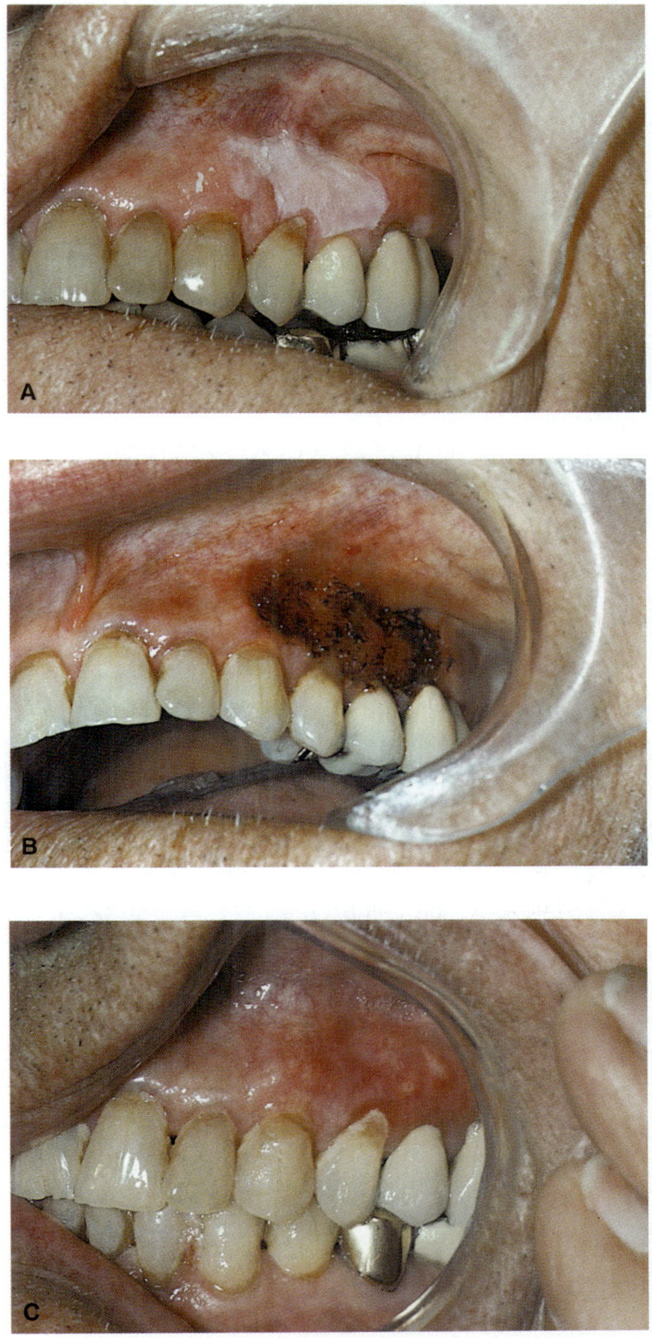

Figure 3–29. Laser removal of leukoplakia associated with mild dysplasia. *A*, Before surgery. *B*, Immediately after surgery. *C*, Healed and asymptomatic at 3 weeks.

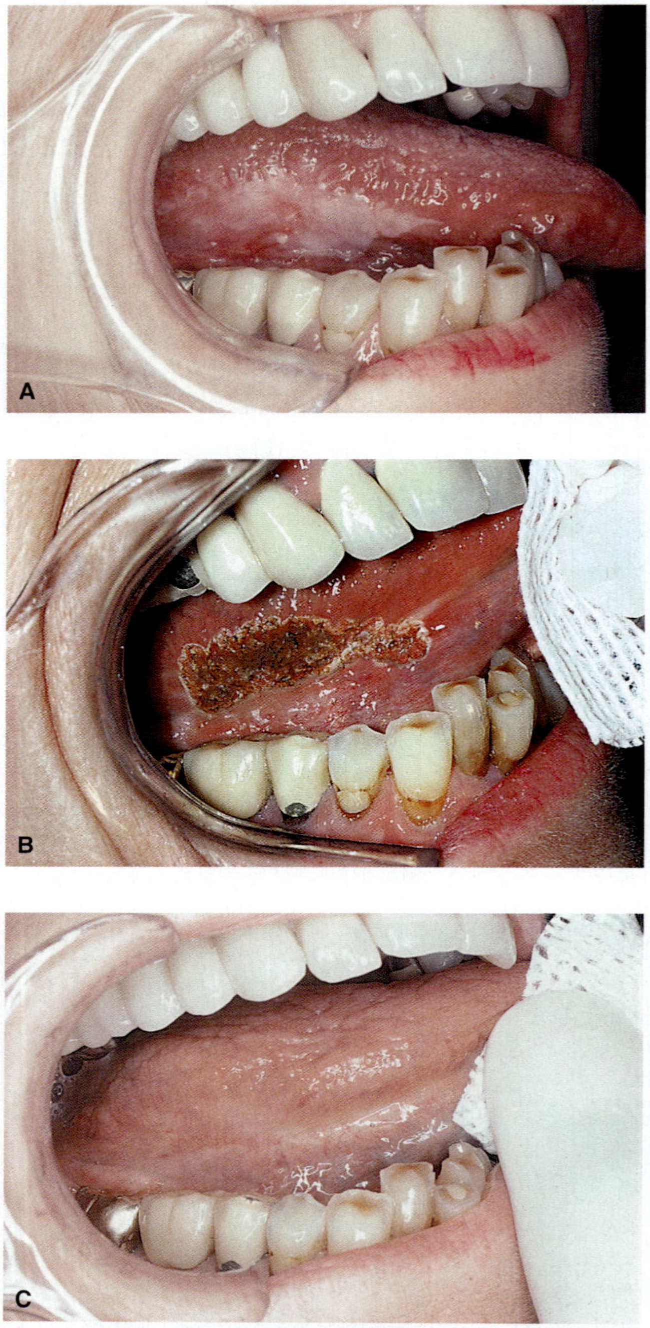

Figure 3–30. Leukoplakia with mild dysplasia. *A,* Before laser surgery. *B,* Immediately after carbon-dioxide laser removal. *C,* Completely healed at 3 weeks. There was no recurrence at 4 years of follow-up.

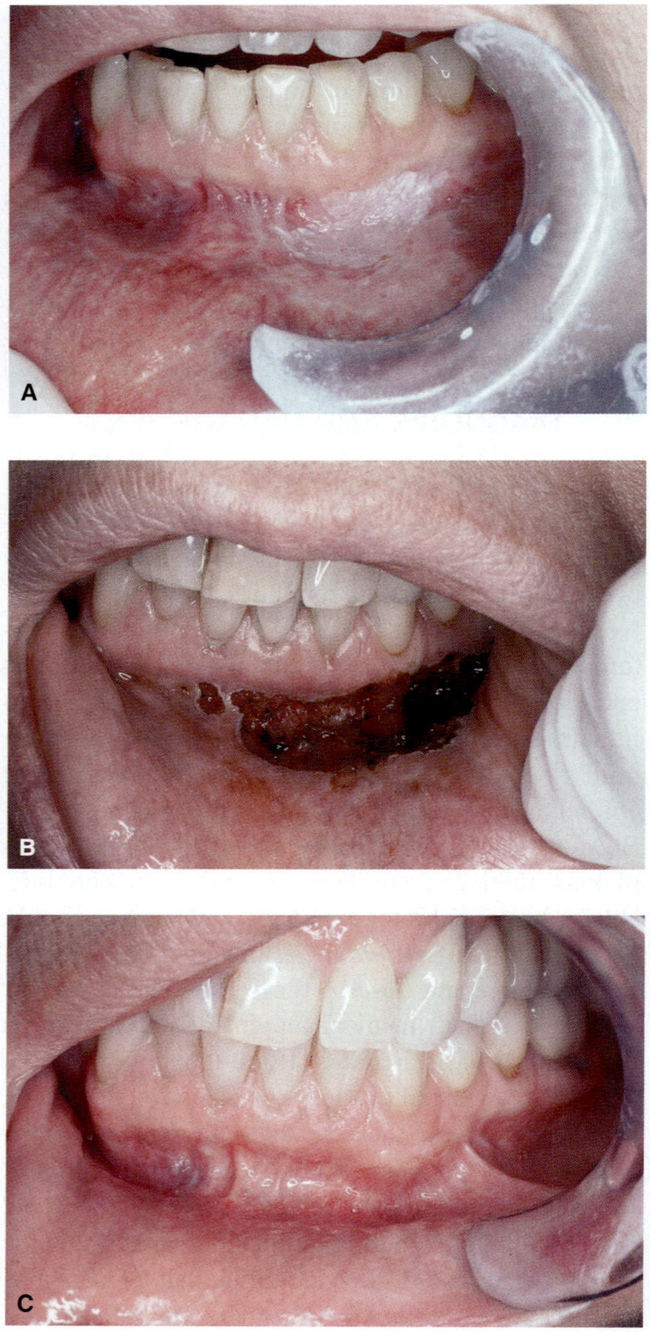

Figure 3–31. *A,* Asymptomatic leukoplakia of several years duration that was spreading. A biopsy showed moderate dysplasia. *B,* Immediately following carbon-dioxide laser removal by vaporization. Healing was complete in 1 month. *C,* At 2 years of follow-up, the patient was asymptomatic and the leukoplakia was controlled.

However, it must be remembered that there is always some degree of risk, not only for recurrences but also for the development of squamous cell carcinoma at the surgical site. Therefore, close follow-up must be emphasized. To help limit recurrences, adjunctive chemotherapy using antiviral drugs and antioxidants is being studied.[22]

Although there might be a "field keratinization," genomic susceptibility for hyperkeratosis, there is some evidence of clonal derivation. This is seen at times when a portion of a leukoplakic lesion is removed and the residual clinical lesion disappears. Electrodesiccation and cryosurgery have not been uniformly effective in permanently removing keratotic lesions. Proteolytic enzymes have been of no value because keratin appears to resist a response at acceptable human dosages.

The use of vitamin A in attempts to control cancer and leukoplakia is often termed "chemoprevention." The potential benefit of vitamin A was postulated from observations of animal studies in which vitamin A deficiencies led to epithelial hyperkeratosis. This led to human trials using vitamin A ester in high dosages (more than 300,000 units per day in troche form), which was effective in some patients in reversing oral leukoplakia associated with hyperkeratosis. The mechanism of action remains unknown but is probably related to effects on epithelial growth and suppressor proteins and cell differentiation. However, on withdrawal of vitamin A, the leukoplakia returns. Vitamin A tolerance is short-lived with the required high dosages because of limited liver storage and subsequent toxicity. The most common adverse side effects are dry skin, rash, and pruritus. One report has shown that oral squamous carcinomas have developed during or shortly following vitamin A regimens in some patients. These reports suggest the possibility that, in some instances, high dosages of vitamin A associated with poorly understood host or other cofactors may increase the risk of carcinogenesis.

In attempts to increase effectiveness and diminish toxicity, an analogue of vitamin A (13-*cis* retinoic acid) was developed.[23] Although intake of moderately high dosages will control some lesions, toxicity still limits its usefulness. Side effects include dry skin, pruritus, rash, cheilitis, photosensitivity, and hypertriglyceridemia. Another retinoid analogue, fenritinide, has also demonstrated the same problems of limited effectiveness and undesirable side effects. Beta carotene, a precursor to vitamin A possessing very few adverse side effects, has not been effective. Additionally, combinations of antioxidant vitamins and nutrients have not been effective in the control of oral leukoplakia.[24] These include beta carotene, vitamin A, ascorbic acid (vitamin C), and α-tocopherol (vitamin E). Their potential biologic actions include (1) quenching of cellular free radicals, which can affect chromosome integrity, mutagenesis, and carcinogenesis, and/or (2) promoting a balanced function between epithelial growth and suppressor proteins. Retinoic acid solution and 13-*cis* retinoic acid (Accutane) have been approved for use in acne. In our experience, daily topical applications of 0.05% retinoic acid solution to oral leukoplakia have achieved partial remissions in some patients. However, applications can produce inflammation and irritation, and the long-term implications are unknown. Also, compliance is a problem, and, as in other forms of vitamin A–type therapy, discontinuation leads to recurrences. Chemoprevention of oral leukoplakia remains experimental (see Chapter 5).

Because many methods of managing leukoplakia are not always feasible or effective, these patients must be observed periodically (Figure 3–32). The follow-up examination includes careful clinical observation and an occasional biopsy. Follow-up biopsy is indicated when changes in signs and/or symptoms occur. Exfoliative cytology using the brush biopsy technique and vital staining with toluidine blue help supplement clinical judgment and serve as an adjunct to biopsy (see Chapter 4). Because the "gold standard" for diagnosis is tissue biopsy, the value of adjunctive techniques is to accelerate microscopic evaluation by indicating the need of biopsy in situations in which a biopsy is delayed or not thought to be indicated or necessary. Negative smears or stains must be balanced with clinical judgment. Therefore, if clinical suspicion persists in a lesion that does not disappear, a biopsy must be considered.

SUMMARY

The risk of malignant transformation in oral leukoplakia always remains. Because leukoplakia and carcinoma can occur simultaneously, and no established prognostic clinical guide exists, all white lesions characterized as leukoplakia must be microscopically diagnosed and either removed or monitored with care. Biopsy is the only definitive way to establish the exact nature of oral leukoplakias.

When seeking dysplastic or malignant areas in leukoplakic lesions, it is important to remember that

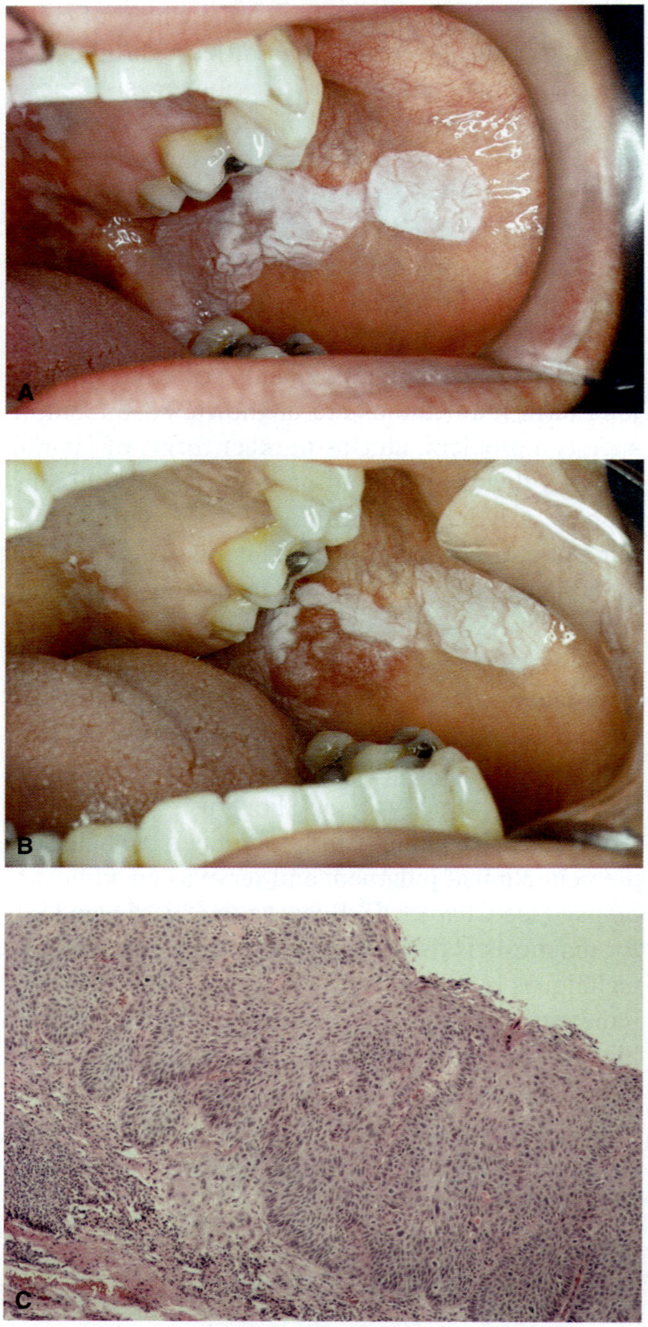

Figure 3–32. *A*, Asymptomatic leukoplakia of many years duration that was slowly enlarging. *B*, Twelve years later, there were marked changes in signs and symptoms: in the posterior left buccal mucosa, the lesion became erythematous and painful. A biopsy from that area revealed a squamous cell carcinoma. The adjacent white areas microscopically remained as benign hyperkeratotic changes. *C*, Biopsy shows early invasive squamous cell carcinoma.

erythematous and speckled regions are more likely to be dysplastic or cancerous than thick and homogeneous white regions. It must also be remembered that the diagnosis of a previously biopsied benign white patch must be periodically reaffirmed because a leukoplakia may unpredictably transform into malignancy. Moreover, although a leukoplakic lesion may regress and disappear when an irritant is reduced or removed, it can recur and may subsequently become cancerous.

In determining the aggressiveness of management, considerations of the following potential risk factors are essential: (1) an erythematous component in a white lesion, (2) microscopic dysplasia, (3) a clinical appearance of proliferative verrucous leukoplakia, (4) associated candidiasis seen microscopically, (5) a nonsmoking patient, (6) pain or irritation (leukoplakia is usually asymptomatic), and (7) a red lesion (erythroplasia, erythroplakia) without a white component, which also may represent a dysplastic or malignant lesion.

REFERENCES

1. Axell T, Pindborg JJ, Smith CJ, et al. Oral white lesions with special reference to precancerous and tobacco-related lesions: conclusions of an international symposium held in Uppsala, Sweden, May 18–21, 1994. J Oral Pathol Med 1996;25:49–54.
2. Bouquot JE, Weiland LH, Kurland LT. Leukoplakia and carcinoma in situ synchronously associated with invasive oral/pharyngeal carcinoma in Rochester, Minn., 1935–1984. Oral Surg Oral Med Oral Pathol 1988;65:199–207.
3. Banoczy J. Follow-up studies in oral leukoplakia. Maxillofac Surg 1977;5:69–75.
4. Shibuya H, Amagasa T, Seto K, et al. Leukoplakia-associated multiple carcinomas in patients with tongue carcinoma. Cancer 1986;57:843–6.
5. Regezi JA, Zarbo RJ, Regev E, et al. p53 protein expression in sequential biopsies of oral dysplasias and in situ carcinomas. J Oral Pathol Med 1995;24:18–22.

5a. Lumerman H, Freedman P, Kerpel S. Oral epithelial dysplasia and the development of invasive squamous carcinoma. Oral Surg Oral Med Oral Pathol Oral Radiol Endod 1995; 79:321–9.

6. Silverman S Jr, Gorsky M, Lozada F. Oral leukoplakia and malignant transformation: a follow-up study of 257 patients. Cancer 1984;53:563–8.
7. Mashberg A, Samit A. Early diagnosis of asymptomatic oral and oropharyngeal squamous cancers. CA Cancer J Clin 1995;45:328–51.
8. Abbey LM, Kaugars GE, Gunsolley JC, et al. Intraexaminer and interexaminer reliability in the diagnosis of oral epithelial dysplasia. Oral Surg Oral Med Oral Pathol Oral Radiol Endod 1995;80:188–91.
9. Sudbo J, Kildal W, Risberg B, et al. DNA content as a prognostic marker in patients with oral leukoplakia. N Engl J Med 2001;344:1270–80.

10. Roed-Petersen B. Cancer development in oral leukoplakia: follow-up of 331 patients. J Dent Res 1971;50:711 (Abstr).
11. Kramer IRH. Precancerous conditions of oral mucosa: a computer-aided study. Ann R Coll Surg Eng 1969;45: 340–56.
12. Waldron CA, Shafer WG. Leukoplakia revisited. A clinicopathologic study of 3,256 oral leukoplakias. Cancer 1975; 36:1386–92.
13. Hansen LS, Olson JA, Silverman S Jr. Proliferative verrucous leukoplakia. Oral Surg Oral Med Oral Pathol 1985;60:285–98.
14. Silverman S Jr, Gorsky M. Proliferative verrucous leukoplakia. A follow-up study of 54 cases. Oral Surg Oral Med Oral Pathol Oral Radiol Endod 1997;84:154–7.
15. Braichotte DR, Wagnieres GA, Bays R, et al. Clinical pharmacokinetic studies of Photofrin by fluorescence spectroscopy in the oral cavity, the esophagus and the bronchi. Cancer 1995;75:2768–78.
16. Fan KFM, Hopper C, Speight PM, et al. Photodynamic therapy using 5-aminolevulinic acid for premalignant and malignant lesions of the oral cavity. Cancer 1996;78:1374–83.
17. Palefsky JM, Silverman S Jr, Abdel-Salaam M, et al. Association between proliferative verrucous leukoplakia and infection with human papilloma virus type 16. J Oral Pathol Med 1995;24:193–7.
18. Zakrzewska JM, Lopes V, Speight P, Hopper C. Proliferative verrucous leukoplakia. Oral Surg Oral Med Oral Pathol Oral Radiol Endod 1996;82:396–401.
19. Femiano F, Gombos F, Scully C. Oral proliferative leukoplakia (PVL): open trial of surgery compared with combined therapy using surgery and methisoprinol in papillomavirus-related PVL. Int J Oral Maxillofac Surg 2001;30:318–22.
20. Chu FWK, Silverman S Jr, Dedo HH. CO_2 laser treatment of oral leukoplakia. Laryngoscope 1988;98:125–30.
21. Schoelch ML, Sekandari N, Regezi JA, Silverman S Jr. Laser management of oral leukoplakias: a follow-up study of 70 patients. Laryngoscope 1999;109:949–53.
22. Shaheen NJ, Straus WL, Sandler RS. Chemoprevention of gastrointestinal malignancies with nonsteroidal antiinflammatory drugs. A review. Cancer 2002;94:950–63.
23. Lippman SM, Spitz M, Zoltan T, et al. Epidemiology, biology, and chemoprevention of aerodigestive cancer. Cancer 1994;74:2719–25.
24. Kaugars GE, Silverman S Jr, Lovas JL, et al. A review of the use of antioxidant supplements in the treatment of human oral leukoplakia. Oral Surg Oral Med Oral Pathol Oral Radiol Endod 1996;81:5–14.

4

Diagnosis

SOL SILVERMAN JR., MA, DDS
NANCY J. FISCHBEIN, MD (Imaging)
WILLIAM P. DILLON, MD (Imaging)

A clinician's dilemma in oral diagnosis stems from the multitude of ill-defined, variable-appearing, controversial, and poorly understood lesions that manifest themselves in the oral cavity. Most of these lesions are benign, and many present changes that may easily be confused with malignancy. Conversely, early malignancy may be mistaken for a benign change (Figures 4–1 to 4–21). Some lesions are considered premalignant because they are statistically correlated with subsequent associated cancerous changes. Inescapably, then, much clinical uncertainty is involved in the early detection of malignancy as well as in the understanding and management of other lesions that may not always remain benign (see Chapter 3, "Leukoplakia and Erythroplasia").

DELAY IN DIAGNOSIS

Both public and professional awareness of oral cancer is fundamental for minimizing the time from onset of signs or symptoms to diagnosis. In most instances, delay is attributable to patients' not seeking consultation. However, in a considerable number of cases, diagnosis has been delayed because a clinician did not suspect the malignant nature of the lesion and treated it by empirical procedures inadequate for cancer control.[1–3] Most reports reveal that patients usually delay seeking professional advice for more than 3 months after having become aware of an oral sign or symptom. Such delays in diagnosis can only lead to local extension of a lesion and increase the risk of metastatic spread (see Chapter 5, "Spread of Tumor, Staging, and Survival").

SIGNS AND SYMPTOMS

Although some patients finally seek consultation only after developing severe and persistent pain, the most frequent chief complaint is that of a "sore" or "irritation" in the mouth. Early carcinoma of the oral cavity may be painless or associated with only a mild irritation. Pain usually occurs when the lesion becomes ulcerated. Sometimes, although rarely, a patient seeks consultation because of a "lump in the neck" that represents a metastasis from an oral lesion of which the patient may be completely unaware. The following are common presenting signs of oral carcinoma:

Ulceration or erosion. Destruction of epithelial integrity owing to discrepancy in cell maturation, loss of intercellular attachments, and disruption of basal lamina (basement membrane).

Erythema. Redness reflecting inflammation, thinness and irregularity of epithelium, and lack of keratinization.

Induration. Hardness owing primarily to an increase in the number of epithelial cells and secondarily to an inflammatory infiltrate.

Fixation. Abnormally dividing cells invading to deeper areas of muscle and bone.

Chronicity. Failure to heal. Cancer is not a spontaneously reversible disease. Therefore, a malignant lesion normally will not disappear in the absence of definitive antitumor therapy. In the world literature, less than 200 cases of spontaneous remission have been reported; only 2 have involved the head and neck region (tongue and laryngeal carcinomas).

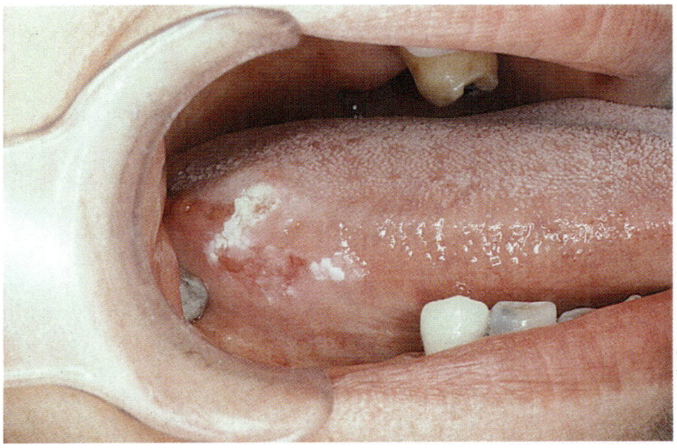

Figures 4–1 to 4–6. Carcinoma of the tongue.
Figure 4–1. Squamous cell carcinoma presenting clinically as erythroleukoplakia and thought to be a benign chronic irritation.

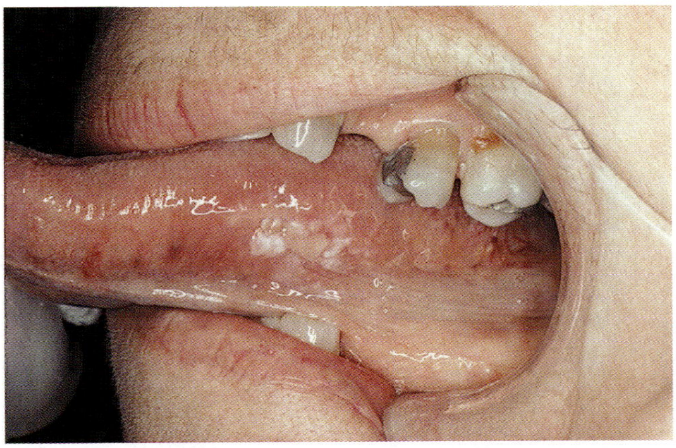

Figure 4–2. Squamous cell carcinoma presenting clinically as a pseudomembrane-covered ulcer with surrounding leukoplakia and thought to be caused by benign trauma from an ill-fitting partial denture.

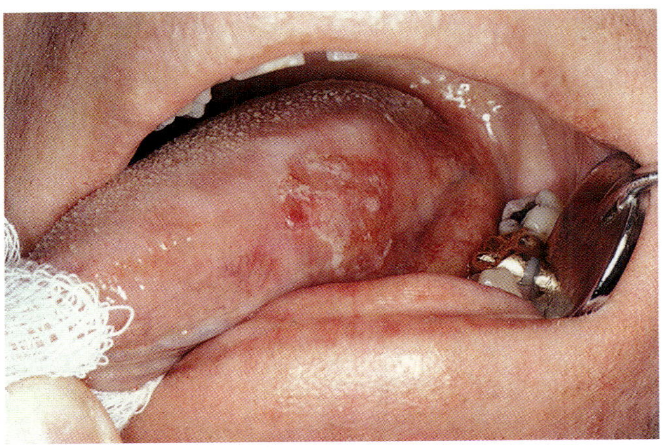

Figure 4–3. Squamous cell carcinoma presenting clinically as erythroleukoplakia and thought to represent a tongue infection.

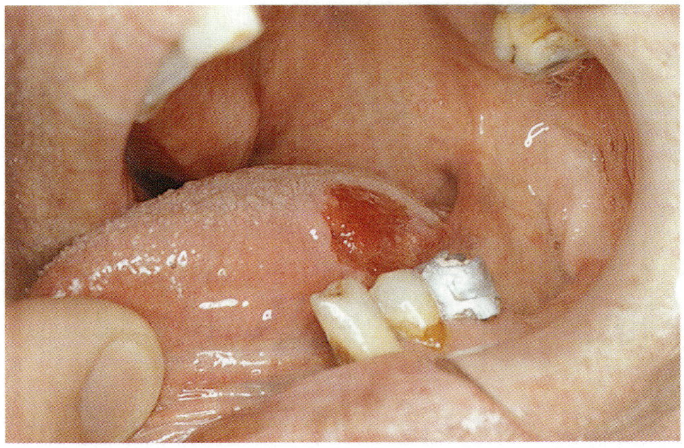

Figure 4–4. Squamous cell carcinoma presenting as erythroleukoplakia and thought to be irritation from a temporary crown.

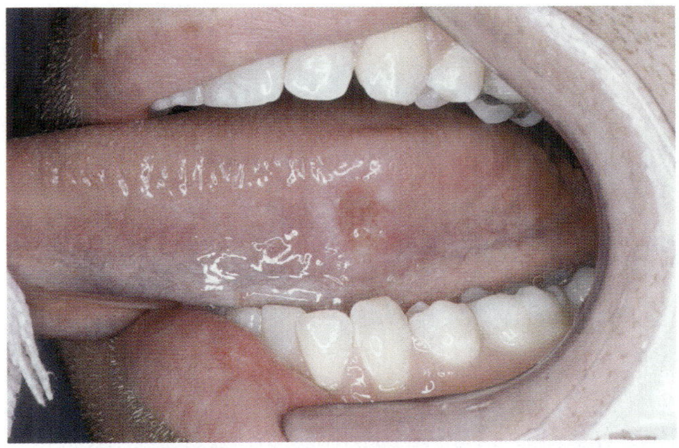

Figure 4–5. Squamous cell carcinoma in a 30-year-old man with no risk factors, at first mistaken for an aphthous ulcer or traumatic lesion.

Spontaneous remissions probably are explained best by immunologic control.

Lymphadenopathy. Hardening and/or enlargement of regional nodes owing to engorgement with neoplastic cells that spread by lymphatic vessels (see Chapter 5). Nodes are usually painless and often become fixed because of capsular erosion and local infiltration. Tumors that involve marked induration, fixation, and lymphadenopathy are signs of advanced cancer.

Leukoplakia. A white patch on the mucosal surface, reflecting excess epithelial keratin production. Hyperkeratosis is often associated with well-differentiated carcinomatous lesions (see Chapter 3).

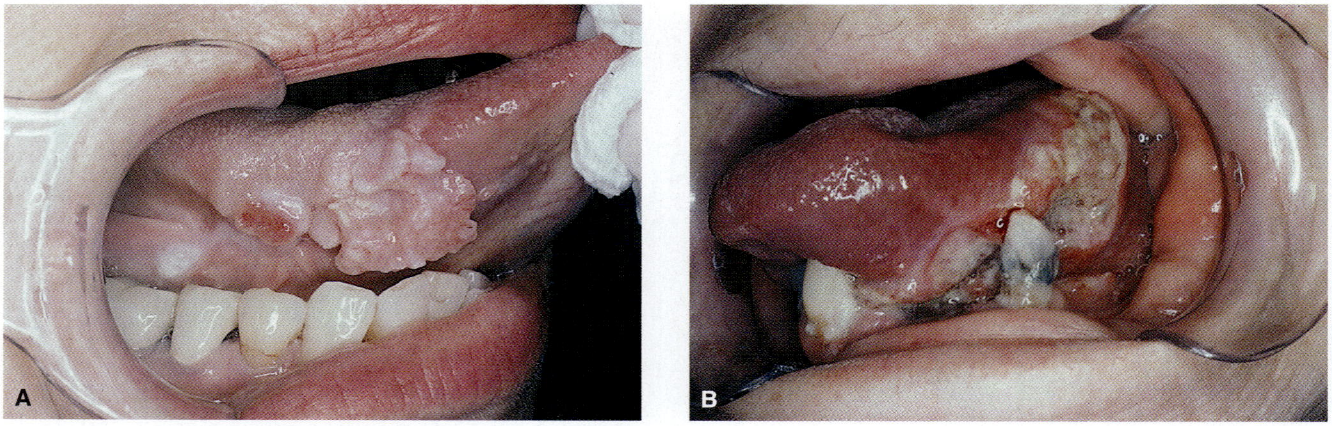

Figure 4–6. *A*, Advanced exophytic carcinoma that had been noticed for more than 6 months. *B*, Advanced ulcerative carcinoma that had been noticed for more than 6 months.

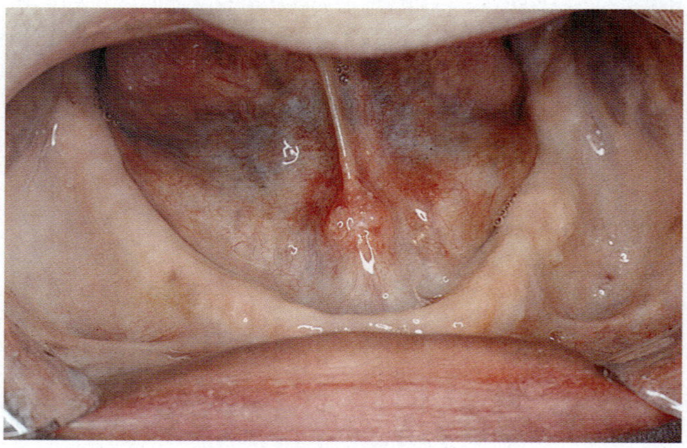

Figures 4–7 to 4–10. Carcinomas of the floor of the mouth.
Figure 4–7. Squamous cell carcinoma presenting clinically as erythema behind the orifices of Wharton's ducts and thought to be inflammatory.

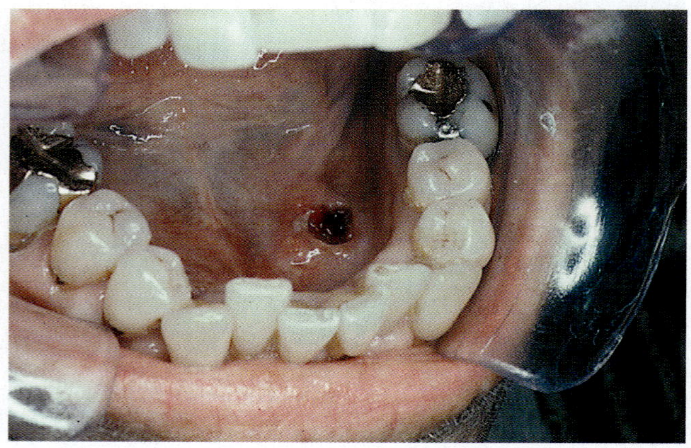

Figure 4–9. Squamous cell carcinoma presenting clinically as an ulcer and thought to be an atypical aphthous ulcer.

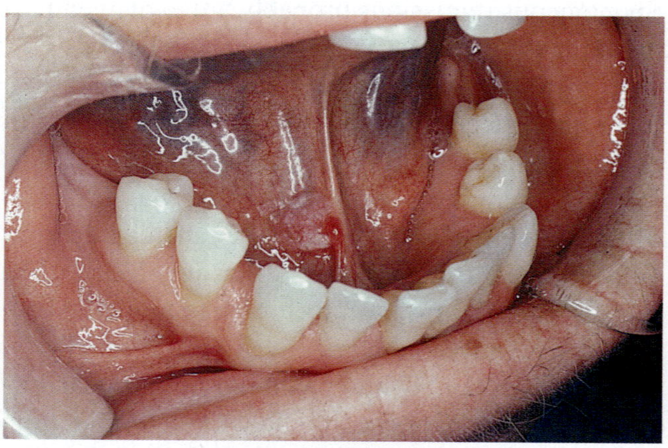

Figure 4–8. Squamous cell carcinoma presenting clinically as leukoplakia and thought to be benign keratosis from smoking.

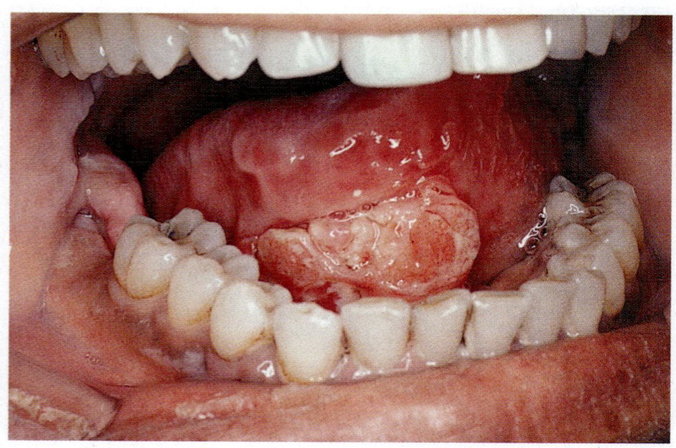

Figure 4–10. Advanced floor of mouth carcinoma noticed for more than 6 months.

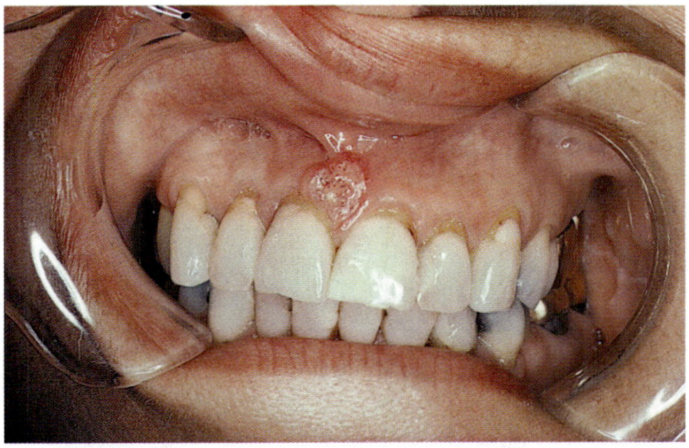

Figures 4–11 to 4–14. Carcinomas of the gingiva.
Figure 4–11. Early carcinoma thought to be an infection (parulis).

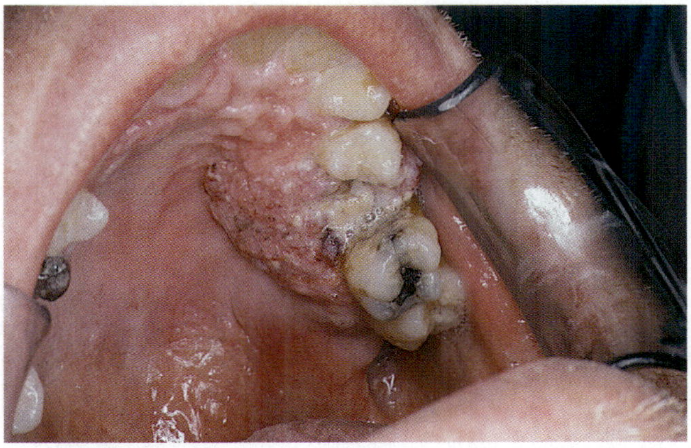

Figure 4–13. Verrucous carcinoma thought to be a squamous papilloma or wart.

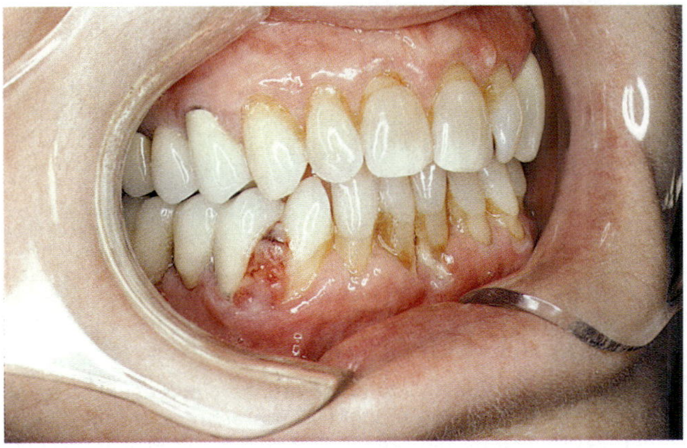

Figure 4–12. Early carcinoma thought to be a pyogenic granuloma from a periodontal infection.

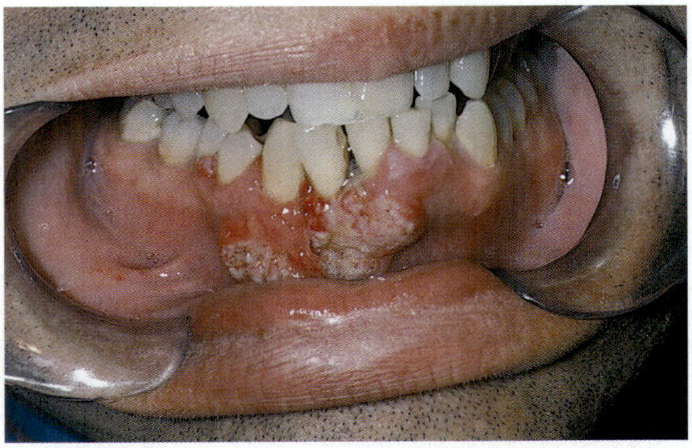

Figure 4–14. Advanced carcinoma treated for months as a periodontal-gingival infection.

Excess keratin also may be produced within the stratified squamous epithelium and can appear as "keratin pearls."

Early carcinomas may appear as small, apparently harmless local changes, frequently lulling the unsuspecting clinician into a false sense of security and empirical treatments, as well as periods of watching. In the premalignant and early cancerous stages, slow cellular proliferation may obscure clinical recognition of neoplastic activity in some cases. Obviously, this can lead to delays in diagnosis, which may dramatically worsen outcomes. All lesions of the oral cavity that persist or do not respond to the usual therapeutic measures must therefore be considered precancerous or malignant until proven otherwise.

An insight into the histopathogenesis of carcinoma may give the clinician a better understanding of presenting signs. Figures 4–22 to 4–25 depict the transformation from normal epithelium to dysplasia and finally to malignancy.

Once dysplasia becomes visible microscopically, there is no way of knowing whether it will reverse itself because there are no clear-cut criteria for determining which dysplasias will transform into carcinoma and which will not (see Chapter 5 regarding advanced diagnostic methods). Therefore, the terms carcinoma in situ or intraepithelial carcinoma refer to severely dysplastic epithelium that most probably will proceed to malignancy. Once the disorderly activity of cells involves disruption of the basal lamina and invasion of the adja-

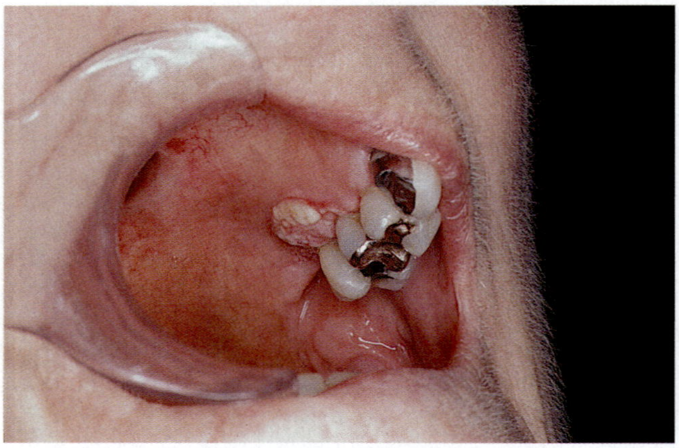

Figures 4–15 to 4–18. Oropharyngeal carcinomas.
Figure 4–15. Carcinoma thought to be a benign palatal papilloma.

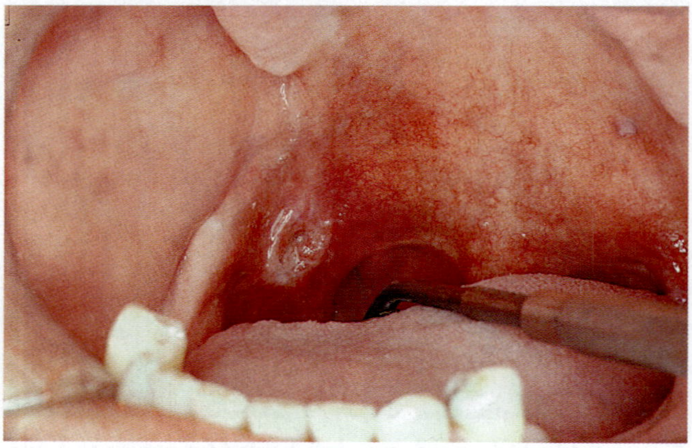

Figure 4–16. Carcinoma of the soft palate thought to be an atypical aphthous-type ulcer.

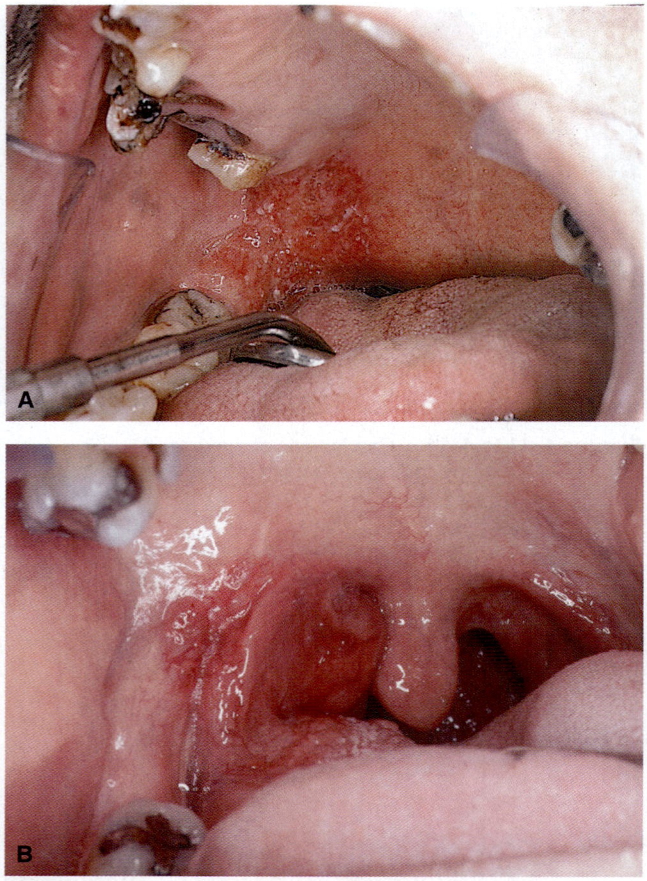

Figure 4–17. *A*, Carcinoma of the oropharynx presenting as an inflammatory lesion and thought to represent a chronic "strep throat." *B*, Squamous cell carcinoma of the right tonsil at first mistaken for an infection.

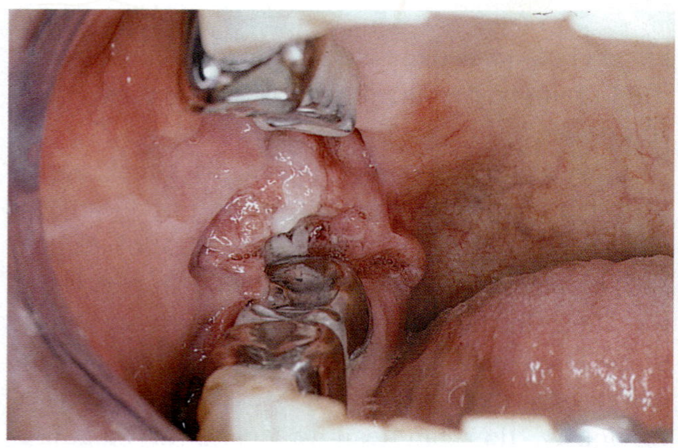

Figure 4–18. Carcinoma of posterior buccal mucosa thought to be an infection from cheek biting.

cent connective tissue, the diagnosis of malignancy can be made unequivocally.

BIOPSY AND EXFOLIATIVE CYTOLOGY

Because of the variability of signs and symptoms, even good clinical judgment and experience will not preclude diagnostic errors. Because oral cancer has such a poor prognosis, early detection and early adequate treatment are essential to the improvement of cure rates. Biopsy is the only method of definitively diagnosing a cancer.

Immediate biopsy of every ill-defined or innocuous-appearing lesion is impractical and not indicated. It is obvious, then, that a simple, reliable, and acceptable technique to support clinical judgment in differentiating benign lesions from early

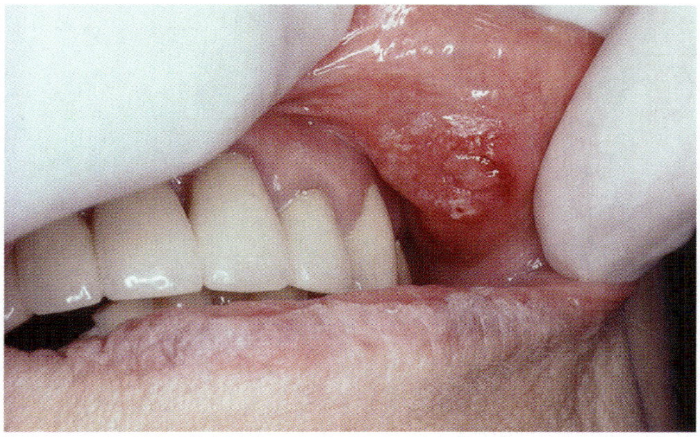

Figures 4–19 to 4–21. Carcinomas of the lip.
Figure 4–19. Squamous cell carcinoma of the upper labial mucosa at first mistakenly thought to be a granulomatous lesion or a traumatized mucocele.

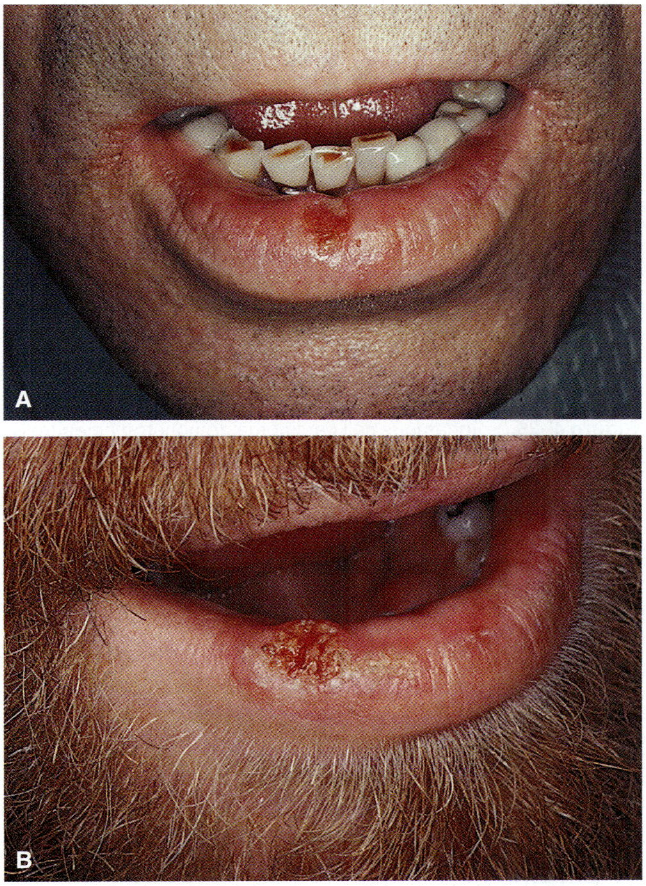

Figure 4–20. *A*, Early carcinoma of the lip thought to be an infection. *B*, Early carcinoma of the lip thought to be a cold sore (herpes).

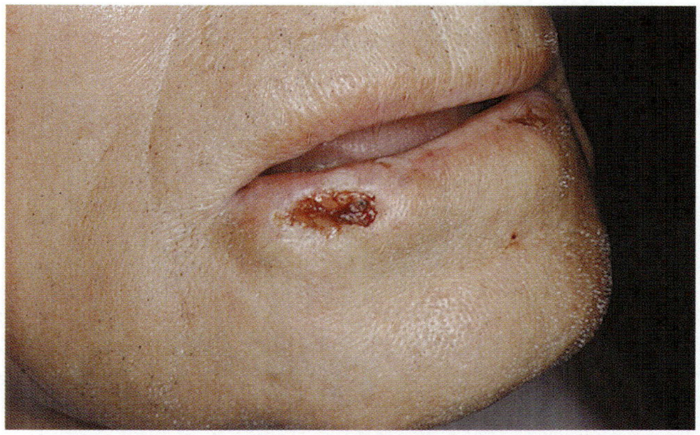

Figure 4–21. Moderately advanced carcinoma of the lip neglected for more than 5 months.

malignant neoplasia is highly desirable. Exfoliative cytology is one technique that serves this purpose, but it must be remembered that cytology is an adjunct to, not a substitute for, biopsy.

CYTOLOGY AND BRUSH BIOPSY

Exfoliative cytology is a technique used for observing the microscopic morphology of individual cells after they have been obtained from a tissue, spread on a slide, fixed, and stained (Table 4–1 and Figures 4–26 to 4–29).[4] Transepithelial sampling using a specially designed brush leads to a high degree of accuracy by obtaining representative cells from all epithelial layers.[5] The usefulness of cytology is augmented in oral cancer detection by the fact that over 90% of oral cancers are epithelial in origin (squamous cell carcinomas) and thereby "surface lesions." Thus, direct brushings allow for representative and accurate samplings of lesions. The availability of the brush biopsy technique and oral cytology examination has aided the evaluation of questionable lesions by accelerating and increasing clinicians' use of scalpel incisional biopsy of lesions that did not clinically appear to be oral cancers. The result has been the early diagnosis of malignancies that would otherwise have remained unsuspected for longer periods of time.

The entire oral cavity is lined with stratified squamous epithelium that varies in thickness and keratinization according to anatomic and functional sites. A thorough examination of the cell sample is made by an automated microscopic system or by a trained cytologist and certified by a pathologist.

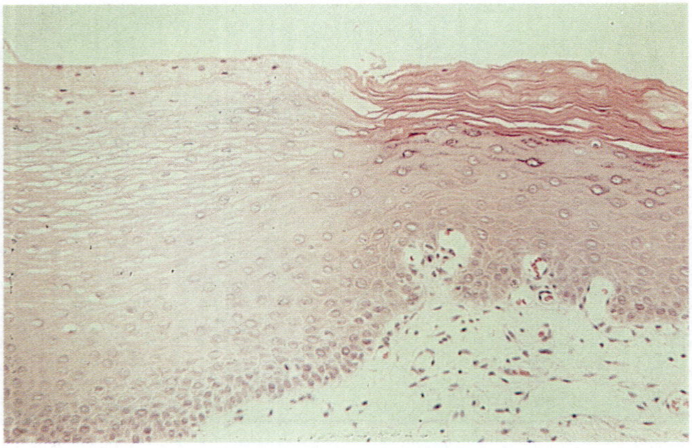

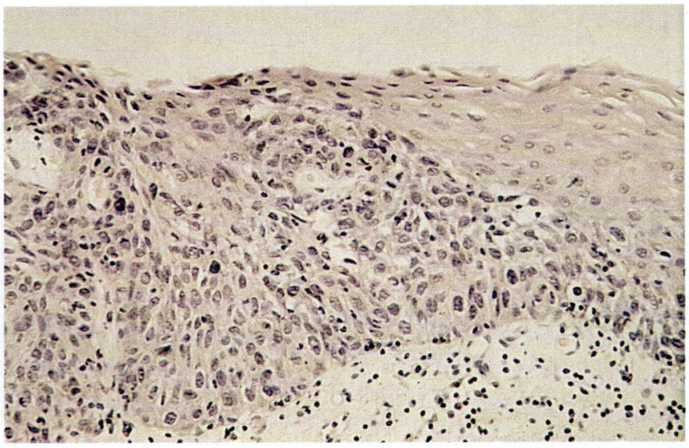

Figures 4–22 to 4–25. Epithelial histology/histopathology.
Figure 4–22. Normal epithelium: transition zone between unkeratinized buccal epithelium and keratinized gingiva (gingivobuccal sulcus area).

Figure 4–24. Severe epithelial dysplasia (carcinoma in situ) demonstrating full thickness discrepancy in epithelial maturation.

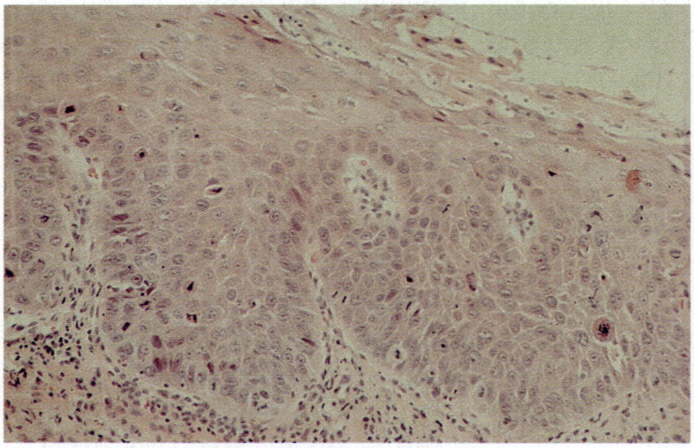

Figure 4–23. Moderate epithelial dysplasia demonstrating some cellular pleomorphism and increased mitosis with a few abnormal mitotic figures (discrepancy in epithelial maturation).

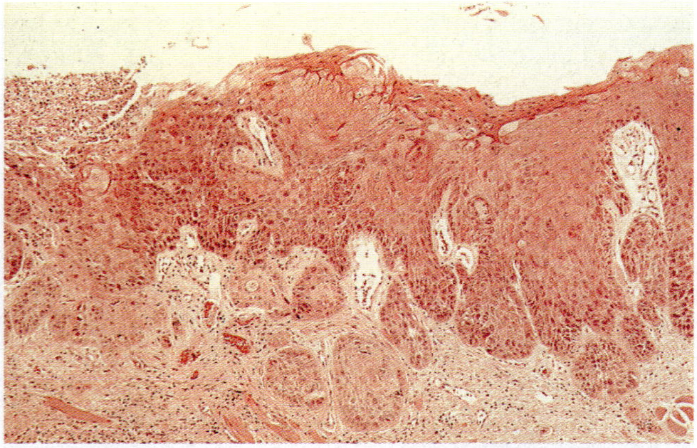

Figure 4–25. Squamous cell carcinoma demonstrating epithelial cell invasion through the basal lamina (basement membrane) into underlying connective tissue.

The general features of normal intraoral squamous cells are as follows (Table 4–2 and Figures 4–30 to 4–31):

1. *Keratinized surface cells (mature or cornified cells).* More flattened and irregular in appearance; small pyknotic nucleus or anucleate; cytoplasm stains pink, yellow, or orange (acidophilic).
2. *Unkeratinized surface cells (intermediate maturity).* May be slightly flattened, with somewhat irregular cytoplasmic morphology; some degree of nuclear contraction; cytoplasm is usually basophilic but may be acidophilic and stain pink or red.
3. *Parabasal and immature prickle cells.* Spherical or cuboidal; centrally placed nucleus with even distribution of chromatin; cytoplasm stains green or blue-green (basophilic).

The following are criteria on which cytologic interpretations of malignant epithelial cells are based (all criteria are not necessarily found in each specimen) (Figures 4–32 and 4–33):

1. Enlarged nuclei
2. Variation in nuclear size and shape (pleomorphism)
3. Prominent and irregular nuclear borders
4. Increased nucleus-to-cytoplasm ratio relative to size
5. Multiple prominent and irregular nucleoli
6. Hyperchromatism (increased nucleoproteins, deoxyribonucleic acid [DNA])

Table 4–1. EXFOLIATIVE CYTOLOGY TECHNIQUE
Collection of smear: Label one end of a glass microscope slide with patient's name, date, and area from which material is to be obtained. Use a clean cotton-tipped applicator or wood spatula for collection of specimen. If the area to be scraped is dry, the applicator or spatula should be moistened. Usually saliva or tissue excretions are sufficient to prevent dehydration. Collect the material from the lesion by using slight rolling and scraping motions. Remember, smears may be inadequate if there is a pseudomembrane covering a lesion, saliva that is too thick, excess bleeding, or no moisture. The scrapings should be immediately smeared on the center area of the slide (approximately 2.5 cm).
Fixation of smear: Alcohol (70%) is adequate for fixation. Commercial spray fixatives or hair sprays are satisfactory and also make it easier to handle the specimen. Do not allow the smear to dry before fixation.
Staining of smear: The smear is stained by a modified Papanicolaou-Traut technique using Mayer's hematoxylin, orange G, eosin, and light green. The slide can be made ready for screening in less than 1 hour.

7. Abnormal chromatin pattern and distribution
8. Discrepancy in maturation (extreme variations)

Cells from benign lesions may have an atypical appearance, but they seldom display enough criteria to cause them to be misinterpreted as malignant (Table 4–3). Classification of benign oral diseases from exfoliative cytologic studies is not yet possible; tissue patterns as seen in biopsies are necessary.

False-positive and false-negative reports have been few. These errors, though undesirable, are not critical because of the manner in which cytologic reports are used and interpreted: (1) if clinical suspicion remains in the face of a negative or atypical report, a biopsy should be performed; (2) a suspicious report indicates a definite need to establish a

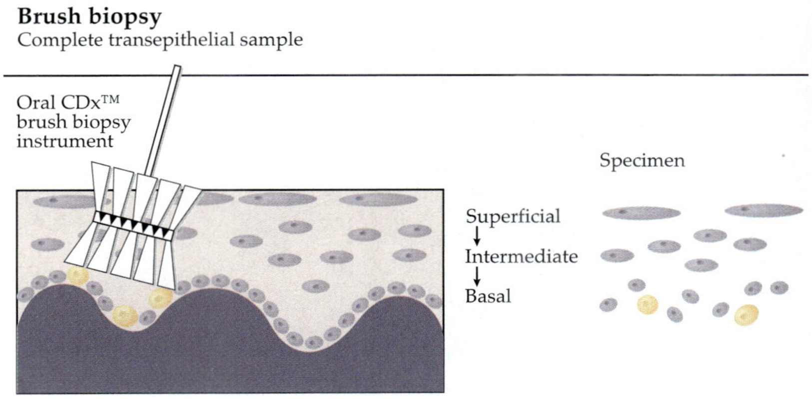

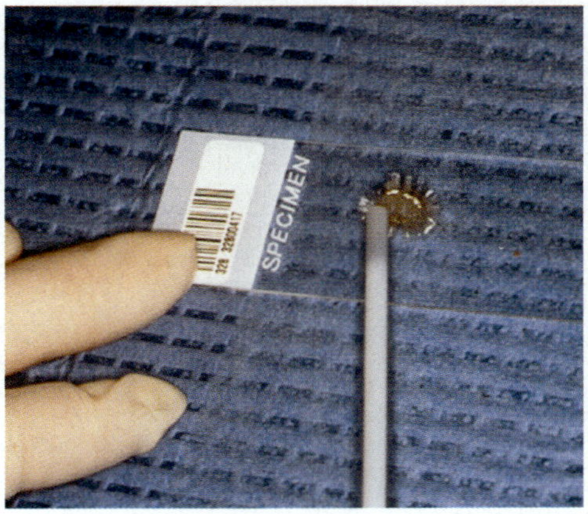

Figures 4–26 to 4–29. Brush biopsy technique.
Figure 4–26. Transepithelial sampling of stratified squamous epithelium.

Figure 4–28. Transferring cells to a glass slide.

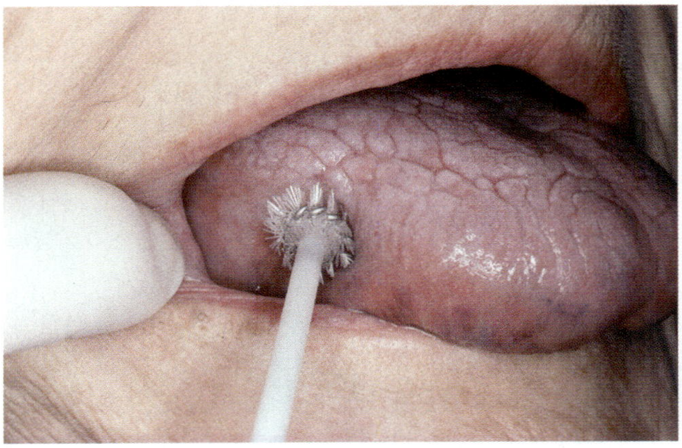

Figure 4–27. Obtaining cells by rotating brush biopsy tool.

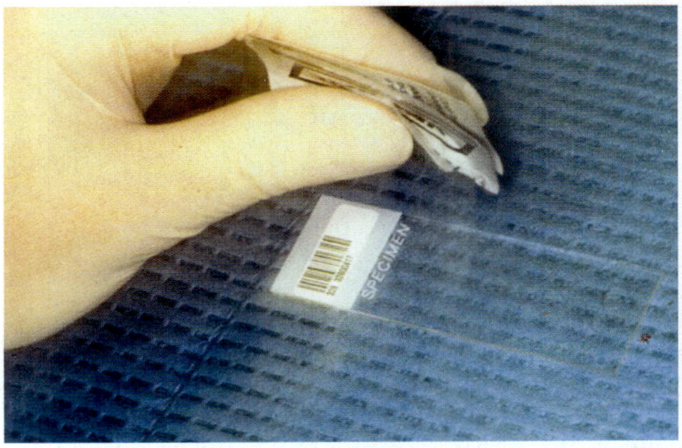

Figure 4–29. Fixing cells to slide using an alcohol/polyethylene glycol fixative.

Table 4–2. APPEARANCE OF SURFACE CELLS IN RELATION TO LOCATION

Hard palate, gingiva, dorsal tongue	Mature cells: High degree of cornification and some cells anucleated
Buccal and labial mucosae	Intermediate maturity: Nucleated basophilic- and acidophilic-staining cells
Floor of mouth, ventral tongue, soft palate, oropharynx	Least maturity: Preponderantly basophilic cells with large nuclei

definitive diagnosis immediately; and (3) when smears contain cells consistent with or suspicious for malignancy, biopsy is mandatory.

Table 4–3. REPORT OF SMEAR

Positive	Criteria for malignant cellular change are observed.
Negative	No malignant cells are observed in the specimen. These cells may appear atypical but do not demonstrate malignant criteria. In the event of continued clinical suspicion or persistence of a lesion, a negative report should not be taken as conclusive. This is particularly true in hyperkeratotic lesions.
Suspicious or inconclusive	Cells seen that do not fulfill the malignant criteria adequately to allow a positive report yet reveal enough deviation from normal to indicate that follow-up studies should be performed.
Inadequate	Either cellular morphology is not preserved adequately for interpretation, or the presented material is too scanty to be a representative specimen.

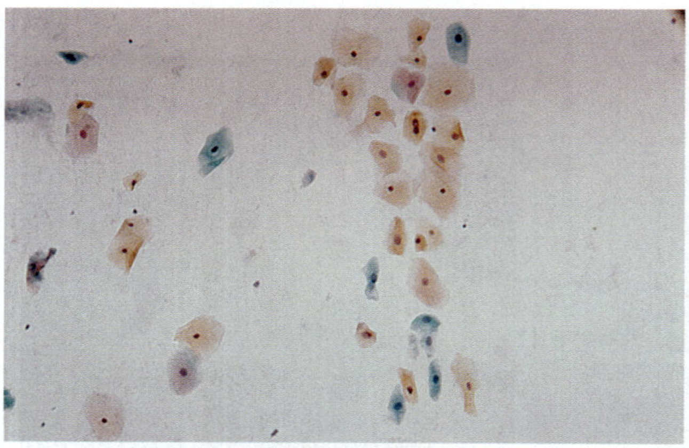

Figures 4–30 to 4–33. Cytologic smears.
Figure 4–30. Normal-appearing cells scraped from buccal epithelium showing a mixture of basophilic- and eosinophilic-staining squamous cells.

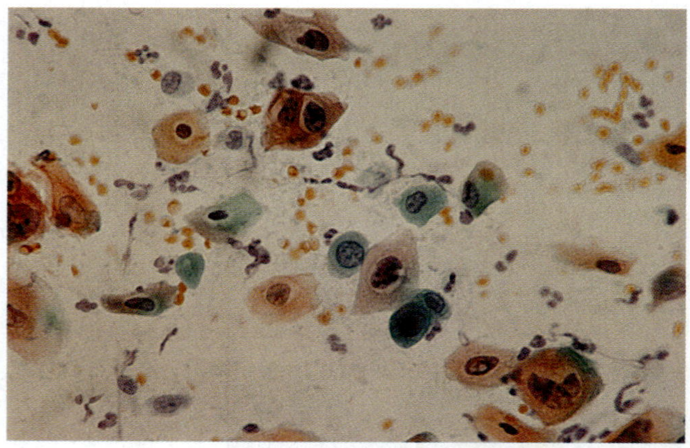

Figure 4–32. Scraping of malignant cells from an oral carcinoma. Note the characteristic pleomorphism reflecting the lack of control in cell maturation.

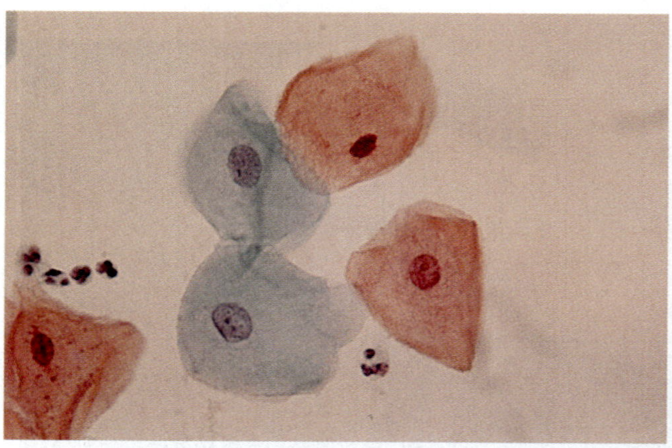

Figure 4–31. Higher power of normal buccal squamous cells. Note the expected small nuclear-to-cytoplasmic ratio and some adjacent polymorphonuclear leukocytes.

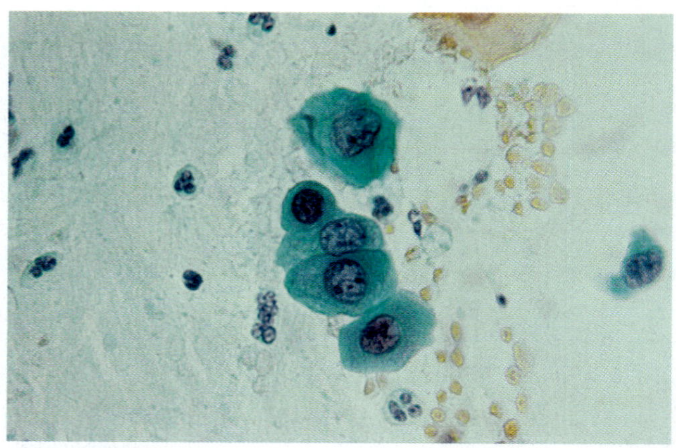

Figure 4–33. Higher power magnification of malignant oral epithelial cells. Note the much smaller adjacent red and white blood cells.

BIOPSY

No oral tumor should be treated without confirmation of the diagnosis by histologic examination. For intraoral malignancies, there is no good evidence from human studies that a properly performed biopsy will encourage the spread of tumor locally or by lymphatic or blood vessels. However, limited studies in animals have shown this spread to be possible. But many biologic (biochemical) factors must be present for circulating malignant cells to attach and grow outside the primary tumor site. The biopsy specimen should be adequate and obtained from a representative portion of the tumor so that the pathologist can examine the tissue appropriately.

It does not matter whether the biopsy procedure is carried out by a dentist or a physician provided that he or she is well qualified in recognizing the potential of the lesion and is capable of obtaining an appropriate and adequate specimen. In general, the most satisfactory biopsy of an intraoral lesion is the incisional biopsy (removal of a small portion). However, incisional biopsy of a small lesion may distort its appearance and consistency, rendering proper evaluation of its extent almost impossible. If cancer is suspected in a very small lesion with a gross appearance that would be altered by biopsy, the clinician/therapist who will apply the definitive treatment must see the lesion before the biopsy specimen is taken to judge the extent of resection or irradiation to be instituted. Tumor boards (treatment planning groups) and

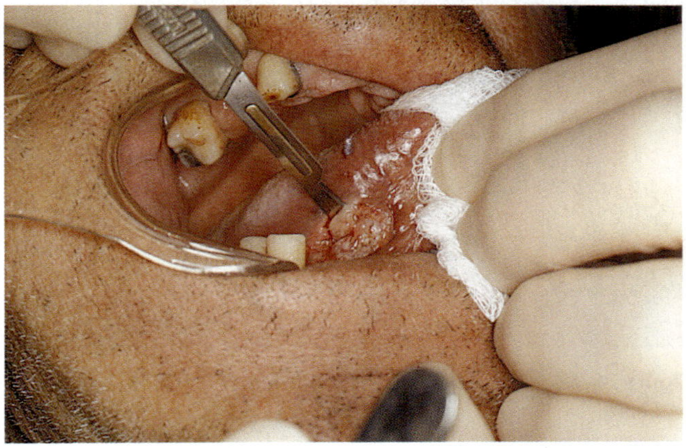

Figures 4–34 to 4–37. Incisional biopsy under local anesthesia using a conventional scalpel for an exophytic carcinoma.
Figure 4–34. Incision under local anesthesia.

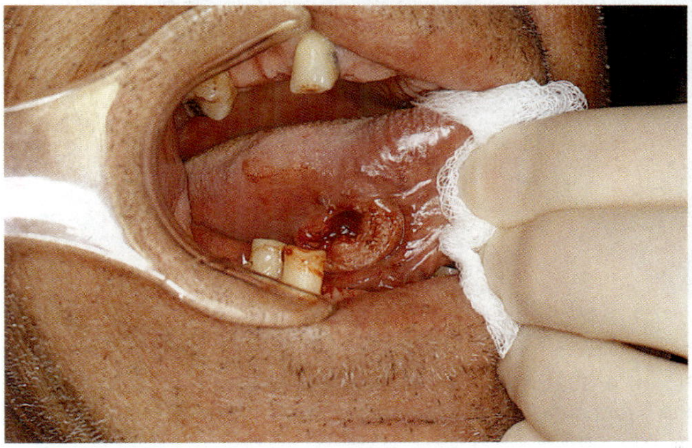

Figure 4–36. Coagulation from gauze pressure.

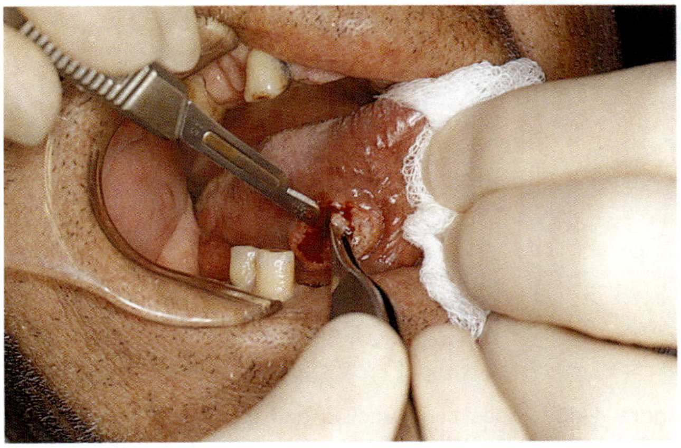

Figure 4–35. Excision of sample.

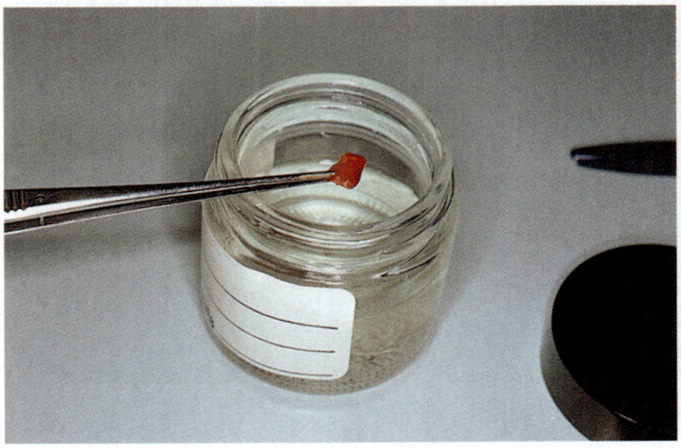

Figure 4–37. Specimen placed in 10% buffered formalin.

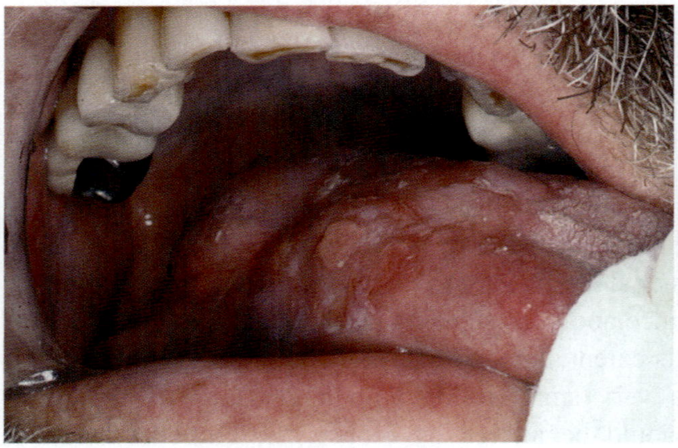

Figures 4–38 to 4–43. Punch biopsy technique.
Figure 4–38. Suspicious lesion, right lateral tongue.

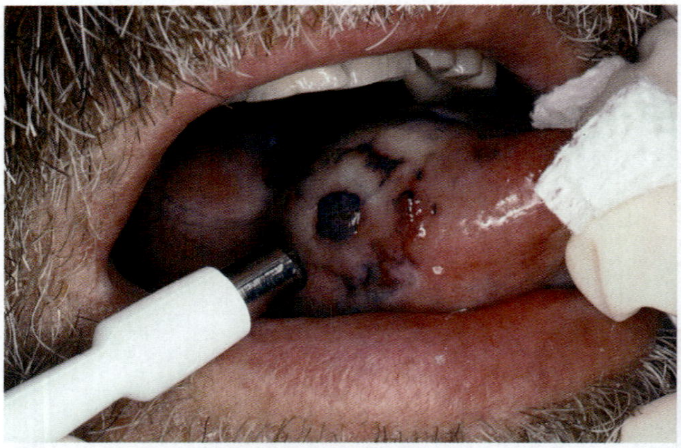

Figure 4–39. Area anesthetized and stained with toluidine blue and 5 mm punch biopsy instrument ready for incision.

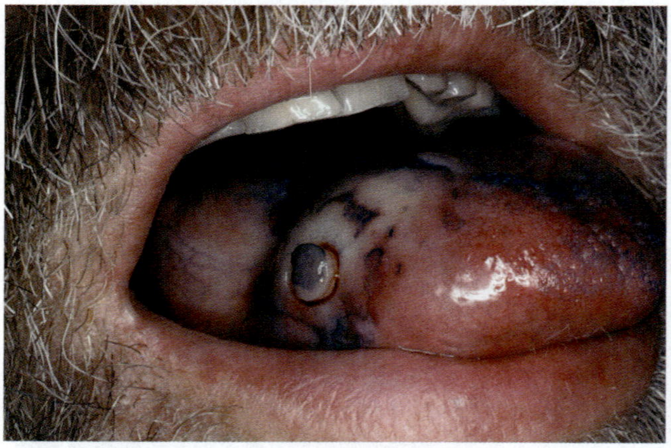

Figure 4–40. Incision made.

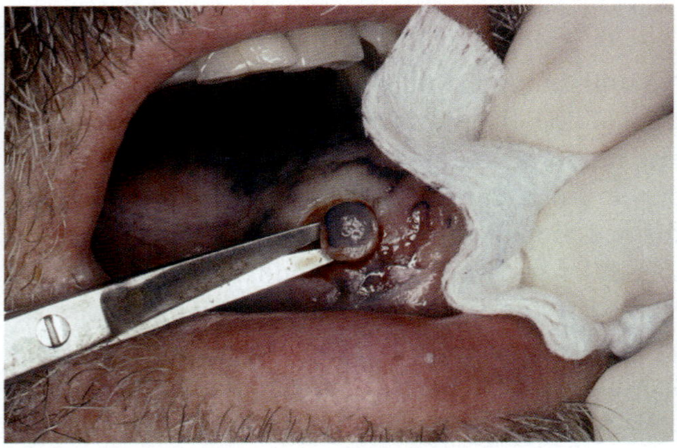

Figure 4–41. Specimen removed with scissors.

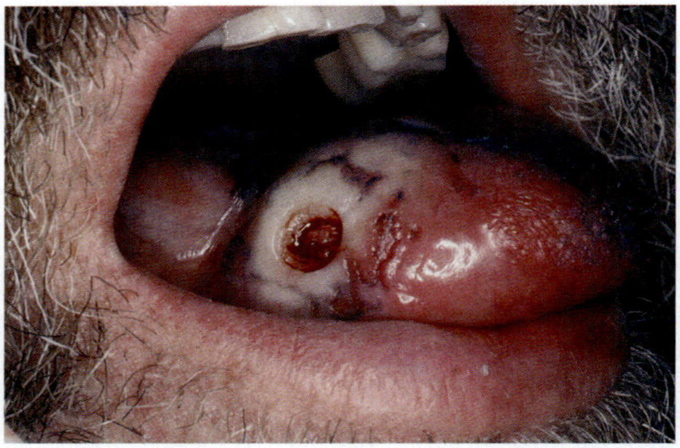

Figure 4–42. Coagulation obtained within minutes by gauze pressure.

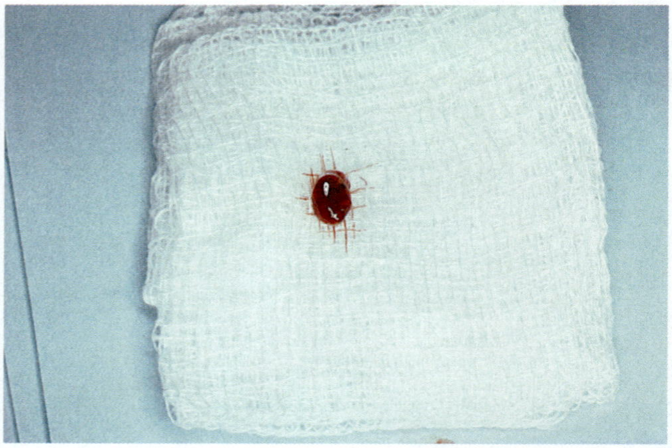

Figure 4–43. Specimen removed and ready for fixation. Note positive toluidine blue stain. Microscopic examination revealed carcinoma in situ.

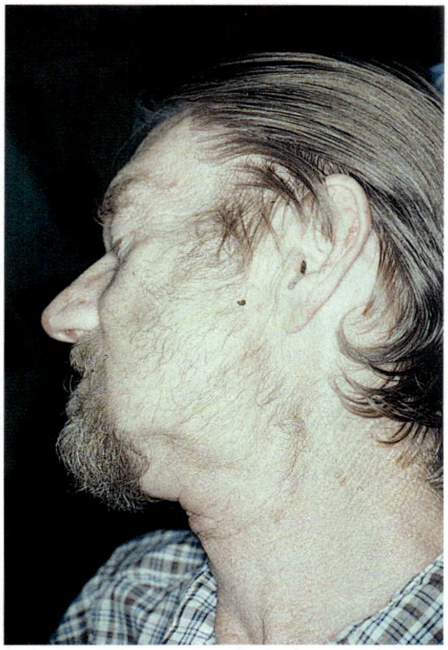

Figures 4–44 to 4–47. Fine-needle aspiration biopsy technique. **Figure 4–44.** A patient presented because of a painful "lump" in the neck. Differential diagnosis included cyst and either a benign or a malignant growth of salivary gland or lymph node.

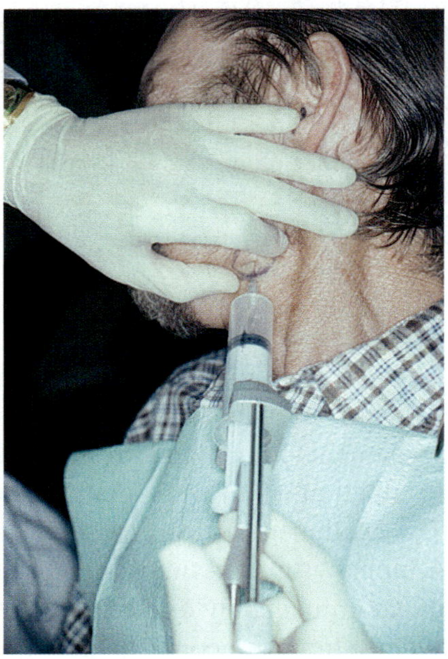

Figure 4–45. Aspiration technique.

advanced imaging techniques are vital in staging and treatment (see this chapter and Chapter 5). Figures 4–34 to 4–43 illustrate several biopsy techniques.

Although biopsies of intraoral lesions ordinarily present no difficult technical problems, biopsies of

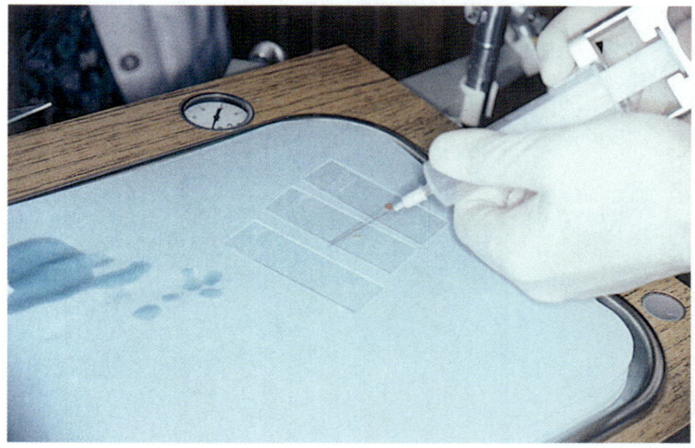

Figure 4–46. Preparing a smear of aspirate prior to staining.

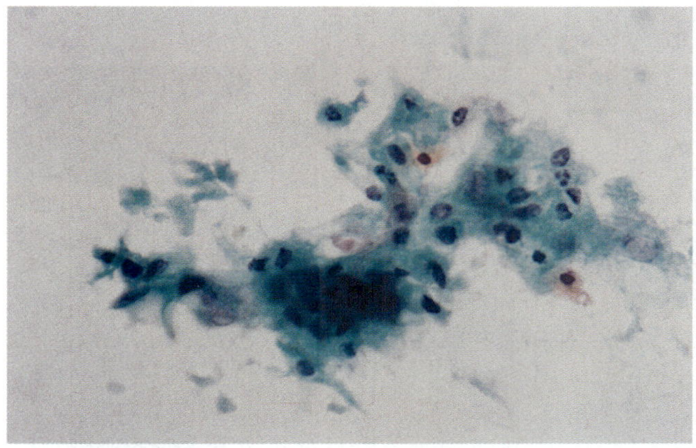

Figure 4–47. Final diagnosis: carcinoma metastatic to lymph node.

tumors in such areas as the base of the tongue and oral pharynx may be difficult to obtain. For tumors or suspected tumors in these sites, it is frequently necessary for referral to a specialist and/or to perform the examination and biopsy with the patient under general anesthesia. Even if cervical lymph nodes are palpable and suspected of being involved in metastatic carcinoma, the biopsy specimen should always be obtained from the primary lesion. Biopsy of the involved bone is rarely indicated. Most often, clinical judgment and imaging techniques can supply the information needed to establish a treatment plan.

Lymph node biopsy is carried out only when the primary lesion cannot be identified or in diseases such as lymphoma. In such instances, the entire lymph node should be excised (excisional biopsy) if at all feasible. Incisional biopsy of a suspicious lymph node should be avoided to prevent contami-

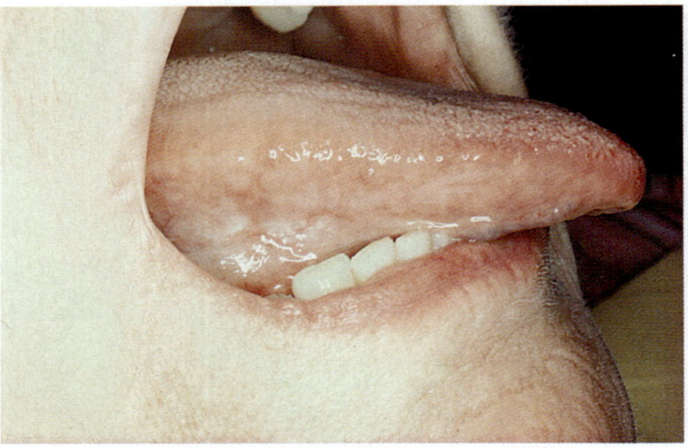

Figures 4–48 to 4–51. Toluidine blue staining technique. **Figure 4–48.** Symptomatic lesion of lateral tongue noticed for more than 3 months.

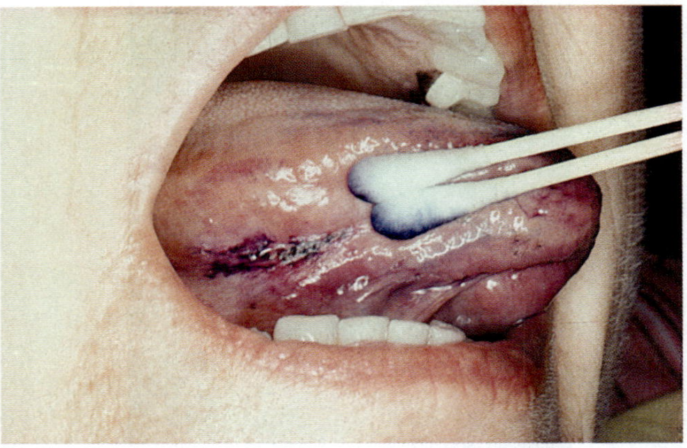

Figure 4–50. Decolorizing with 1% acetic acid.

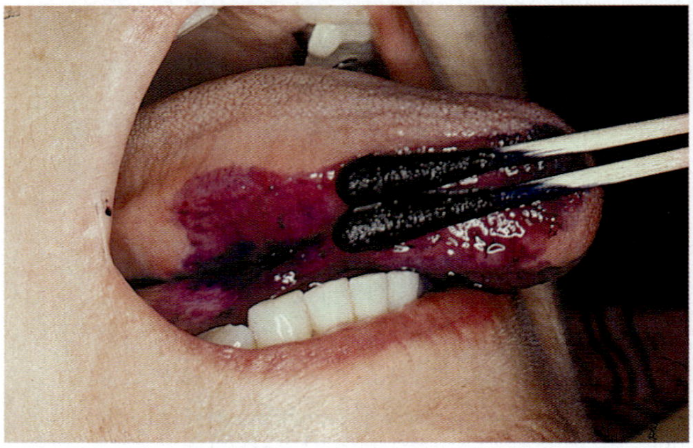

Figure 4–49. Applying 1% aqueous toluidine blue.

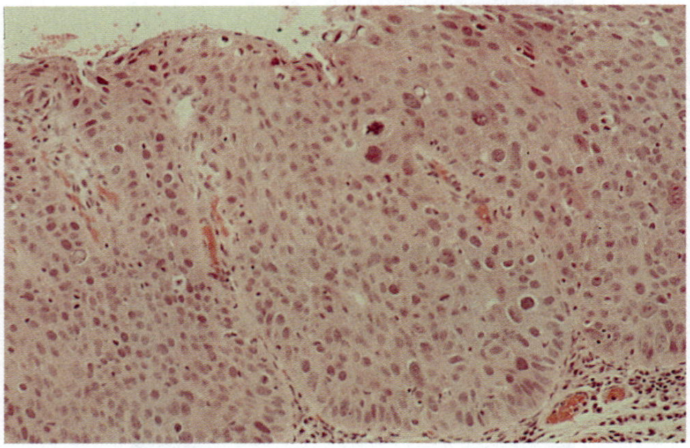

Figure 4–51. Biopsy from the retained blue dye area revealed severe dysplasia (carcinoma in situ).

nation of the biopsy site by tumor cells. Such a spillage of cells might worsen the prognosis in patients who otherwise might be curable.

In patients with cervical lymphadenopathy in whom a primary tumor cannot be identified, the location in the neck of the enlarged lymph node is of considerable help in identifying the site of origin of the metastasis (see Chapter 5). However, it must be remembered that tumors can metastasize to almost any node.

Fine-Needle Aspiration

Fine-needle aspiration (FNA) biopsy is a highly acceptable and accurate technique for differentiating benign from malignant lesions involving lymph nodes.[6] Use of this minimally invasive technique accelerates diagnosis and treatment and improves overall management. This technique also has greatly aided the evaluation of salivary gland lesions (see Chapter 10, "Malignant Salivary Gland Tumors"). Thus, FNA biopsy is a safe, quick, and reliable procedure that can immediately differentiate inflammatory, reactive, cystic, and neoplastic processes.

FNA biopsies are preferred over incisional biopsies when lymph nodes and major salivary glands are suspected of being neoplastic because they do not tend to spread tumor or disrupt the field for ideal surgical dissection. The armamentarium includes a 22-gauge needle and a special holder for a 10 or 20 mL syringe to obtain optimal suction and cytologic material. Anesthesia is usually not required,

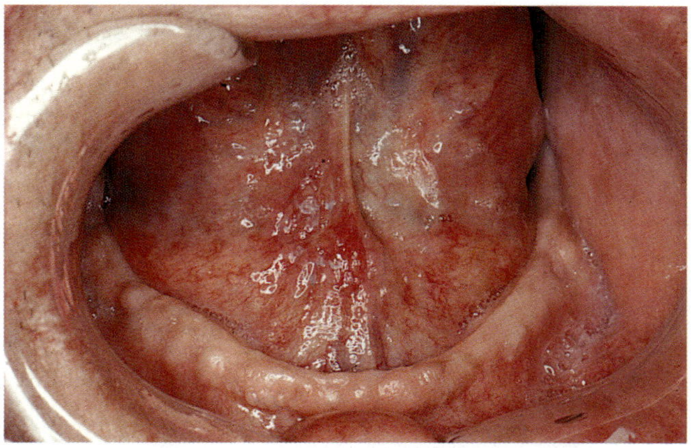

Figures 4–52 to 4–55. Early carcinoma, floor of the mouth.
Figure 4–52. Irritation of the floor of the mouth noticed for about 2 months.

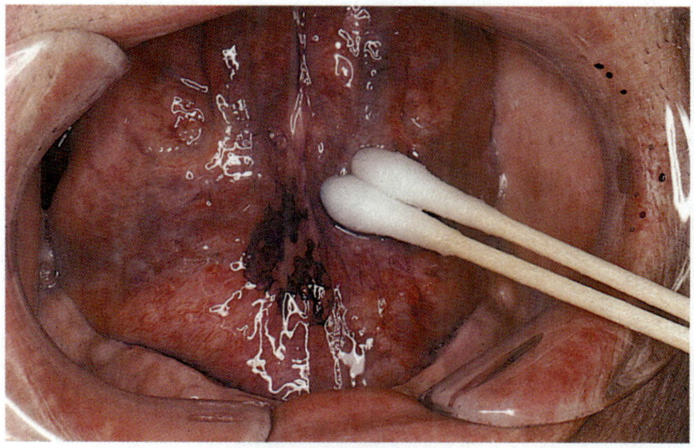

Figure 4–54. Decolorization with 1% acetic acid; note persistent binding of the toluidine blue dye.

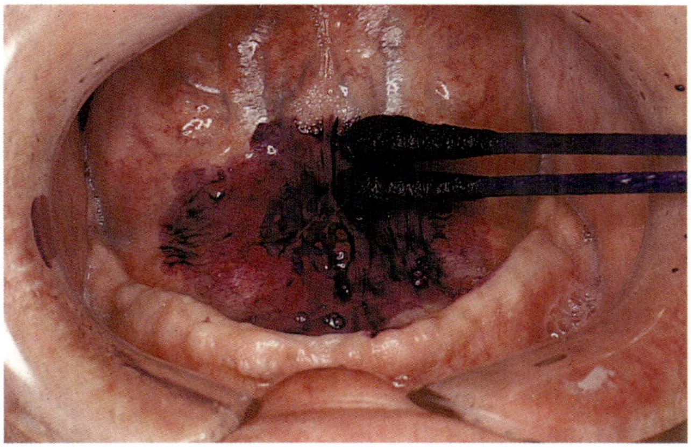

Figure 4–53. Application of 1% aqueous toluidine blue.

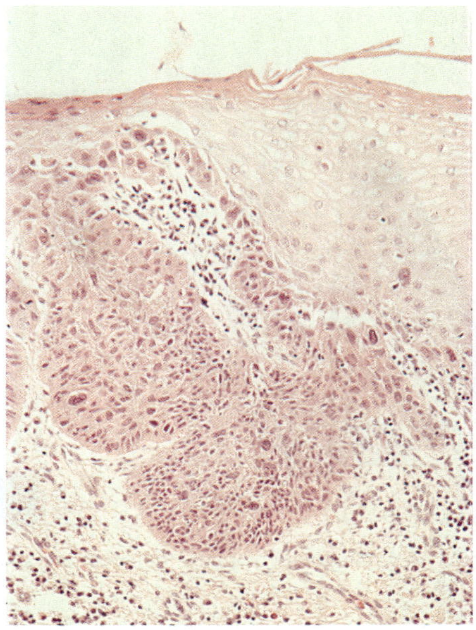

Figure 4–55. Biopsy revealed early squamous cell carcinoma.

and specimens are prepared by cytologic techniques (Figures 4–44 to 4–47).

TOLUIDINE BLUE

Because epithelial dysplasia and early squamous cell carcinoma vary considerably in appearance and often resemble certain benign lesions, clinical identification is difficult, and biopsy is frequently delayed by attempts at empirical remedies. Vital staining with toluidine blue has been shown to aid early recognition and accelerate biopsy, diagnosis, and treatment.[7–9] Toluidine blue is a metachromatic dye of the thiazine group that has been effectively used as a nuclear stain because of its binding to DNA.

In our oral medicine clinic, the reliability of this vital staining technique was tested in 169 consecutive patients suspected of having malignant or precancerous oral lesions by comparing clinical toluidine blue dye uptake with results of a simultaneous biopsy (Figures 4–48 to 4–61). The histopathologic diagnosis confirmed 62 squamous carcinomas, 13 epithelial dysplasias, and 94 benign mucosal changes (Table 4–4). Overall accuracy of the toluidine blue uptake was 93%. Other recent studies have similarly confirmed the specificity and sensitivity of toluidine blue detection of cancer and precancer.

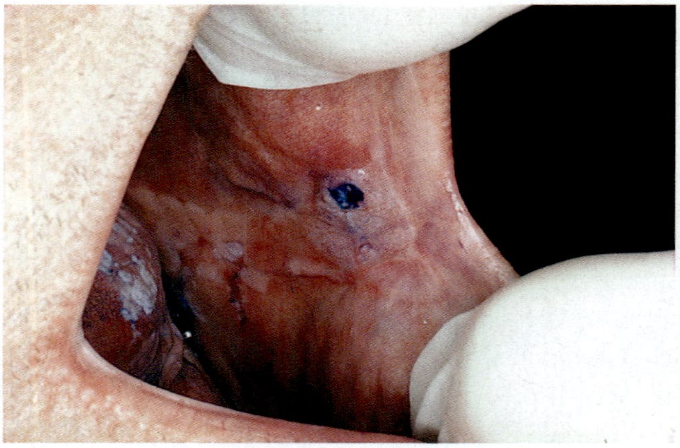

Figures 4–56 to 4–61. Unsuspected asymptomatic early squamous cell carcinoma in a 72-year-old woman.

Figure 4–56. Note toluidine blue–positive staining in a small, longstanding area of leukoplakia. The patient was being seen on a routine follow-up visit.

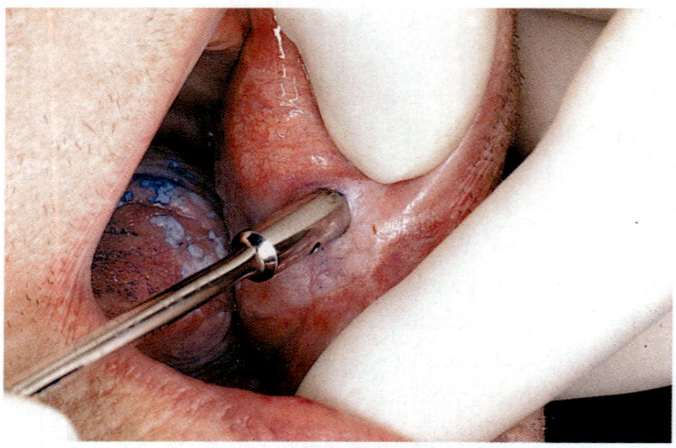

Figure 4–57. A 5 mm punch biopsy under local anesthesia.

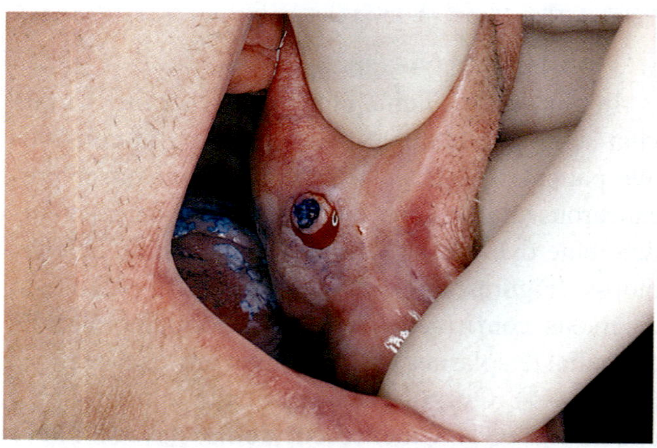

Figure 4–58. Immediately after punch incision.

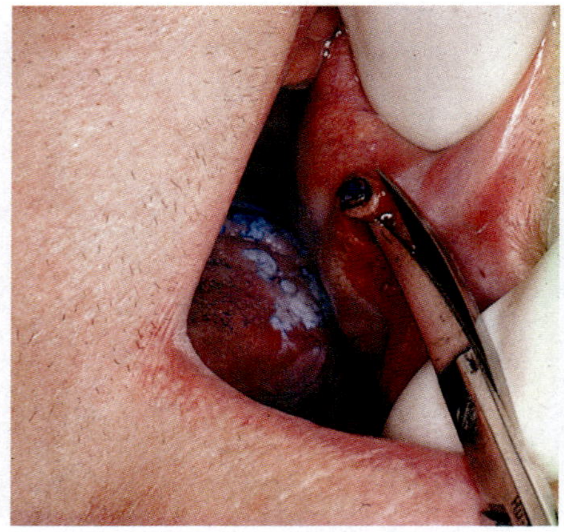

Figure 4–59. Removing the specimen with scissors.

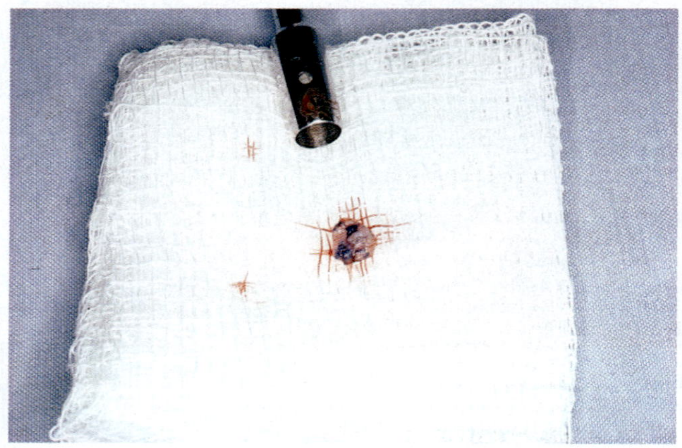

Figure 4–60. The specimen. Note surface dye retention.

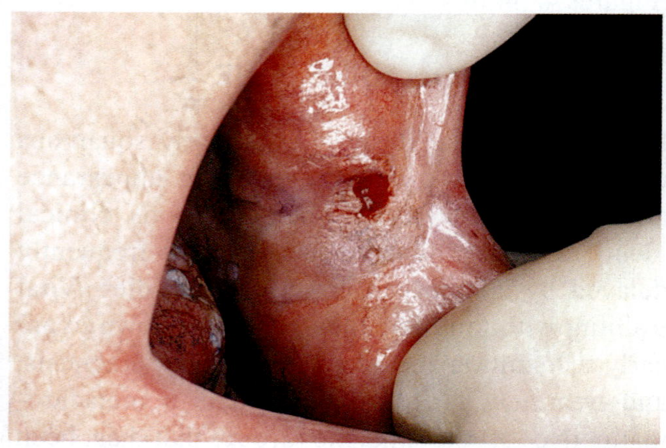

Figure 4–61. Coagulation of blood following 3 minutes of pressure with gauze.

Table 4–4. TOLUIDINE BLUE STAINING (TB)

Biopsy Diagnosis	n	TB+	TB–	Correct
Carcinoma	62	58	4	93.5%
Dysplasia	13	11	2	84.6%
Benign	94	6	88	93.6%
Total	169	75	94	92.9%

TB+ = dye uptake; TB– = no dye uptake

The accuracy of the toluidine blue technique supports its clinical use to confirm clinical impressions further regarding tissues at risk of malignancy, as well as to assist the clinician in choosing biopsy sites within suspected lesions and surgical margins. Clinicians should be aware, however, that false-positive reactions can result from dye retention by filiform papillae and ulcerations, as well as mechanically in fissures. The mechanism for this reaction has several explanations, but it might be related to a high rate of protein synthesis and/or binding by sulfated mucopolysaccharides. Because toluidine blue is regarded as a nuclear stain, selective dye uptake by dysplastic and malignant cells, which contain quantitatively more nucleic acids than normal tissue, is plausible. Another explanation of binding in vivo by precancerous and cancerous tissue is the immediate binding by sulfated mucopolysaccharides, which are found in higher quantities in tissues that are actively growing, such as tumors and tissues that have a high turnover rate. Additionally, it has been shown that toluidine blue binds to negatively charged mitochondrial membranes, which occur more prominantly in dysplastic and malignant cells.

It can be concluded that toluidine blue staining is a useful adjunct to careful examination, clinical judgment, and biopsy. There is abundant evidence that toluidine blue dye used in this diagnostic manner is neither mutagenic nor carcinogenic.

MONOCLONAL ANTIBODIES

No matter what diagnostic technique is used, the possibility of a false-negative response exists. The development of monoclonal antibodies that have high sensitivity and specificity for epithelial dysplastic and malignant cells would enhance accuracy of diagnosis in some cases in which the usual or typical cellular characteristics of precancer or cancer are not apparent. Such antibodies could also possibly minimize errors regarding "tumor-free" margins of surgical resections, thus reducing a potential source of recurrence. In addition, logical and possible sequelae for improving cancer control would be to bind cancer cell antibodies to cytotoxic chemotherapeutic agents. Because these agents would be directed to the cancer by the monoclonal antibodies, normal cells would be spared. Some of these monoclonal antibodies have been developed, studied, and reported. However, the cumbersome techniques entailed time, expense, and questions regarding specificity and have limited large studies and use in diagnostic laboratories. This technique could be applied to cytology as well as biopsy specimens. Numerous biomarkers now being developed and studied will yield additional information regarding cellular neoplastic potential and even the risks of metastases (see Chapter 5 regarding modern molecular analysis of oral cancer).

Neoplasms of the oral cavity and oropharynx are usually discovered by clinical examination and confirmed by FNA or surgical biopsy. Imaging studies may then be employed to map the extent of disease, detect bone invasion and cervical adenopathy, and evaluate adherence of tumor to the carotid artery. Occasionally, a patient may present with cervical nodal metastases without a clinically evident primary lesion. In this setting, cross-sectional imaging obtained prior to panendoscopy and biopsy is useful to locate submucosal tumor and direct biopsies to possible targets. The detection of recurrent disease following therapy may also be facilitated by cross-sectional imaging. The advanced imaging techniques presently available include computed tomography (CT), magnetic resonance imaging (MRI), and positron emission tomography (PET). Ultrasonography, often in conjunction with FNA biopsy, is used in some European centers to evaluate neck disease, but this technique has not found wide acceptance in the United States. The limitations and the strengths of the more commonly used modalities will be addressed.

Imaging Techniques

Computed Tomography

The CT image is a computer-generated cross-sectional representation of anatomy that is created by analysis of the attenuation of an x-ray beam passed through a section of the body (Figure 4–62). As the x-ray source, collimated to the desired slice thickness, rotates around the patient, sensitive x-ray detectors aligned 180 degrees from the x-ray source detect those x-rays that have passed through and been variably attenuated by the patient's body tissues. A computer then calculates a "back-projected" gray-scale image from the 360-degree x-ray attenuation profile. Greater attenuation of x-rays by dense structures such as bone is represented by increasing "whiteness" on the gray-scale image, whereas soft tissue structures that attenuate the x-ray beam to a lesser degree (ie, are lower density) are more black. Air, as in the lungs or pharynx, is completely black. The resolution of an image depends on the radiation dose, collimation (slice thickness), field of view, and matrix size of the display. Neck CT images are usually performed with a slice thickness of 2.5 to 3.75 mm and a 512 × 512 reconstruction matrix. It is easy to see why powerful computers are required to deal with this great volume of data and why these scans are best viewed interactively on a PACS system rather than film. The radiation dose to the patient varies with the particular imaging technique used and the extent of coverage, with higher doses required to obtain thin, high-matrix slices with adequate signal-to-noise ratio. A typical CT of the neck results in an effective dose of approximately 4 mSv to the patient.

CT has recently reached a new level of technologic capability with the development of fast detectors, "helical" scanning, and multislice acquisition. In helical mode, a volume of data is acquired by having the table move continuously through the rotating x-ray beam. This volume of data can then be reconstructed into individual slices, allowing increased speed, decreased motion artifact, and thin slices. A multislice scanner allows simultaneous acquisition of interleaved volumes of data, further increasing speed of acquisition and further decreasing motion artifacts. With the

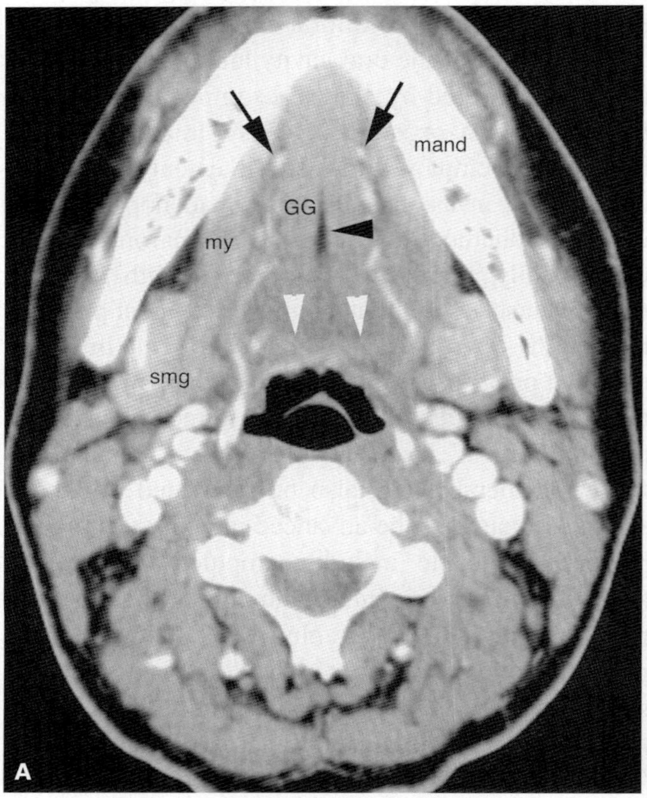

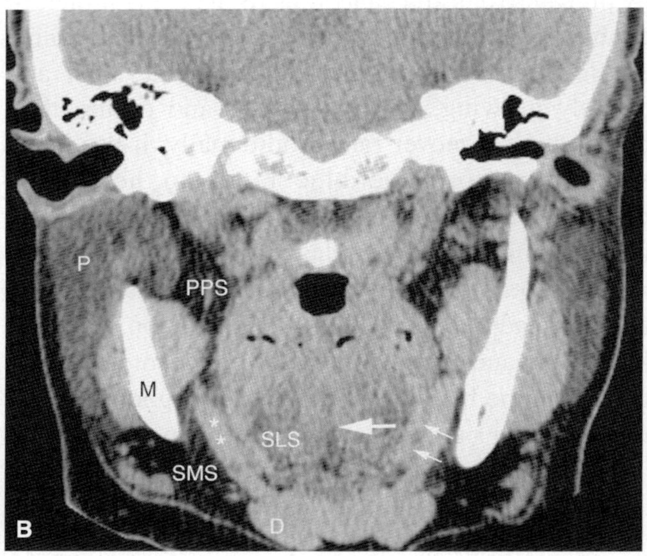

Figure 4–62. Normal computed tomographic scans through the oral cavity. *A*, Axial 3 mm study through the lower mandible (mand) and floor of the mouth during intravenous infusion of contrast. The midline fat-filled lingual septum (*black arrowhead*) is an important landmark. On either side of the septum, the paired genioglossus (GG) muscles are seen coursing from the genu of the mandible to insert into the intrinsic tongue muscles. The lingual tonsil (*white arrowheads*) appears as a slightly more dense band of tissue lining the anterior aspect of the oropharyngeal airway. Also seen is the submandibular gland (smg) and mylohyoid muscle (my). Lingual vessels coursing in the sublingual space are opacified by the intravenous contrast (*black arrows*). *B*, Coronal 3 mm study without intravenous contrast. The mylohyoid muscle (*asterisks*) divides the submandibular space (SMS) from the sublingual space (SLS). The fatty lingual septum is seen (*large white arrow*), as is the hyoglossus muscle (*small white arrows*) and the anterior belly of the digastric muscle (D). The fat-filled parapharyngeal space (PPS) extends from the posterior aspect of the SMS to the skull base. The parotid gland (P) is usually rather fatty in the adult and is seen to be intermediate in density between muscle and fat.

newest modern CT scanners, an examination of the neck, from skull base through the aortic-pulmonic window, can be performed within 1 to 2 minutes. In addition, rapid image acquisition allows one to image very effectively during bolus administration of intravenous contrast material, resulting in excellent opacification of vessels and facilitating their distinction from normal soft tissue structures and masses. A noncontrast CT of the neck may be performed if one is seeking a radiodense structure, such as a salivary calculus, that might be obscured on a postcontrast scan, but otherwise, unless there is a contraindication to iodinated contrast material (allergy, renal insufficiency), intravenous contrast material is infused for all CT scans of the neck (Figure 4–63).

Although the soft tissue contrast resolution of CT is less than that achievable with MRI, the fast scan time essentially freezes motion and has greatly improved imaging of the oral cavity and neck. In addition, the thin slices that are now routinely performed allow fine-detail assessment of the cervical lymph node chain and other structures. Other advantages of CT include excellent patient tolerance, relatively low cost ($300 to 800 per examination), and superior osseous detail compared with MRI. CT examination of the head and neck still requires the rapid administration of intravenous iodinated contrast material during scanning to differentiate vessels from lymph nodes, as mentioned above, but the now widespread use of nonionic contrast media has greatly reduced the incidence of contrast reactions. In addition, the amount of contrast required has been significantly reduced by the faster scan times and helical scan modes, which make far more efficient use of the contrast bolus.

CT quality may be degraded by dental appliance artifacts (Figure 4–64).[10] In some cases, the CT gantry can be angled or the patient's position can be altered so that images are oriented to avoid the teeth, and this may be useful in assessing lesions of the parotid glands and floor of the mouth.

Magnetic Resonance Imaging

MRI techniques also continue to evolve and improve, and MRI can offer important information regarding

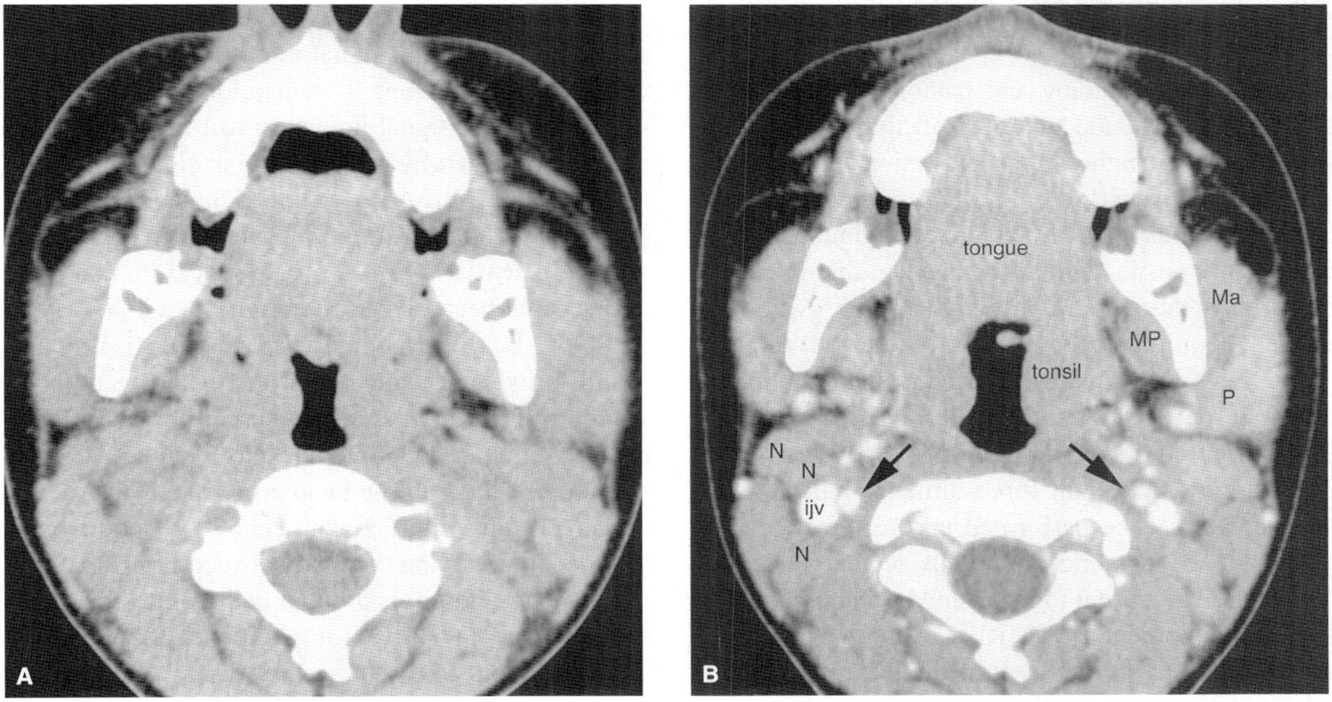

Figure 4–63. Axial 3 mm computed tomographic scans through the oropharynx and oral cavity of a child, without (*A*) and with (*B*) intravenous contrast. On the noncontrast scan, it is difficult to separate lymph nodes from vessels. Following contrast, the internal jugular vein (ijv) and internal carotid artery (*black arrow*) are well seen, as are lymph nodes (N). Distinction among other soft tissue structures is also improved.

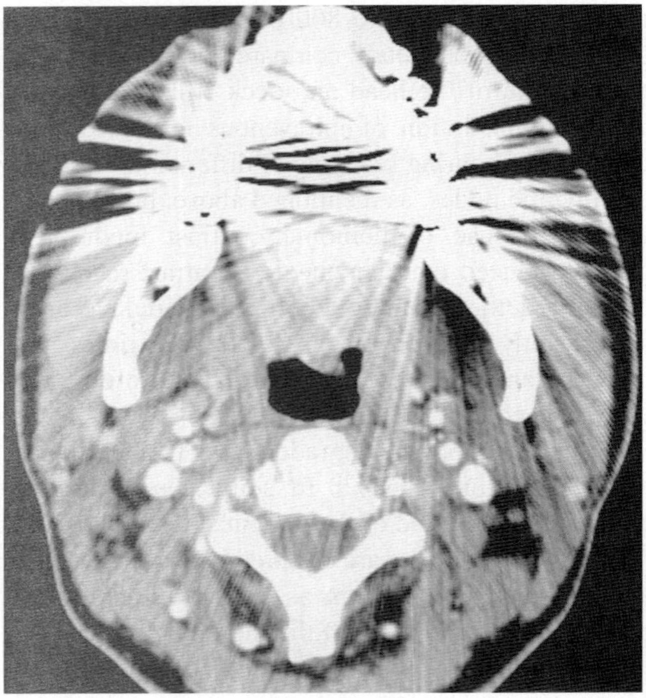

Figure 4–64. Axial 3 mm computed tomographic (CT) scan through the lower mandible demonstrates marked artifact from dental amalgam obscuring the anatomy of the tongue and floor of the mouth. This is a frequent problem with CT scanning through the oral cavity and can be reduced to some degree by altering the angle at which the scan is performed and by acquiring coronal as well as axial scans. Magnetic resonance imaging is less compromised in general by artifact related to dental amalgam.

head and neck anatomy and pathology. The advantages of MRI include superior soft tissue resolution, which results in high-contrast definition between neoplasms and adjacent muscle. MRIs can be generated in sagittal, axial, and coronal planes without changing the patient's position, an advantage that often helps in radiation treatment planning, especially with the advent of intensity-modulated radiation therapy (IMRT) for head and neck cancer and monitoring tumor response following therapy. Each plane of acquisition requires a separate sequence lasting 4 to 7 minutes. Although three-dimensional volume acquisitions can be performed and reformatted into any plane on a workstation, this technique is not widely used at present for head and neck applications.

The phenomenon of MRI is a complex interaction between protons within biologic tissues, a strong static magnetic field, superimposed varying gradient magnetic fields, and energy in the form of radiofrequency waves of set frequency (RF pulses), the latter usually introduced by coils placed around or adjacent to the body part of interest. The energy state of the hydrogen protons within tissues is transiently elevated by the RF pulse. The subsequent return to equilibrium (relaxation) of the protons results in a release of RF energy (the echo) that can be measured by coils placed over regions of interest. After Fourier transformation of the frequencies, computer processing can generate a gray-scale image of the anatomic region of interest.

T_1 and T_2 relaxation times. The rate of return to equilibrium of excited protons is called the relaxation rate. The relaxation rate is different for various normal and pathologic tissues. The relaxation rate of a hydrogen proton in a tissue is influenced by its surrounding molecular environment and atomic neighbors. Two rates of relaxation, designated T_1 and T_2, are measurable. The intensity of the signal and the image contrast can be modulated by altering imaging parameters, such as the interval between RF pulses (TR) and the time between the RF pulse and the signal reception (TE). So-called "T_1-weighted images" (T_1WIs) are produced by keeping the TR and TE relatively short. In T_1WIs, contrast between structures is based primarily on their T_1 relaxation differences. Fat, which has a short T_1 relaxation time, appears high in signal intensity, whereas fluid, which has a very long T_1 relaxation time, is represented by lower signal intensity; soft tissues such as muscle are generally intermediate in signal intensity (Figure 4–65, A). A T_2-weighted image (T_2WI) is produced with long TR and TE times. T_2WIs are usually more sensitive to pathologic processes that produce edema because fluid is bright on a T_2WI (Figure 4–65, B). In head and neck imaging, T_2WIs are usually produced using a fast spin echo technique, which minimizes magnetic susceptibility effects related to the air and bone interfaces with soft tissue that are prevalent in the head and neck. Because fat remains bright on a fast spin echo T_2WI and would thereby diminish the contrast between bright fat and typically bright tumors or other pathologic processes, a "fat saturation" pulse is applied, which suppresses the signal from fat and renders it dark.[11] So for head and neck imaging, the preferred T_2-weighted sequence is a fast spin echo T_2WI with fat saturation. As tumors of the head and neck generally have long T_1 and T_2 relaxation rates, they are typically low in signal intensity on T_1WI and high in signal intensity on T_2WI (see Figure 4–65).

MR contrast material. The heavy metal gadolinium is a paramagnetic substance, having the effect of shortening the T_1 and T_2 relaxation times of nearby water protons. When administered during an MR sequence, gadolinium leads to more efficient relaxation of nearby water protons and therefore high signal intensity on T_1WI. The metal ion is chelated to a carrier molecule such as diethylenetriamine pentaacetic acid (DTPA), which allows for renal excretion and essentially no toxicity. Usually, 0.2 mL/kg is administered intravenously, or 10 to 15 cc of contrast material for the average-sized adult. Although patent vessels have absent signal or "signal void" within their lumen on MRI, allowing ready distinction from lymph nodes and other structures without administration of contrast material (unlike CT), MR contrast is very useful to assess the enhancement characteristics of patho-

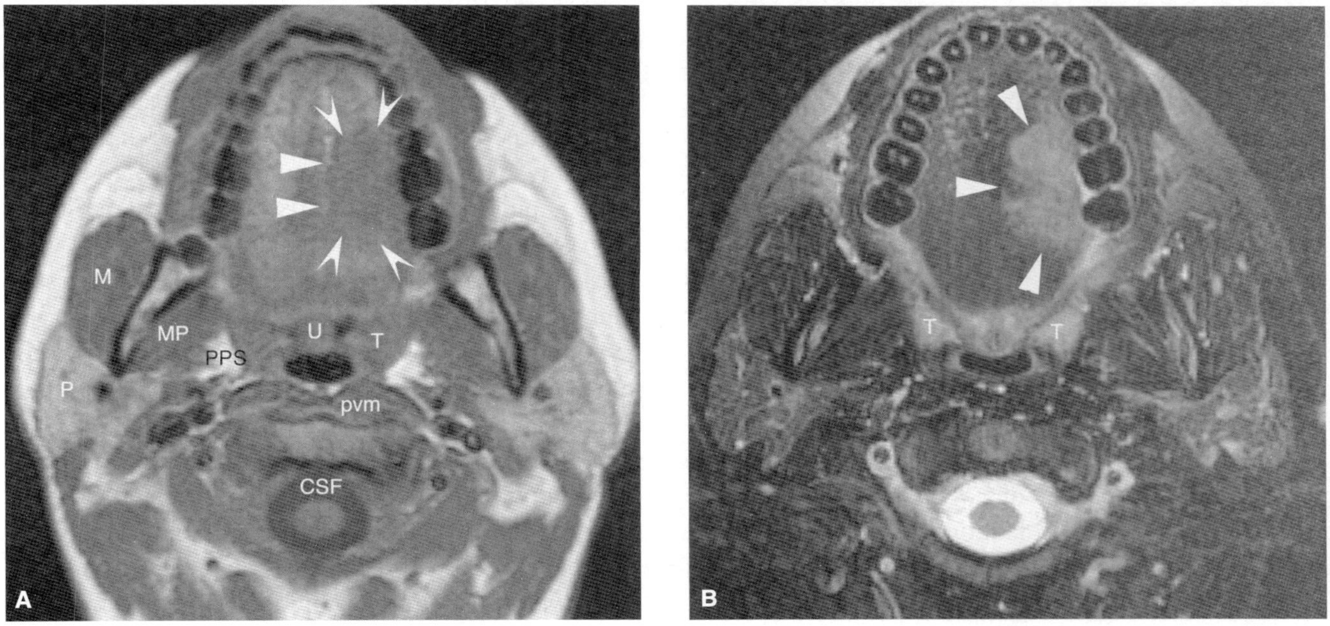

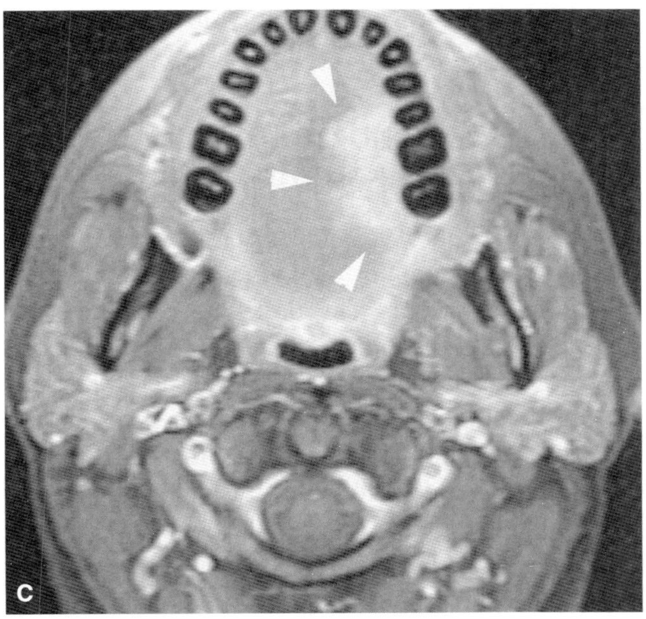

Figure 4–65. Squamous cell carcinoma of the oral tongue. *A*, Axial T_1-weighted magnetic resonance image through the oral cavity demonstrates a low signal intensity mass (*curved arrowheads*) infiltrating the left tongue. The midline lingual septum (*flat arrowheads*) is slightly displaced to the right, but the tumor does not appear to infiltrate the right hemitongue. Note that on a T_1-weighted image, subcutaneous fat is very bright, whereas fluid (such as the cerebrospinal fluid (CSF, around the spinal cord) is dark. Normal anatomic structures include the masseter muscle (M), medial pterygoid muscle (MP), parotid gland (P), parapharyngeal space (PPS), tonsil (T), uvula (U), and prevertebral muscle (pvm). *B*, Axial T_2-weighted fast spin echo image with fat saturation more clearly demonstrates the irregularly marginated infiltrative tongue mass (*white arrowheads*). On T_2-weighted images, the signal intensity of muscle decreases, and the signal intensity of fat is decreased owing to the application of the fat saturation pulse. Tumor is bright because of its relatively increased water content. Lymphoid tissue, as in the tonsils (T), is also mildly hyperintense. *C*, Axial postgadolinium T_1-weighted image with fat saturation shows improved delineation of the tumor (*white arrowheads*) from adjacent soft tissues compared with the unenhanced T_1-weighted image.

logic processes, helping to tailor a differential diagnosis and also to characterize the internal architecture of lymph nodes and to assess cranial nerve, cavernous sinus, or meningeal involvement by neoplastic or inflammatory processes. Gadolinium administration adds approximately $80 to the cost of an MR examination. Allergic reactions to gadolinium chelates have been described but are extremely rare compared with iodinated contrast material, and these agents are considered safe to administer even to very young children.

Alternative contrast media are under development for the head and neck, and one of these is superparamagnetic iron oxide particles (SPMIO).[12] Iodinated contrast agents for CT and gadolinium-based contrast agents for MRI are useful in detecting areas of nodal necrosis (seen as peripheral enhancement with a central area of nonenhancement) that are characteristic of metastatic squamous cell carcinoma,[13] but the absence of nodal necrosis does not exclude nodal metastasis, and both CT and MRI are relatively insensitive to small foci of tumor in normal-sized, non-necrotic lymph nodes. Small iron oxide particles are taken up by macrophages within lymph nodes after intravenous administration, which results in reduced signal intensity of the normally functioning nodes owing to their magnetic susceptibility and T_2 relaxation shortening effects. Metastatic nodes that are partially or completely replaced by tumor cells do not possess the same levels of phagocytic activity as normal nodes and maintain the same signal intensity on post-SPMIO MRIs. A downside of this technique is that it requires a baseline imaging study and a postinjection imaging study approximately 24 hours apart.

Routine MR protocol. Our routine MR protocol includes sagittal, axial, and coronal T_1WIs. Post-gadolinium T_1WIs are obtained in the axial and coronal planes, and a fat suppression pulse is applied to maximize the contrast of pathologic processes with normal structures. If fat suppression is not used, it is often difficult to distinguish pathologically enhancing processes from the large amount of intrinsically high signal intensity fat on a T_1-based image. A fast spin echo T_2WI with fat suppression is also acquired, usually in the axial plane, but coronal imaging may be useful for the palate, skull base, and other selected areas. Slice thickness is usually on the order of 4 to 5 mm. Within the oral cavity, notably for buccal lesions, it may be useful to have the patient "puff out" his or her cheeks during CT or MRI to separate the lesion from other soft tissues (tongue, gingiva) that might be resting against the lesion in the resting, closed-mouth position.[14]

As with CT, MRI also has some limitations in the evaluation of the head and neck region. MR acquisitions take minutes per sequence rather than the seconds per slice of CT, so patient motion is a more significant problem. Approximately 10% of patients cannot tolerate the confining MRI environment owing to claustrophobia, and some patients have absolute contraindications to MRI studies, such as the presence of a cardiac pacemaker or a ferromagnetic intracranial aneurysm clip. MRI studies are presently expensive (minimum $800 to $1,100 per study), and whereas soft tissue contrast is superb with MRI, fine bone detail is inferior on MRI compared with CT. MRI is generally preferred for assessment of the skull base, nasopharynx, oropharynx, hypopharynx, and oral cavity. Both CT and MRI perform well with laryngeal and lymph node imaging.

Advanced applications of MR technology are also being applied to the head and neck, although they remain in the research/experimental stage at this time. MR spectroscopy results using hydrogen and phosphorus 31 techniques suggest that markers may exist for predicting tumor response to radiation therapy. In the future, such new functional techniques may improve our ability to predict tumor behavior accurately.

NORMAL MR AND CT ANATOMY OF THE ORAL CAVITY AND THE OROPHARYNX

The oral portion of the upper aerodigestive tract is divided into two major components: the oral cavity and the oropharynx. The oral cavity includes the anterior two-thirds of the tongue, the buccal mucosa, and the floor of the mouth and is bordered laterally by the mandible and portions of the maxilla. The floor of the mouth is beneath the oral tongue and is supported by the mylohyoid muscle. The oropharynx includes the posterior third of the tongue (tongue base), the palatine tonsils and pillars, the soft palate, the oropharyngeal mucosa, and the pharyngeal constrictor muscles from the level of the soft palate to the top of the epiglottis.[15]

The oral tongue consists of three intrinsic bundles of muscle separated by fat planes (Figure 4–66, A). It is attached in part to the floor of the mouth and has several extrinsic muscles that insert into it and help control its motion. It actually can be considered as two halves fused in the midline, each with its own neurovascular supply. A neurovascular bundle containing the lingual artery and vein and the hypoglossal nerve, as well as the submandibular duct, is located in the sublingual space on each side of midline. The base of the tongue extends inferiorly and posteriorly to attach near the hyoid bone. The floor of the mouth includes a mucosa-covered group of extrinsic muscles and the neurovascular bundles. In the midline, a fatty septum separates the genioglossus muscles and extends up into the midline of the intrinsic tongue, serving as an important midline landmark (Figure 4–66, B and C). The floor of the mouth includes two important nonmucosal spaces: the sublingual and submandibular spaces. These are separated from each other by the mylohyoid muscle, a curvilinear muscle that extends medially from the mandibular bodies and forms the supporting structure of the floor of the mouth (Figure 4–66, D and E). The sublingual space contains the sublingual salivary glands and the submandibular duct, as well as neurovascular structures. The submandibular space contains the submandibular gland, as well as lymph nodes and branches of the facial artery. The submandibular duct exits the medial aspect of the gland and courses within the floor of the mouth in the sublingual space. Posterior and superior to the sublingual and submandibular spaces is the parapharyngeal space, a fat-filled space that extends from the skull base down to the level of the superior cornu of the hyoid bone (see Figure 4–66, C and E). The inferior aspect of the parapharyngeal space communicates freely with the posterior aspect of the submandibular space, providing a route for pathology to spread from the oral cavity to the skull base.

Four major types of soft tissue are present in the normal oral cavity and oropharynx: muscle, lymphoid tissue, salivary glandular tissue, and fat. These tissues demonstrate MR signal intensities that differ depending on the imaging parameters selected. Fat has a short T_1 relaxation time, resulting in high signal intensity on T_1WIs, whereas muscle and lymphoid tissue have low-to-intermediate signal intensity on T_1WIs. Salivary glandular tissue has intermediate to slightly high signal intensity on T_1WIs. Lymphoid tissue has a relatively long T_2 relaxation time and therefore increases in signal intensity relative to muscle on T_2WIs (Figure 4–66, F and G). T_1-weighted sequences afford the best contrast between fat and muscle, whereas T_2-weighted sequences demonstrate the best contrast between muscle and lymphoid tissue. On CT, many of these tissue types are similar in density (see Figure 4–63), making distinction among them more difficult. Salivary tissue has signal characteristics between those of muscle and lymphoid tissue. Tumors generally have relatively increased water content, which prolongs relaxation times and results in relatively higher signals on T_2WIs.[16]

The extrinsic muscles in the floor of the mouth are separated by fat planes. T_1-weighted axial and coronal images demonstrate this anatomy most clearly.[17] The most prominent landmark in the floor of the mouth is the midline fat-filled lingual septum, which separates the paramedian genioglossus muscles. Deviation or obliteration of this septum is abnormal. The submandibular gland, located inferior to the mylohyoid muscle beneath the mandible, has intermediate signal intensity between muscle and fat on T_2WIs (see Figure 4–66, F). The proximal 3 to 4 mm of the submandibular duct may normally be seen on T_2WIs as a high signal intensity structure leaving the deep portion of the gland, just medial to the mylohyoid muscle. The duct may be obstructed by carcinomas of the floor of the mouth (Figure 4–67). This may result in swelling of the gland and enlargement of the duct. The sublingual gland occupies the anterior third of the lateral floor of the mouth in a position superomedial to the mylohyoid muscle. As it is mildly hyperintense on T_2WI, it can be difficult to separate from tumor on T_2WI.

The oropharynx includes the base of the tongue, the pharyngeal constrictor muscles surrounding the airway, the palatine tonsils, and lymphoid tissue at the base of the tongue, as well as the oral surface of the soft palate. The centrally located parapharyngeal space is an important fat-filled landmark located deep to the mucosal space. It is best defined on T_1WIs. Displacement of the parapharyngeal fat often indicates deep invasion of neoplasm (Figure 4–68). Tumor that abuts lymphoid tissue in the palatine and lingual tonsils cannot always be reliably differentiated from this tissue on the basis of signal intensity, but MRI, in general, better distinguishes tumor from these other tissues than does CT.

NEOPLASMS

The most common tumor involving the oral cavity and oropharynx is squamous cell carcinoma. Squamous cell carcinomas have T_1 relaxation times similar to lymphoid tissue and muscle and therefore may be difficult to differentiate from these structures on T_1WIs. However, displacement or obliteration of fat planes by these infiltrating neoplasms facilitates a diagnosis on CT or T_1-weighted MRI studies (Figure 4–69, A). On T_2-weighted MRI sequences, the signal intensity of neoplastic tissue generally increases owing to increased water content. This usually affords excellent contrast between the tumor and the adjacent tissues it infiltrates (Figure 4–69, B).

Because the musculature of the oral cavity and oropharynx offers little resistance to the spread of

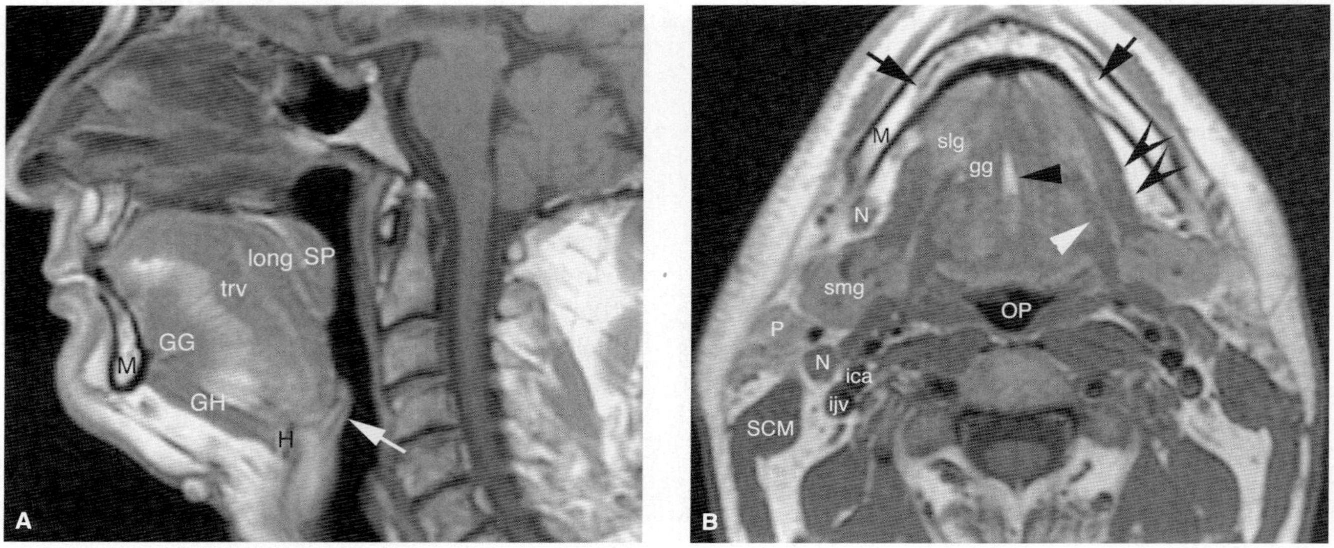

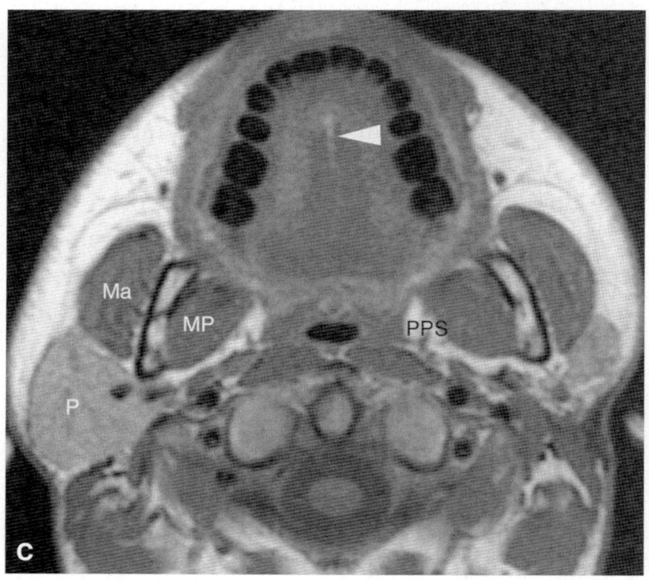

Figure 4–66. Normal magnetic resonance anatomy of the oral cavity and oropharynx. *A*, Sagittal T_1-weighted image through the midline demonstrates the geniohyoid muscle (GH) extending from the genu of the mandible (M) to the hyoid bone (H). Above this, the genioglossus (GG) muscle fans out from the genu of the mandible to insert on the intrinsic tongue musculature, represented by transverse (trv) and longitudinal (long) fibers. The soft palate (SP) is seen, as is the epiglottis (*white arrow*). *B*, Axial T_1-weighted image through the floor of the mouth demonstrates the genioglossus muscles (gg) on either side of the fat-filled lingual septum (*black arrowhead*). The hyoglossus (*white arrowhead*) and mylohyoid (*curved black arrowheads*) muscles are indicated. The submandibular (smg) and parotid (P) glands are slightly brighter than muscle. Lymph nodes (N) are intermediate in signal, whereas flow voids in the internal carotid artery (ica) and internal jugular vein (ijv) are black. The oropharyngeal airway (OP) is indicated. *Black arrows* demonstrate the inferior alveolar canals in the mandible (M). *C*, A more superior axial T_1-weighted image through the upper oral cavity again shows the midline fatty lingual septum (*white arrowhead*). The masseter (Ma) and medial pterygoid (MP) muscles are seen, as is fat in the parapharyngeal space (PPS). The parotid gland (P) is intermediate in signal between fat and muscle. *(continued)*

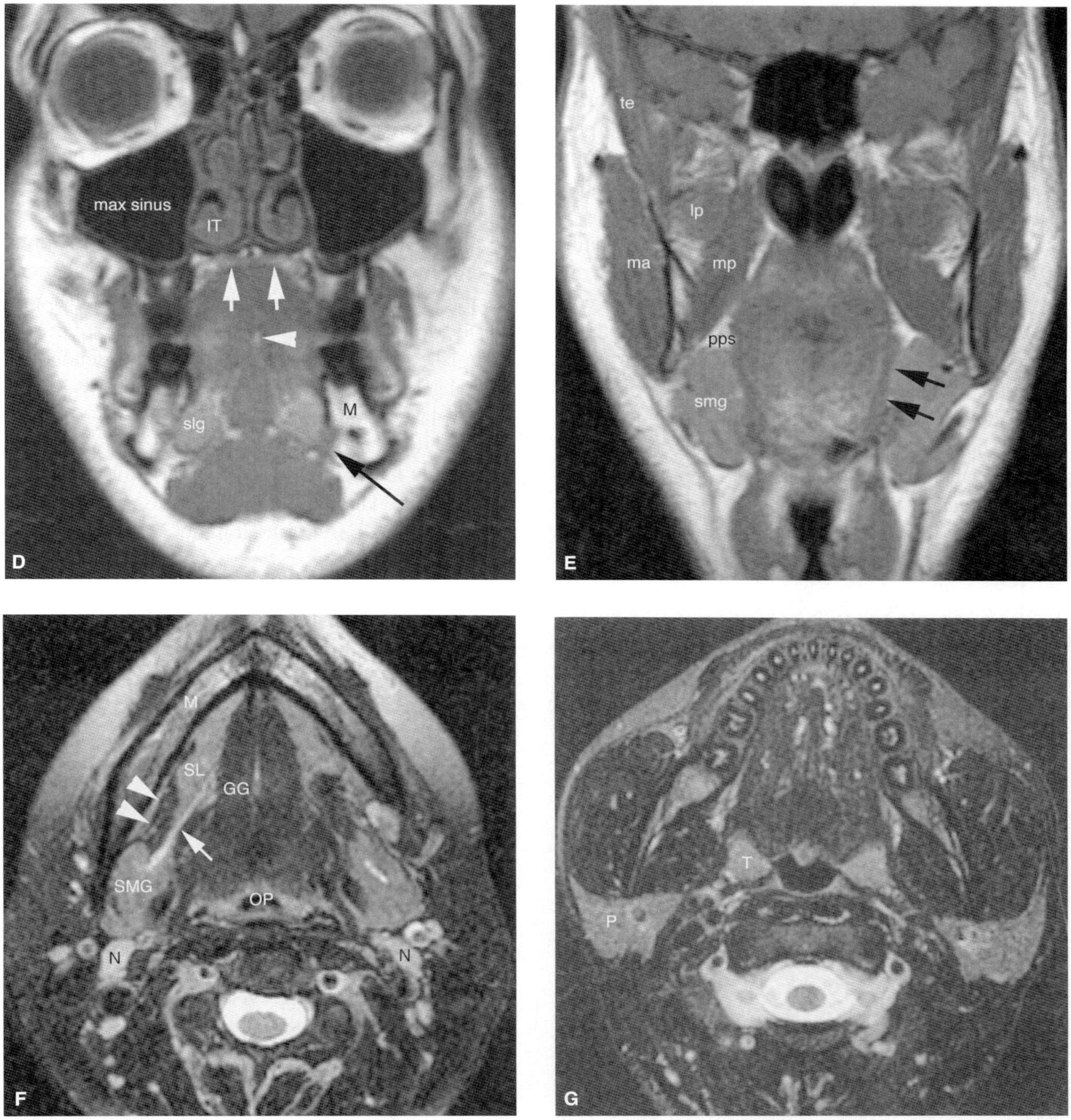

Figure 4–66 *continued.* *D*, A coronal T_1-weighted image through the anterior oral cavity demonstrates the mylohyoid muscle (*black arrow*) separating the sublingual space from the submandibular space. The sublingual gland (slg) is mildly hyperintense to muscle. Again seen is the midline septum (*white arrowhead*). The hard palate is indicated (*white arrows*), as is the mandible (M), the inferior turbinate (IT), and the maxillary sinus. *E*, A more posterior coronal T_1-weighted image demonstrates the submandibular gland (smg) inferior and lateral to the hyoglossus muscle (*black arrows*). The fat-filled parapharyngeal space (pps) is well seen, as are the muscles of mastication: masseter (ma), medial pterygoid (mp), lateral pterygoid (lp), and temporalis (te). *F*, Axial fast spin echo T_2-weighted image with fat saturation through the floor of the mouth demonstrates the genioglossus muscle (GG) and mylohyoid muscle (*white arrowheads*), which are low in signal intensity. Salivary tissue, notably the sublingual (SL) and submandibular (SMG) glands, is slightly bright, as is normal lymphoid tissue in cervical lymph nodes (N). The submandibular duct (*white arrow*) is fluid containing and therefore quite bright. Also indicated are the mandible (M) and the oropharyngeal airway (OP). *G*, A more superior axial fast spin echo T_2-weighted image with fat saturation demonstrates the mildly hyperintense palatine tonsils (T) and parotid tissue (P).

carcinoma, both measurement of surface extension and palpation of extent of induration may underestimate the extent of squamous cell carcinoma based on physical examination. Radiologic delineation of tumor extent and nodal involvement prior to surgery offers some key advantages in planning therapeutic strategies and tailoring the extent of surgical and/or radiation therapy.

CT has historically served as the staging modality of choice in evaluating tumors of the oral cavity and oropharynx. However, MRI provides superior contrast between normal soft tissue anatomy and pathology, without the need for iodine-based intravenous contrast agents. More accurate detection of tumor extent across the midline of the tongue and into the tongue base, floor of the mouth, and deep fascial spaces is therefore possible, as is detection of perineural spread of disease (Figure 4–70). The presence of flow void in vascular structures on MRI permits easy differentiation of vessels from surrounding tumor and cervical adenopathy without intravenous contrast agents. This is particularly helpful for assessing carotid artery invasion by tumor. In the tongue, the anatomic proximity of tumor to the contralateral lingual artery is particularly important in planning surgical or radiation therapy. Multiplanar MRI has improved the estimation of tumor volume with sagittal and coronal images, and a calculation of tumor volume may influence choices regarding surgical versus radiation therapy. Finally, dental artifacts produced by CT scans through the oral cavity are greatly diminished by MRI in most instances as dental amalgam is generally not ferromagnetic (Figure 4–71).[10]

A relative drawback of MRI, and a more significant drawback of CT, in the upper aerodigestive tract is the lack of contrast between tumor and lymphoid tissue. This is particularly true in and around the soft palate, base of the tongue, and palatine ton-

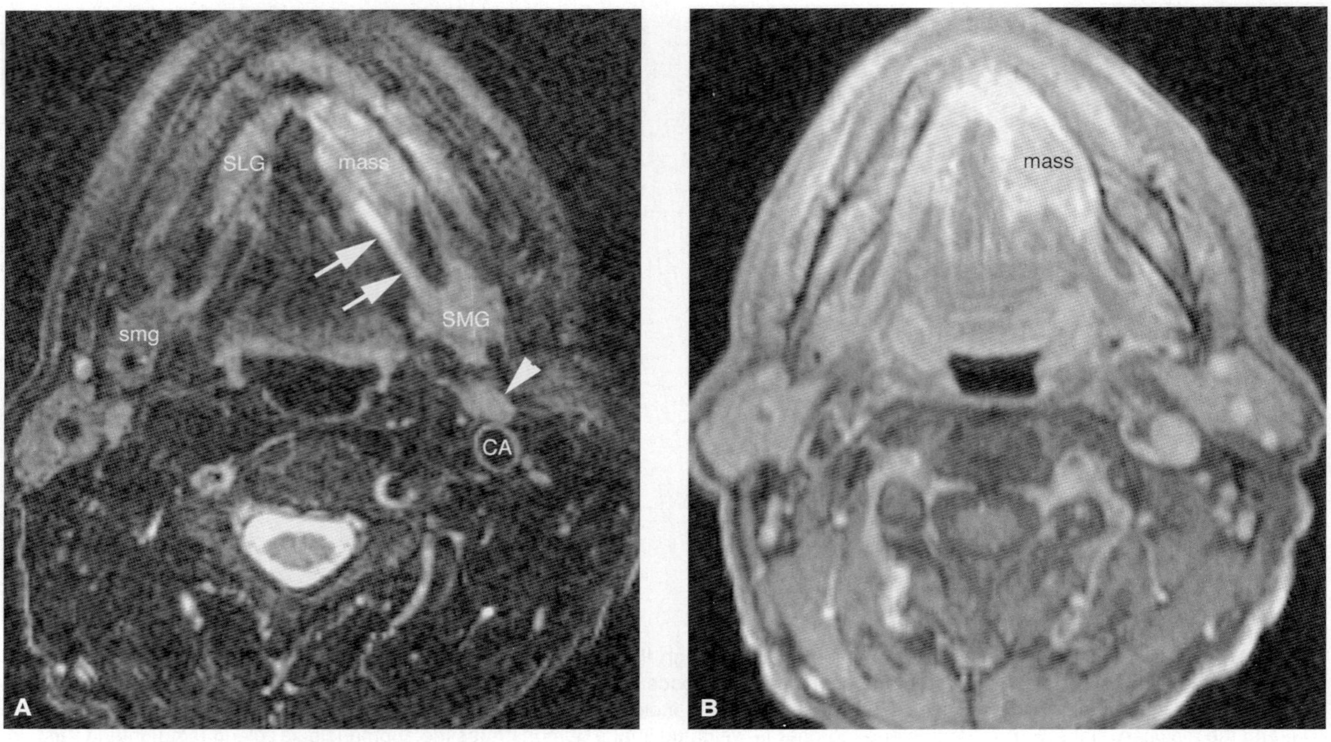

Figure 4–67. Squamous cell carcinoma of the anterior floor of the mouth, with obstruction of the submandibular duct. *A*, Axial fast spin echo T_2-weighted image with fat saturation through the lower mandible demonstrates a mass in the left anterior floor of the mouth, consistent with the patient's known squamous cell carcinoma. The left submandibular duct is dilated (*white arrows*), and the left submandibular gland (SMG) is bright compared with the normal right gland (smg), presumably owing to obstruction and inflammation of the left gland. A lymph node (*arrowhead*) is seen anterior to the carotid artery (CA) but is indeterminate for the presence of metastatic tumor. *B*, Axial postgadolinium T_1-weighted image with fat saturation at a slightly higher level demonstrates homogeneous enhancement of the irregularly marginated, infiltrative tumor.

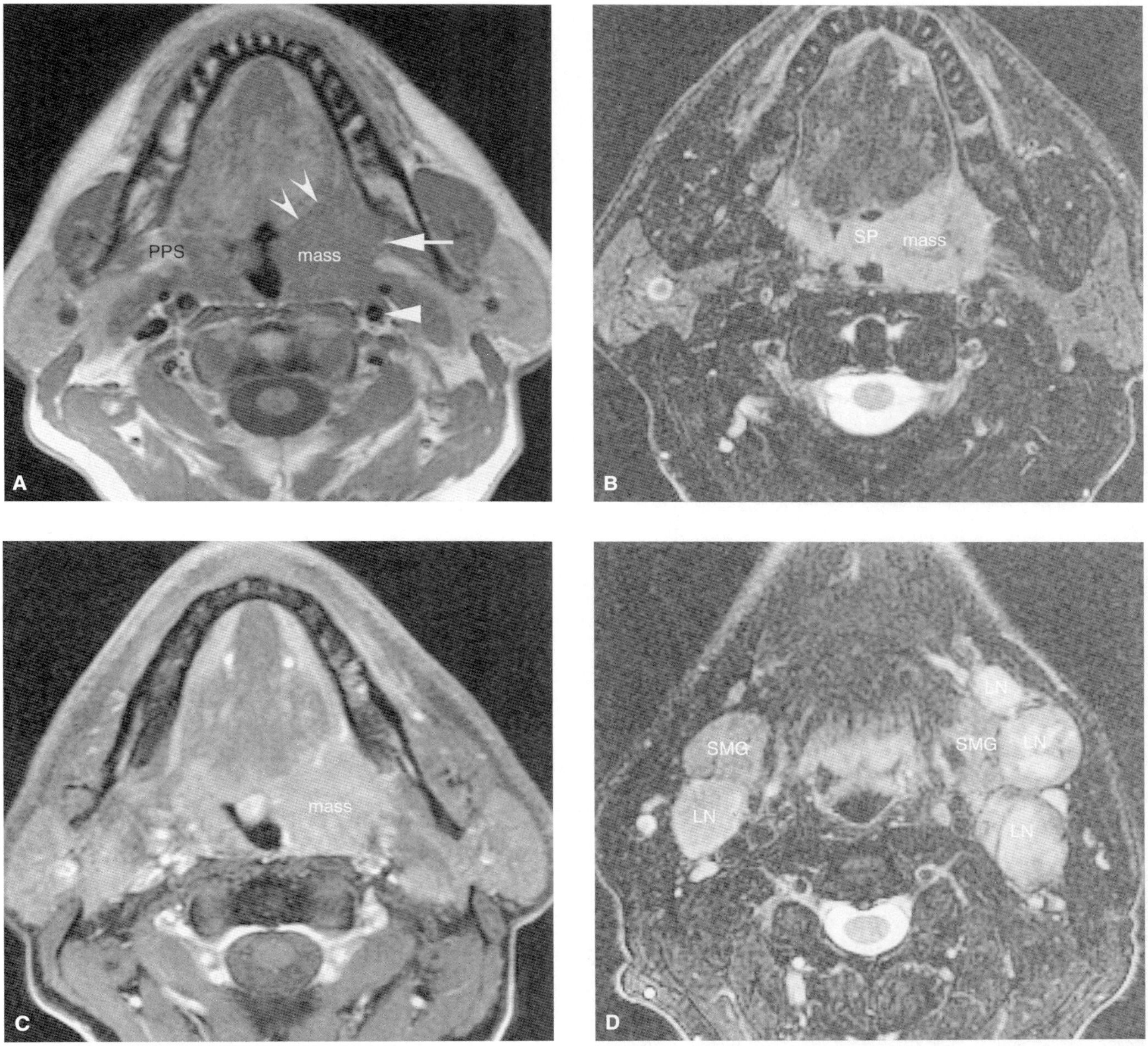

Figure 4–68. Squamous cell carcinoma of the tonsil. *A*, Axial T_1-weighted image shows the large mass deviating the left base of tongue (*curved arrowheads*) but not invading it. The mass does infiltrate the left parapharyngeal fat (*white arrow*), and this is best appreciated by comparing the volume and appearance of fat in the normal right parapharyngeal space (PPS). The internal carotid artery (*arrowhead*) is displaced posteriorly but not encased or narrowed. *B*, A slightly more superior axial fast spin echo T_2-weighted image with fat saturation shows that the mass is hyperintense to muscle and extends medially into the soft palate (SP). The exact margins of the lesion are difficult to define. *C*, Axial postgadolinium T_1-weighted image with fat saturation demonstrates moderate homogeneous enhancement of the tumor mass. *D*, A slightly more inferior axial fast spin echo T_2-weighted image with fat saturation demonstrates multiple large metastatic lymph nodes (LN) adjacent to the submandibular glands (SMG). Note that bilateral pathologic lymphadenopathy is not uncommon with cancers of the oral cavity and oropharynx, and both necks should be carefully assessed in all patients with head and neck cancer.

sils, where the signal intensity of normal tissues is similar to most malignant tumors on both T_1WIs and T_2WIs. Close examination may demonstrate subtle intensity differences, but, in these regions, noting morphologic changes such as asymmetric enlargement of a tonsil or infiltration of the surrounding deep fat planes is probably the most useful way to detect a lesion. This also emphasizes the importance of strong clinical-radiologic correlation as the radiologist will best be able to detect subtle

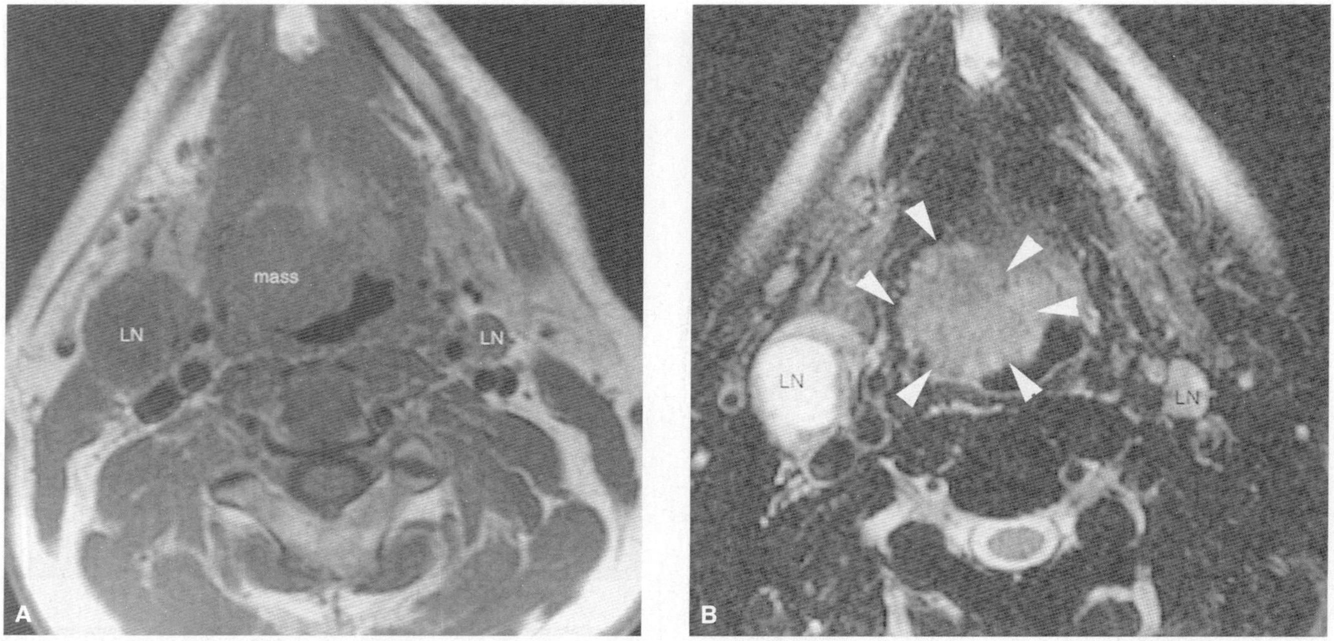

Figure 4–69. Squamous cell carcinoma of the right base of the tongue. *A*, Axial T_1-weighted image demonstrates an exophytic lesion involving the right base of tongue. Extension of tumor anteriorly into the floor of the mouth can be appreciated by obliteration of adjacent fat planes and displacement of adjacent structures. Also seen are metastatic lymph nodes (LN). *B*, Axial fast spin echo T_2-weighted image with fat saturation shows the tumor in more clear contrast to adjacent muscle. Also better appreciated are areas of necrosis (seen as very bright signal) in the metastatic lymph nodes.

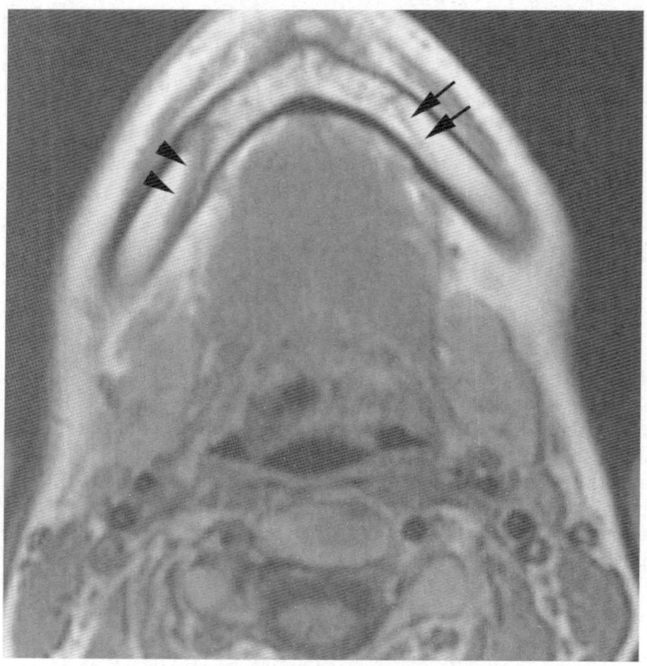

Figure 4–70. Axial T_1-weighted image through the lower mandible in a patient with a history of squamous cell carcinoma of the gingivobuccal sulcus and new right chin numbness. Asymmetric enlargement of the right inferior alveolar nerve (*black arrowheads*) compared with the left (*black arrows*) is highly suspicious for perineural spread of disease. This was confirmed at the time of surgery.

changes if he or she understands the clinical location and extent of disease.

Both T_1WIs and T_2WIs are necessary in the evaluation of cancer of the oral cavity and oropharynx. Axial and sagittal MR planes are the most useful in delineating oropharyngeal pathology. Axial images define the posterior and lateral extent of pathology, whereas sagittal images are helpful in defining invasion of the tongue base, preepiglottic space, and the posterior pharyngeal wall. Imaging in the coronal plane also proves useful when evaluating the inferior extension of tumor into the floor of the mouth and mandible (Figure 4–72).

MRI and CT improve the ability to stage a primary tumor accurately by assessing the deep extent of a lesion, which cannot always be predicted on the basis of clinical examination. If a biopsy is performed prior to an imaging study, the edema generated by the biopsy may simulate tumor infiltration. Therefore, if the patient is to have an imaging study, particularly in search of an unknown primary lesion, it is most important to perform it prior to deep biopsies.

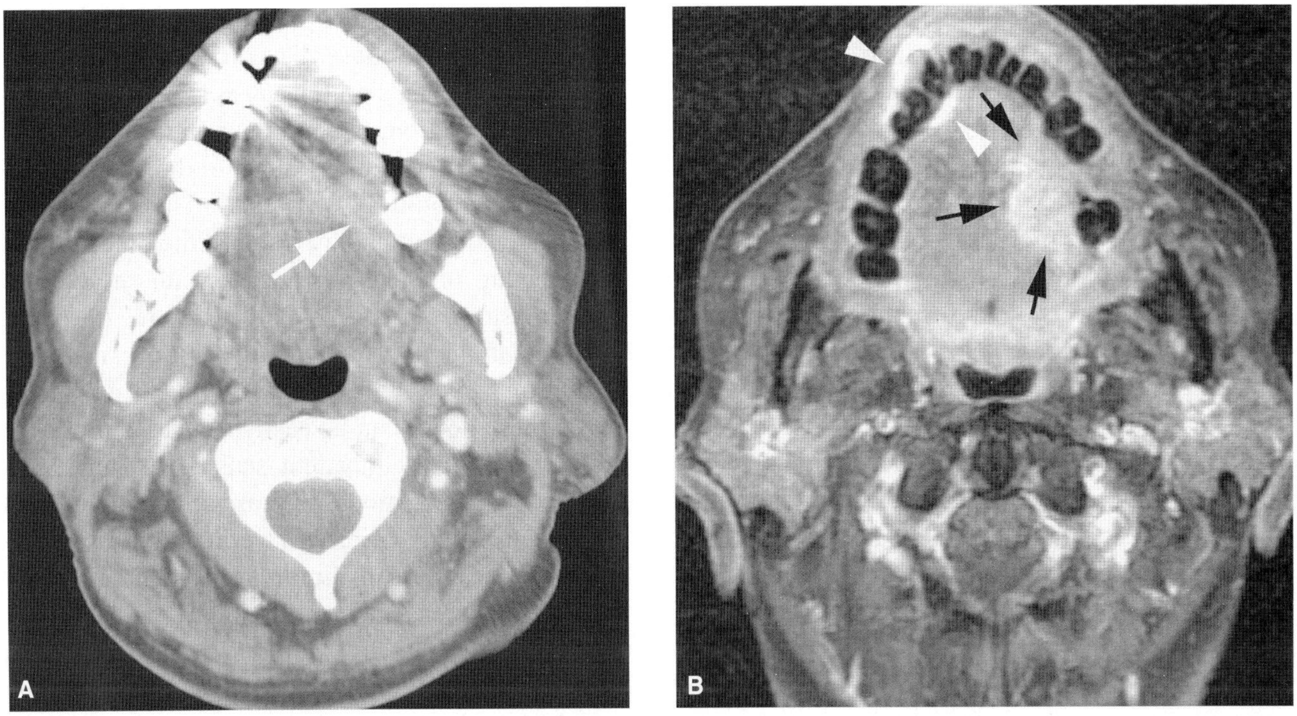

Figure 4–71. *A*, Axial contrast enhanced 3 mm computed tomographic (CT) image in a patient with known squamous cell carcinoma of the left tongue. The presence of extensive streak artifact from the patient's dental work makes his left-sided lesion (*white arrow*) difficult to appreciate. *B*, Axial postgadolinium T_1-weighted image with fat saturation in the same patient demonstrates the tongue lesion (*black arrows*) to far better advantage. The dental artifact (*white arrowheads*) is minimal compared with the CT scan.

The pathways of extension of a neoplasm are usually predictable. A careful search for subtle tumor extension along regional nerves and muscles and into regional nodes is necessary to derive the most information from the MRI or CT study. Skull-base erosion or intracranial extension may occur if perineural tumor reaches the sphenoid bone. Adenoid cystic carcinoma is notorious for extending along the regional nerves a distance away from the primary lesion, but all soft tissue tumors have the potential for perineural spread, and a detailed search for this pathway of spread is necessary in every case.

Mandibular involvement by squamous cell carcinoma alters the management of patients with oral carcinoma. Both MRI and CT offer advantages over plain film assessment of the mandible. Whereas MRI is more sensitive to tumor extension into the medullary cavity of the mandible, CT probably offers greater sensitivity to cortical bone erosion and should be used when doubt exists regarding the integrity of the mandible adjacent to a neoplasm. Noncontrast T_1WI and contrast-enhanced fat-saturated T_1WI in the coronal and axial planes have

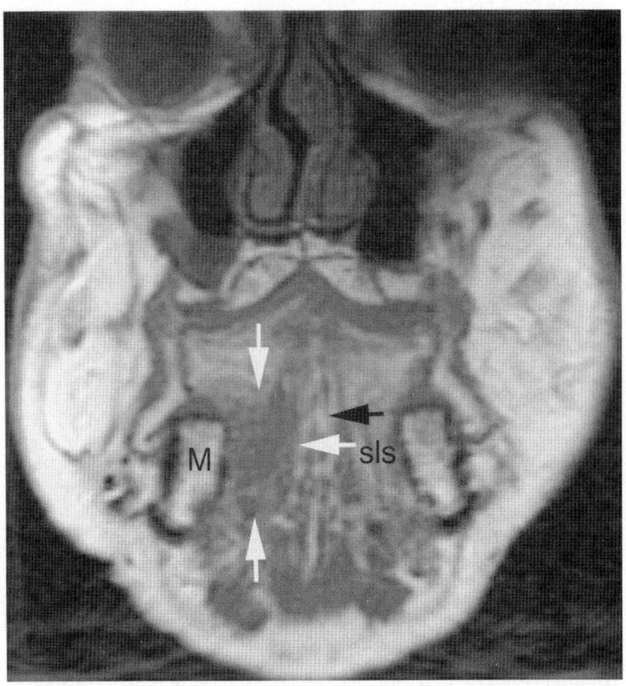

Figure 4–72. Coronal T_1-weighted image in a patient with squamous cell carcinoma of the right floor of the mouth demonstrates infiltration into the right sublingual space (*white arrows*). The lingual septum (*black arrow*) is well seen, indicating that this lesion does not cross the midline. Normal high signal intensity of the left sublingual space (sls) is seen, as is normal fatty marrow in the mandible (M).

proven most useful in the detection of malignant involvement of the mandibular marrow cavity. MRI is also useful in the evaluation of patients with osteoradionecrosis (Figure 4–73).

The detection of metastatic adenopathy is an important goal in the staging of patients with oral cavity tumors. The presence of metastatic adenopathy from an oral tongue carcinoma decreases the 5-year survival by 50%. Many centers advocate routine elective neck dissections in patients with T_2 or greater oral tongue lesions as the risk of microscopic nodal metastases is upward of 30 to 40%. With this approach, imaging has less impact on therapeutic decision making. However, the detection of nodal disease in the clinically N0 neck may alter the treatment modality in many centers that advocate either observation ("watchful waiting") or radiation therapy.

Squamous cell carcinoma of the head and neck generally involves the draining nodes in an orderly fashion, infiltrating the more proximal regional nodes prior to the more distal nodes in the chain. Therefore, a focused search can be directed at nodes in a specific region, although the entire neck, from the retropharyngeal nodes down to the supraclavicular fossa, should be surveyed. Up to 30% of metastatic nodes are not palpable at the time of diagnosis owing to their position beneath the sternocleidomastoid muscle or adjacent to the submandibular glands. Patient body habitus can also be a limiting factor with regard to clinical palpation. All of these nodes can be easily evaluated by CT or MRI, with fairly equivalent sensitivity and specificity of these two modalities, assuming attention to good technique.[18] Criteria have been developed to help identify tumor infiltration of lymph nodes. On CT or MRI, metastatic nodal involvement is suggested if the minimal axial diameter is greater than 7 mm. The presence of focal necrosis surrounded by peripheral enhancement is diagnostic of metastatic lymphadenopathy. On MRI, metastatic nodes often but not always have heterogeneous signal intensity on both T_2WIs and T_1WIs. However, metastatic nodes containing small tumor deposits may appear normal in their MR signal. Gadolinium-based contrast agents, administered intravenously during the scan procedure, may increase the specificity of MRI in the detection of these small metastatic nodes by allowing the detection of nodal necrosis. Obtaining postgadolinium images in the head and neck requires the use of a fat-suppression technique to distinguish contrast enhancement from the high signal of surrounding fat.

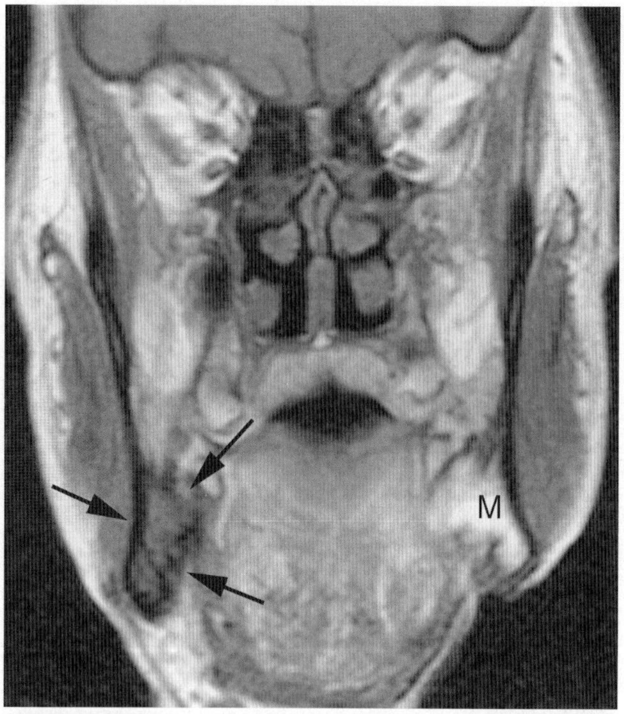

Figure 4–73. Coronal T_1-weighted image in a patient with a remote history of prior radiation, chemotherapy, and neck dissection for squamous cell carcinoma of the tonsil demonstrates replacement of the normal fatty marrow in the mandible (M) with low signal intensity soft tissue (*black arrows*). No associated soft tissue mass is seen. This is consistent with osteoradionecrosis, although a component of infiltrative tumor cannot necessarily be excluded by imaging alone, and clinical correlation is required.

The role of MRI and CT in the workup of the unknown primary tumor has been fairly well established. One study examining the sensitivity of CT in this setting concluded that CT was useful in locating the tumor or directing a biopsy in 30% of the 15 patients studied.[19] A similar study of MRI has not been published, but, anecdotally, the potential for even greater detection rates exists. For this reason, at our institution, we use high-resolution MRI prior to biopsy in patients with an unknown primary tumor. This does not delay the diagnostic or therapeutic workup and has the potential to direct biopsies during subsequent panendoscopy. Nodal staging can be accomplished at the same time.

POSITRON EMISSION TOMOGRAPHY

PET using ^{18}F-2-fluoro-2-deoxy-D-glucose (FDG) has demonstrated utility in head and neck cancer for staging of nodal disease, detection of residual or recurrent disease following therapy, and detection of occult primary lesions, as well as detection of synchronous primary lesions and the presence of distant metastases.[20] In a patient with an unknown primary site of tumor, FDG-PET should be performed prior to panendoscopy and biopsy so that sites of biopsy will not lead to a false-positive study. FDG-PET may yield useful information regarding a primary site in as many as 65% of cases (Figure 4–74).[21] When a previously radiated patient is suspected of having residual or recurrent disease, FDG-PET can be very useful but is most reliable if at least 3 or 4 months have elapsed since completion of radiation therapy. An alternative method, FDG-SPECT (FDG single-photon emission computed tomography), makes use of the more widely available gamma cameras that are present in every nuclear medicine department. The FDG-SPECT images, however, are generally of inferior quality compared with images produced by dedicated FDG-PET scanners, particularly if they are done using "high-resolution" machines. FDG-PET can also be useful in nodal staging, performing with sensitivity ranging from 72 to 91% and specificity ranging from 88 to 100%.[22–24] FDG-PET is particularly useful in the identification of subclinical sites of nodal disease, and the identification of these sites may significantly alter therapy and prognosis. Unexpected metastatic disease may also significantly alter the therapeutic plan (Figure 4–75). A recent development, PET-CT, can obtain both FDG-PET images and CT images on a patient without moving the patient. This facilitates anatomic correlation of FDG-PET findings and also facilitates directed biopsies in questions of unknown primary lesions and residual/recurrent disease.[25]

Accurate detection of recurrent squamous cell carcinoma remains a significant problem despite the advances in CT and MRI because these anatomically based modalities are limited by postsurgical and postradiation scarring and obliteration of normal tissue planes.[26,27] FDG-PET has shown promise in the detection of residual or recurrent disease because it detects abnormal tumor metabolism rather than relying on anatomy. FDG-PET has detected recurrent disease with sensitivities and specificities in the 86 to 100% range (Figure 4–76), allowing more timely diagnosis and institution of salvage therapy if such therapy is available. Furthermore, a negative FDG-PET study can be highly reassuring to both physician and patient as the negative predictive value of a high-quality scan approaches 100% (Figure 4–77). Note that an FDG-PET scan can be falsely negative if less than 3 or 4 months have elapsed postcompletion of radiation therapy. FDG-PET can also be used to monitor tumor response to therapy, the aim being that a nonresponding patient could be triaged to a different therapeutic modality.[28]

Other nuclear medicine–based techniques are also being evaluated in the management of patients with oral cancer. Performing gamma probe–directed biopsy of the sentinel node has become quite common for melanoma and has been investigated for patients with oral squamous cell carcinoma.[29] This technique requires the injection of unfiltered technetium 99m sulfur colloid in quadrants around the primary tumor

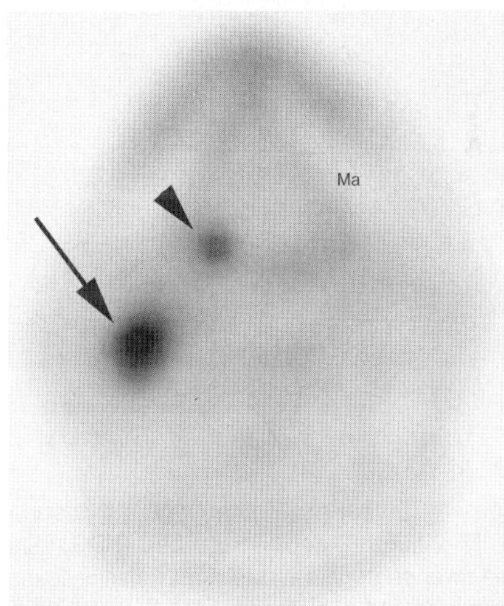

Figure 4–74. Axial image from an ^{18}F-2-fluoro-2-deoxy-D-glucose (FDG) positron emission tomographic (PET) scan in a patient who presented with a right neck mass that was found to be metastatic squamous cell carcinoma at fine-needle aspiration. The head and neck examination was negative for a primary site of disease, as was a magnetic resonance scan. The FDG-PET scan demonstrates the known right neck node (*black arrow*), as well as a focus of activity at the right base of the tongue (*black arrowhead*). The mandible (Ma) is seen as a photopenic area. During subsequent panendoscopy, a subtle focus of irregularity was seen at the right base of the tongue, and biopsy confirmed squamous cell carcinoma.

A B

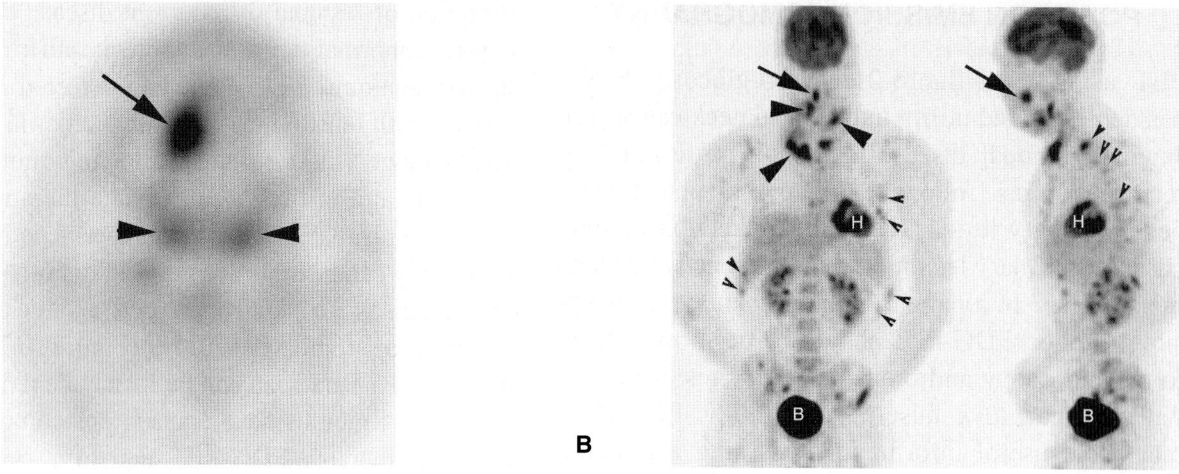

Figure 4–75. A ^{18}F-2-fluoro-2-deoxy-D-glucose (FDG) positron emission tomographic (PET) scan in a 40-year-old patient with T1N0 squamous cell carcinoma of the right tongue who has no history of tobacco or alcohol use. Because of his young age and lack of risk factors, a baseline FDG-PET scan was requested to stage the neck and to establish a comparison for follow-up studies. *A*, Axial image demonstrates intense uptake of FDG at the right tongue primary site of disease (*black arrow*). Mild activity is seen in the tonsils bilaterally (*black arrowheads*). *B*, Frontal and lateral whole-body views demonstrate the patient's primary lesion (*black arrow*), as well as unexpected nodal metastases (*large black arrowheads*) and extensive bony metastases (*small arrowheads*; note that only a few of the patient's innumerable lesions are marked).

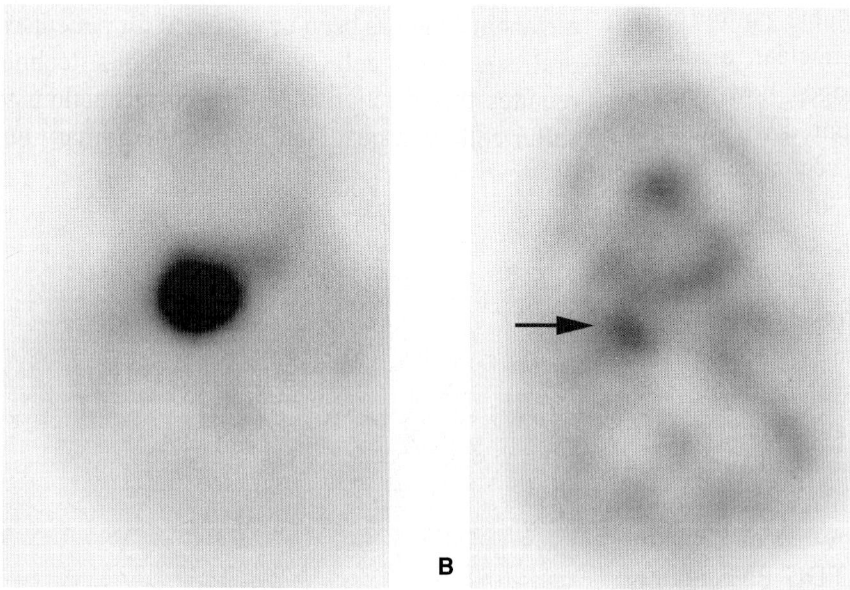

A B

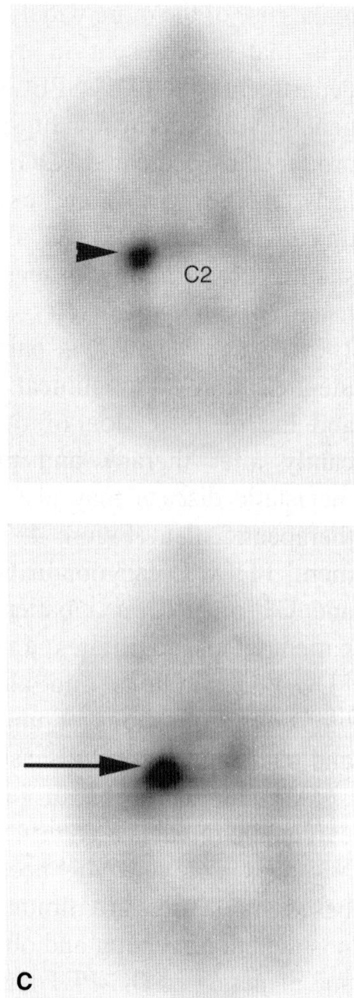

C

Figure 4–76. A 75-year-old woman with T3N0 squamous cell carcinoma of the right tonsil. *A*, Baseline ^{18}F-2-fluoro-2-deoxy-D-glucose (FDG) positron emission tomographic (PET) scan demonstrates intense uptake in the right tonsillar fossa. The scan was otherwise negative, and the patient was treated with radiation and chemotherapy. *B*, A follow-up FDG-PET scan performed 4 months after completion of radiation therapy demonstrates a diffuse increase in soft tissue uptake of FDG, as is commonly seen following irradiation, and markedly reduced activity in the right tonsillar fossa (*black arrow*). The residual activity was interpreted as residual tumor versus post-treatment inflammation, and it was elected to follow the patient as her clinical examination and magnetic resonance (MR) scan showed no definite evidence of persistent or recurrent disease. *C*, A follow-up FDG-PET scan 5 months later, at which time the patient has right throat pain and otalgia. The activity in the right tonsillar region is increased compared with the prior (*black arrow*), and a new focus of activity is present just below the skull base at the C2 level (*arrowhead*). An MR scan was suspicious for recurrent tumor, and this was confirmed with fine-needle aspiration. The patient unfortunately died of massive oral bleeding before further intervention could be performed.

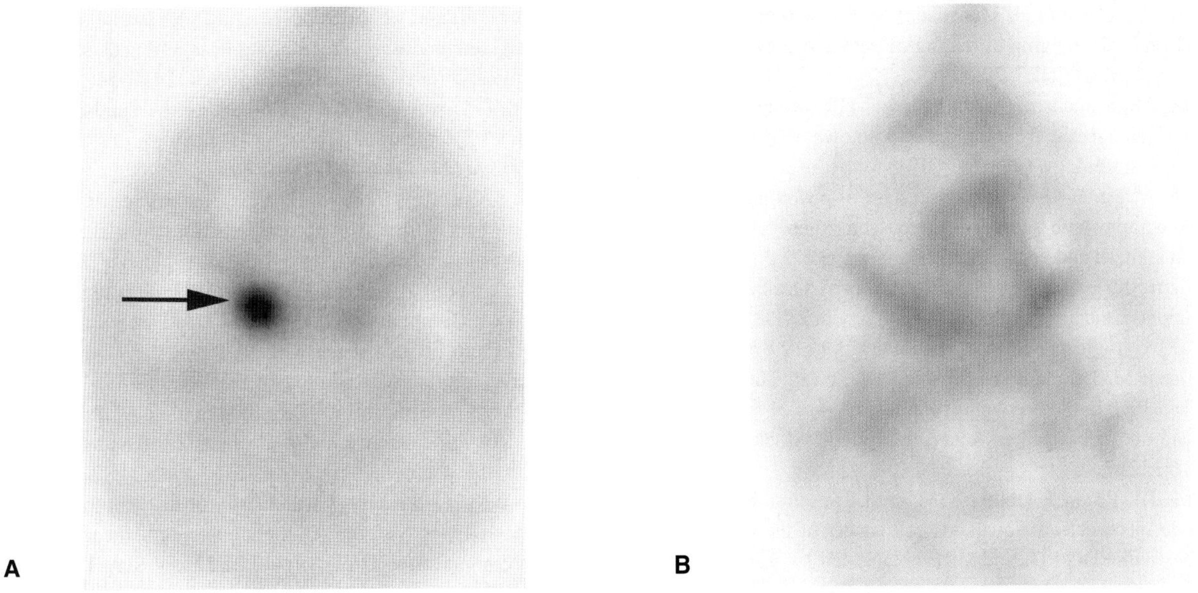

Figure 4–77. A 55-year-old man with T1N0 squamous cell carcinoma of the right tonsil. *A*, A ^{18}F-2-fluoro-2-deoxy-D-glucose (FDG) positron emission tomographic (PET) scan obtained for staging showed activity confined to the right tonsillar fossa (*black arrow*). *B*, A follow-up FDG-PET scan obtained 4 months postcompletion of radiation therapy shows mild generalized uptake of FDG consistent with prior radiation but no asymmetric activity. The patient has been followed with serial FDG-PET scans and has shown no evidence of residual or recurrent disease.

site followed by lymphoscintigraphy to identify the dominant lymphatic patterns of drainage. Open biopsy of the sentinel node is then performed. Preliminary results in patients with oral squamous cell carcinoma suggest that the technique is feasible, but its reliability has not yet been established.

REFERENCES

1. Horowitz AM, Nourjah P, Gift HC. U.S. adult knowledge of risk factors and signs of oral cancers: 1990. J Am Dent Assoc 1995;126:39–45.
2. Slavkin HC. The war on oral cavity and pharyngeal cancer. J Am Dent Assoc 1996;127:517–20.
3. Yellowitz JA, Goodman HS. Assessing physicians' and dentists' oral cancer knowledge, opinions and practices. J Am Dent Assoc 1995;126:53–60.
4. Silverman S Jr. Oral cavity. In: Bibbo M, editor. Comprehensive cytology. 2nd ed. Philadelphia: WB Saunders; 1997. p. 403–12.
5. Christian DC. Computer-assisted analysis of oral brush biopsies at an oral cancer screening program. J Am Dent Assoc 2002;133:357–62.
6. Scher RL, Oostingh PE, Levine PA, et al. Role of fine-needle aspiration biopsy in the diagnosis of lesions of the oral cavity, oropharynx, and nasopharynx. Cancer 1988;62:2602–6.
7. Mashberg A, Samit A. Early diagnosis of asymptomatic oral and oropharyngeal squamous cancers. CA Cancer J Clin 1995;45:328–51.
8. Portugal LC, Wilson KM, Biddinger PW, Gluckman JL. The role of toluidine blue in assessing margin status after resection of squamous cell carcinomas of the upper aerodigestive tract. Arch Otolaryngol Head Neck Surg 1996;122:517–9.
9. Warnakulasuriya KAAS, Johnson NW. Sensitivity and specificity of Orascan toluidine blue mouthrinse in the detection of oral cancer and precancer. J Oral Pathol Med 1996;25:97–103.
10. Hinshaw DB Jr, Holshouser BA, Engstrom HI, et al. Dental material artifacts on MR images. Radiology 1988;166:777–9.
11. Tien RD, Robbins KT. Correlation of clinical, surgical, pathologic, and MR fat suppression results for head and neck cancer. Head Neck 1992;14:278–84.
12. Anzai Y, Prince MR. Iron oxide-enhanced MR lymphography: the evaluation of cervical lymph nodes metastases in head and neck cancer. J Magn Reson Imaging 1997;7:75–81.
13. Yousem DM, Som PM, Hackney DB, et al. Central nodal necrosis and extracapsular neoplastic spread in cervical lymph nodes: MR imaging versus CT. Radiology 1992;182:753–9.
14. Weissman JL, Carrau RL. "Puffed-cheek" CT improves evaluation of the oral cavity. AJNR Am J Neuroradiol 2001;22:741–4.
15. Harnsberger HR. Head and neck imaging. St. Louis: Mosby Yearbook; 1990.
16. Schaefer SD, Maravilla KR, Suss RA, et al. Magnetic resonance imaging vs. computed tomography. Comparison in imaging oral cavity and pharyngeal carcinomas. Arch Otolaryngol 1985;111:730–4.
17. Unger JM. The oral cavity and tongue: magnetic resonance imaging. Radiology 1985;155:151–3.

18. Curtin HD, Ishwaran H, Mancuso AA, et al. Comparison of CT and MR imaging in staging of neck metastases. Radiology 1998;207:123–30.
19. Muraki AS, Mancuso AA, Harnsberger HR. Metastatic cervical adenopathy from tumors of unknown origin: the role of CT. Radiology 1984;152:749–53.
20. Rege S, Maass A, Chaiken L, et al. Use of positron emission tomography with fluorodeoxyglucose in patients with extracranial head and neck cancers. Cancer 1994;73:3047–58.
21. Mukherji SK, Drane WE, Mancuso AA, et al. Occult primary tumors of the head and neck: detection with 2-[F-18]fluoro-2-deoxy-D-glucose SPECT. Radiology 1996;199:761–6.
22. Benchaou M, Lehmann W, Slosman DO, et al. The role of FDG-PET in the preoperative assessment of N-staging in head and neck cancer. Acta Otolaryngol (Stockh) 1996; 116:332–5.
23. Braams JW, Pruim J, Freling NJM, et al. Detection of lymph node metastases of squamous cell cancer of the head and neck with FDG-PET and MRI. J Nucl Med 1995;36:211–6.
24. Laubenbacher C, Saumweber D, Wagner-Manslau C, et al. Comparison of fluorinc-18-fluorodeoxyglucose PET, MRI and endoscopy for staging head and neck squamous cell carcinomas. J Nucl Med 1995;36:1747–57.
25. Beyer T, Townsend DW, Blodgett TM. Dual-modality PET/CT tomography for clinical oncology. Q J Nucl Med 2002;46:24–34.
26. Anzai Y, Carroll WR, Quint DJ, et al. Recurrence of head and neck cancer after surgery or irradiation: prospective comparison of 2-deoxy-2-[F-18]fluoro-D-glucose PET and MR imaging diagnosis. Radiology 1996;200:135–41.
27. Lapela M, Grenman R, Kurki T, et al. Head and neck cancer: detection of recurrence with PET and 2-[F-18]fluoro-2-deoxy-D-glucose. Radiology 1995;197:205–11.
28. Haberkorn U, Strauss LG, Dimitrakoupulou A, et al. Fluorodeoxyglucose imaging of advanced head and neck cancer after chemotherapy. J Nucl Med 1993;34:12–7.
29. Koch WM, Choti MA, Civelek AC, et al. Gamma probe-directed biopsy of the sentinel node in oral squamous cell carcinoma. Arch Otolaryngol Head Neck Surg 1998;124: 455–9.

5

Spread of Tumor, Staging, and Survival

SOL SILVERMAN JR., MA, DDS
NANCY LEE, MD
ALAN M. KRAMER, MD (Chemoprevention)
RICHARD C. K. JORDAN, DDS, PHD (Modern Molecular Analysis)

Squamous cell carcinoma (SCC) of the oral cavity spreads primarily by local extension and by lymphatic permeation. The extent of tumor spread can quite accurately be assessed and measured by modern imaging techniques using computed tomography (CT), magnetic resonance imaging (MRI), and positron emission tomography (PET) (see Chapter 4, "Diagnosis"). Hematogenous spread (by blood vessels) occurs rarely with oral malignancies but is important in the development of distant metastases.

LOCAL EXTENSION

Direct extension locally into surrounding tissue depends a great deal on the anatomic location of the tumor (Figure 5–1). Muscle is easily invaded. The periosteum offers a good barrier but is eventually destroyed, and the tumor may proceed into the osseous tissue (Figure 5–2). Obviously, the unknown biologic characteristics that determine tumor aggressiveness (ie, the differentiation, mitotic index, and biochemical properties of neoplastic cells and extracellular matrix, as well as host immune responses) are major determinants.

LYMPHATIC SPREAD

Lymphatic spread is the most important and the most frequent pathway for the spread of oral malignancies (Figure 5–3). Tumor cells usually involve the lym-

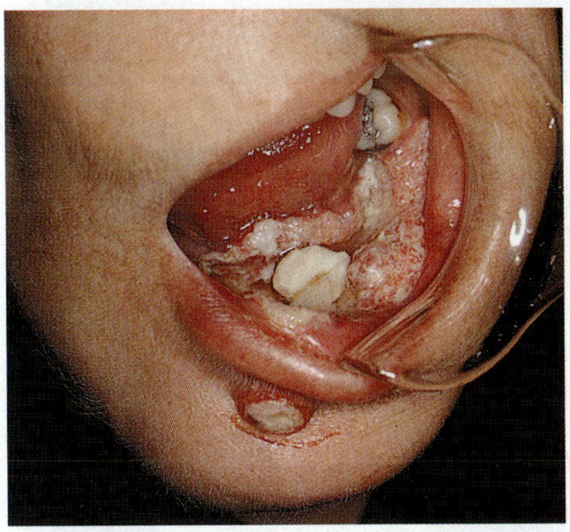

Figure 5–1. Advanced squamous cell carcinoma that had been present for 6 months before the patient sought consultation. The malignancy that had started as an ulceration in the floor of the mouth now extended to the tongue, mandible, and through the skin of the chin.

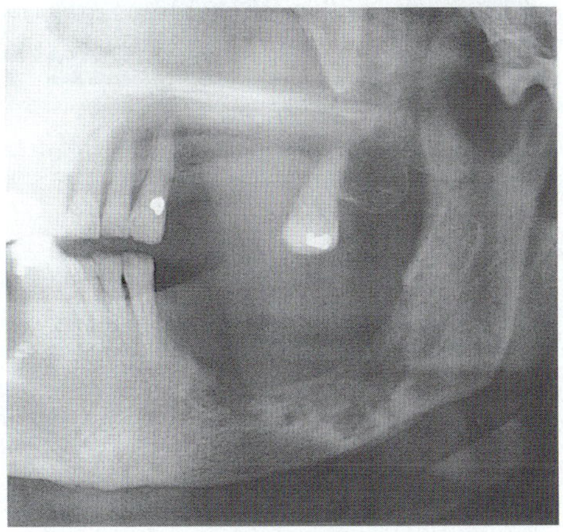

Figure 5–2. Squamous cell carcinoma of the floor of the mouth and gingiva that has penetrated the periosteum and is destroying the mandibular bone.

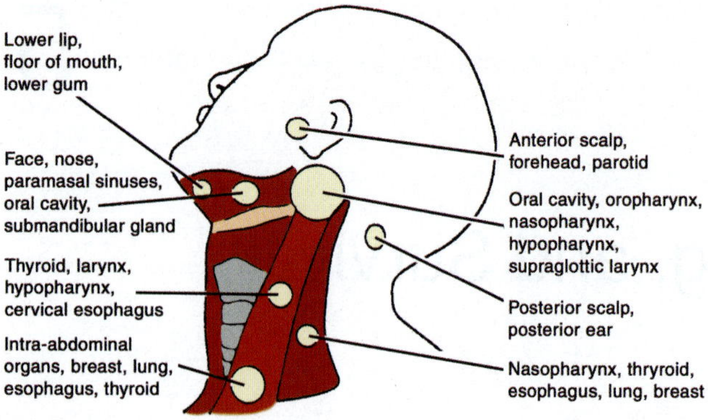

Figure 5–3. Likely sites of involved cervical lymph nodes from the spread of primary head and neck squamous cell carcinomas.

phatic channels and nodes by embolization. When lymph nodes are invaded, they gradually become replaced by tumor tissue and may attain a considerable size and hardness (induration) (Figure 5–4, A–C). The involved lymph nodes are freely movable at first, but as the tumor breaks through the capsule, the nodes become fixed to vital structures such as the carotid artery. The extent of lymph node involvement has been categorized in a staging system, which, in turn, is related to survival. When the spread of tumor involves lymph nodes, the prognosis is significantly reduced, and treatment becomes more aggressive. Infection in the primary lesion may also give rise to enlarged lymph nodes, which become palpable even though they do not contain cancer.

The usual pattern of findings from palpation of enlarged lymph nodes is described in Table 5–1; however, the clinician must realize that various combinations may exist. These findings are helpful in patient management but are not diagnostic. Sometimes it is extremely difficult to distinguish by palpation a metastatically involved submandibular lymph node from an enlarged submandibular salivary gland that has become infected or inflamed secondarily to obstruction of Wharton's duct. Conversely, at times, tumor-involved cervical nodes are so small that clinical recognition is uncertain. MRI and/or fine-needle

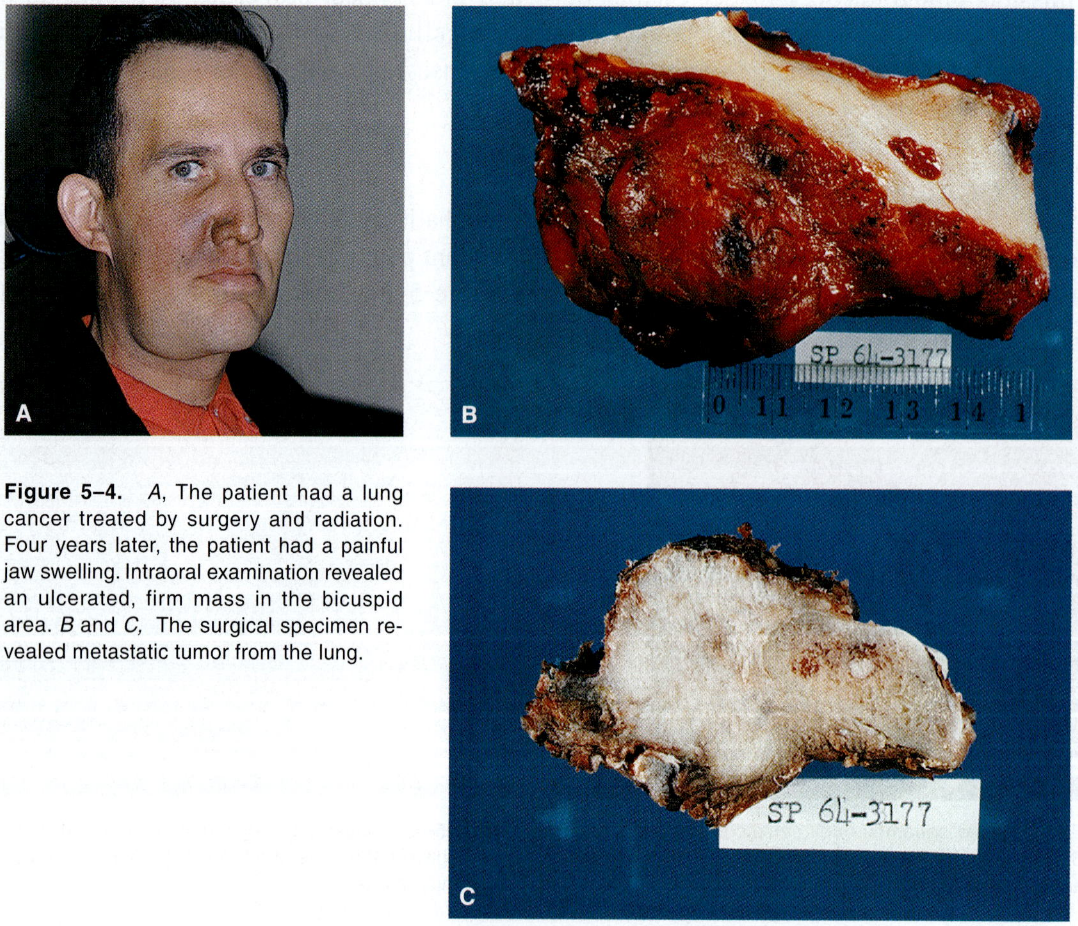

Figure 5–4. *A*, The patient had a lung cancer treated by surgery and radiation. Four years later, the patient had a painful jaw swelling. Intraoral examination revealed an ulcerated, firm mass in the bicuspid area. *B* and *C*, The surgical specimen revealed metastatic tumor from the lung.

Table 5–1. LYMPH NODE PALPATION FINDINGS

Cause of Lymphadenopathy	Texture	Sensitivity	Mobility
Acute infection or malignancy	Soft	Tender	Movable
Malignancy	Firm	Nontender	Movable or fixed

aspiration (see Chapter 4) may help to establish the diagnosis. PET may also be helpful in the detection of subclinical lymph node involvement.

The frequency of metastatic involvement of lymph nodes correlates with the size and depth of invasion, the site of origin, the degree of differentiation of the primary tumor, and cell surface molecules that interact with the extracellular matrix. In general, the frequency of lymph node metastasis increases with the size, depth of penetration, and duration of the lesion. This, however, does not preclude the occasional involvement of lymph nodes from a very small primary tumor. The more posterior the location of the primary lesion in the oral cavity and pharynx, the greater is the risk for lymphatic spread. Thus, the risks are greater for spread from tonsillar lesions than for floor of the mouth lesions. This increased risk may be attributable to a delay in diagnosis and to richer lymphatic drainage. The more poorly differentiated tumors also have greater risk.

Lymphatic spread of intraoral carcinoma usually occurs in an orderly manner, involving first the uppermost, then the middle, and finally the lower cervical nodes. About half of all oral cancer patients have metastatic cervical nodes at the time of diagnosis or follow-up.

When lymph nodes are only microscopically involved by metastatic carcinoma, they may not be detectable clinically or even by MRI. Because of this possibility, clinical prophylactic irradiation or surgical neck dissection is performed (see Chapter 6). The risk of subclinical disease in the lymph nodes in patients with no clinical evidence of lymphadenopathy may be determined as follows: careful follow-up of patients with necks that are initially negative then become positive when the neck is not treated or by examination of the incidence of positive nodes found in elective neck dissection specimens. The incidence of subsequent lymphadenopathy in patients with untreated necks that were initially negative has been estimated to be in the range of 20 to 35% for carcinoma of the floor of the mouth, 38 to 52% for the oral tongue, 17% for the gingiva, 22% for the hard palate, and 16% for the buccal mucosa. The incidence of positive nodes in elective neck dissection has been reported to be in the range of 40 to 50% for carcinoma of the floor of the mouth, 25 to 54% for the oral tongue, and 19% for the gingiva.

Occasionally, patients have a positive node in the neck when a primary site cannot be found.[1] Most lymph node metastases from an unknown primary site occur in the neck. The most common occult primary sites, often in the head and neck area, include the nasopharynx, tonsil, base of the tongue, and hypopharynx.

HEMATOGENOUS SPREAD

Manipulation of a malignant tumor, for example, during palpation and biopsy, often causes hematologic dissemination of tumor cells. However, studies to evaluate the relationship between prognosis and the appearance of tumor cells in venous blood after manipulation have been equivocal.

From the Stanford University Hospital in California, a study reported that 14% of 217 patients with oral carcinoma had distant metastases clinically or at autopsy. Most of these patients had advanced tumors. The lungs, bone, and liver were the most common metastatic sites. Data from the M. D. Anderson Cancer Center in Houston, Texas, revealed that 11% of 5,019 patients with SCCs of the upper respiratory and digestive tracts developed distant metastases. A majority of these patients had advanced tumors.

In summary, the risk for distant metastasis increases significantly with advanced lesions. Because it appears that the disease remains localized above the clavicles for a period of time and thus remains accessible to the surgeon or radiation oncologist, early diagnosis and treatment are of utmost importance in preventing the spread of tumor.[2,3]

METASTASIS TO THE MOUTH

The oral cavity is infrequently the site of spread from other primary tumors. When this occurs, it is chiefly from breast cancers, and the mandible is the most common metastatic site. Oral signs and symptoms from a metastatic lesion indicate a grave prognosis, and, at times, but rarely, they may precede recognition of distant primary sites. Metastatic lesions to the oral cavity can mimic benign tumors and infections. Therefore, even though metastatic neoplasias occur infrequently, they should be considered in the differential diagnosis of unusual and unexplainable oral lesions (Figures 5–5 to 5–7).

SURVIVAL

The survival rates for oral cancer depend on several factors: the stage of the disease (size of the primary lesion, local extension, lymph node involvement, distant metastasis), the site of the primary tumor (in general, the more posterior the site, the more negative the prognosis), the adequacy of initial treatment, the Karnofsky performance status (a patient's functional status), and the histologic differentiation of the malignancy.[4–6] The patient's general health, habits (especially tobacco and alcohol use), and predisposition toward multiple oral malignancies are important secondary factors.

Survival rates are reported in the following manner: the observed rate, which is based on the proportion of patients alive in a period of time after diagnosis, and the relative rate, which adjusts the cancer survival rates, taking into account deaths expected from other causes.

STAGING AND CLASSIFICATION

Staging of tumors (Tables 5–2 and 5–3) depends on the size of the primary tumor and extent of spread. Staging is important because treatment modalities, prognosis, and accurate reporting of end results depend on a uniform description of the malignancy and mucosal sites.

SCCs may also be graded according to Broders' classification:

GX: Grade cannot be assessed
G1: Well differentiated
G2: Moderately well differentiated
G3: Poorly differentiated
G4: Undifferentiated

However, the criteria for this cytologic assessment, as well as therapeutic and prognostic significance, are uncertain.

END RESULTS

The staging of an untreated tumor is usually directly related to the length of time it has been present.

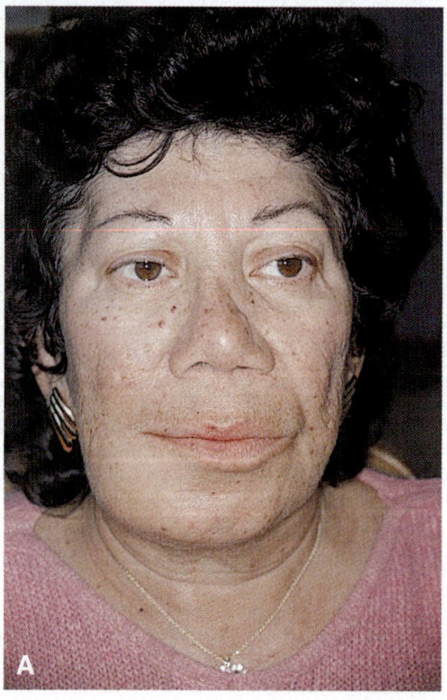

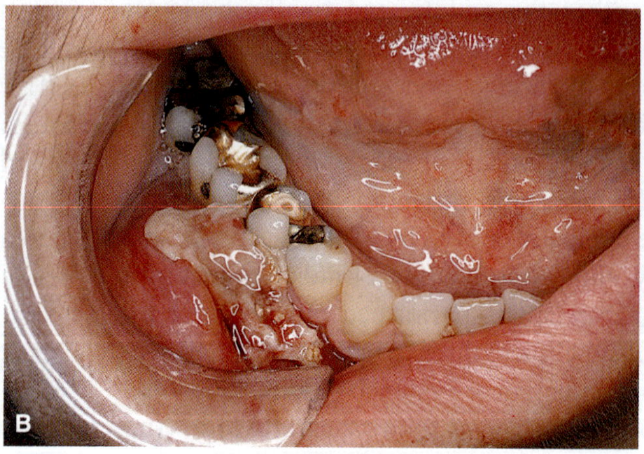

Figure 5–5. *A*, The patient had a lung cancer treated by surgery and radiation. Four years later, the patient had a painful jaw swelling. *B*, Intraoral examination revealed an ulcerated, firm mass in the bicuspid area. A biopsy showed metastatic tumor from the lung.

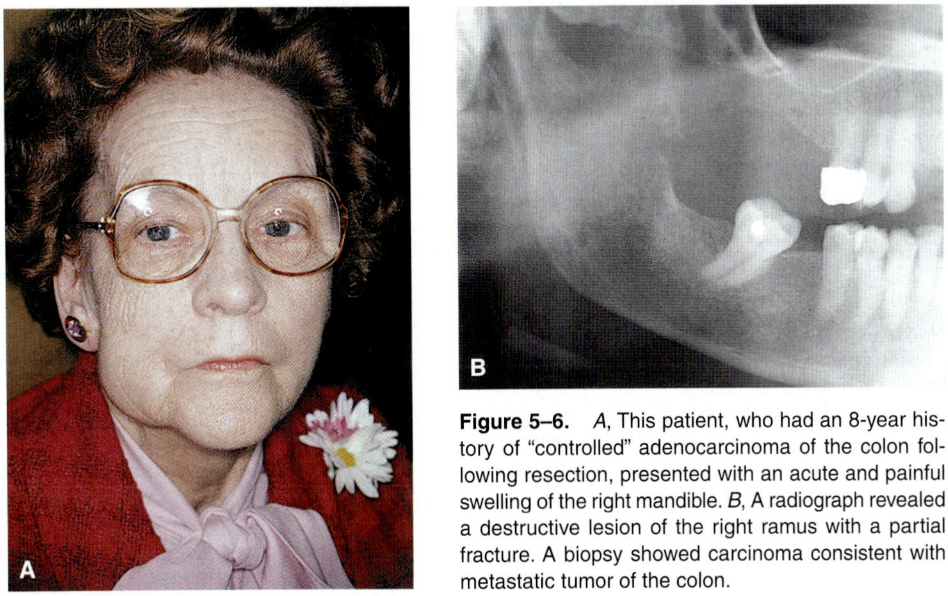

Figure 5–6. *A*, This patient, who had an 8-year history of "controlled" adenocarcinoma of the colon following resection, presented with an acute and painful swelling of the right mandible. *B*, A radiograph revealed a destructive lesion of the right ramus with a partial fracture. A biopsy showed carcinoma consistent with metastatic tumor of the colon.

Therefore, both early detection and adequate treatment are extremely important to improve the chances for survival by diagnosing and treating cancers at earlier (more localized) stages.

Detection of cancer at an early stage is absolutely critical to reduce mortality. By means of survival data obtained from more than 24,000 oral cancer patients entered in nine cancer registries, the National Cancer Institute's (NCI) SEER (Surveillance, Epidemiology, and End Results) Program showed the minimally improved survival for the leading sites of oral cancer over two time periods, comparing 1973 to 1984 with 1985 to 1996 for white and black men and women (Table 5–4; see also Table 1–7). Table 5–5 compares relative 5-year survival rates for localized (stages I and II) lesions with advanced (stages III and IV) lesions for white and black Americans for the period 1992 to 1997 (see Table 1–4 for all races).

Other reports from large treatment centers confirm similar survival rates when localized lesions (stages I and II) are compared with those that show metastases or are very extensive (stages III and IV). Because most patients at the time of diagnosis have

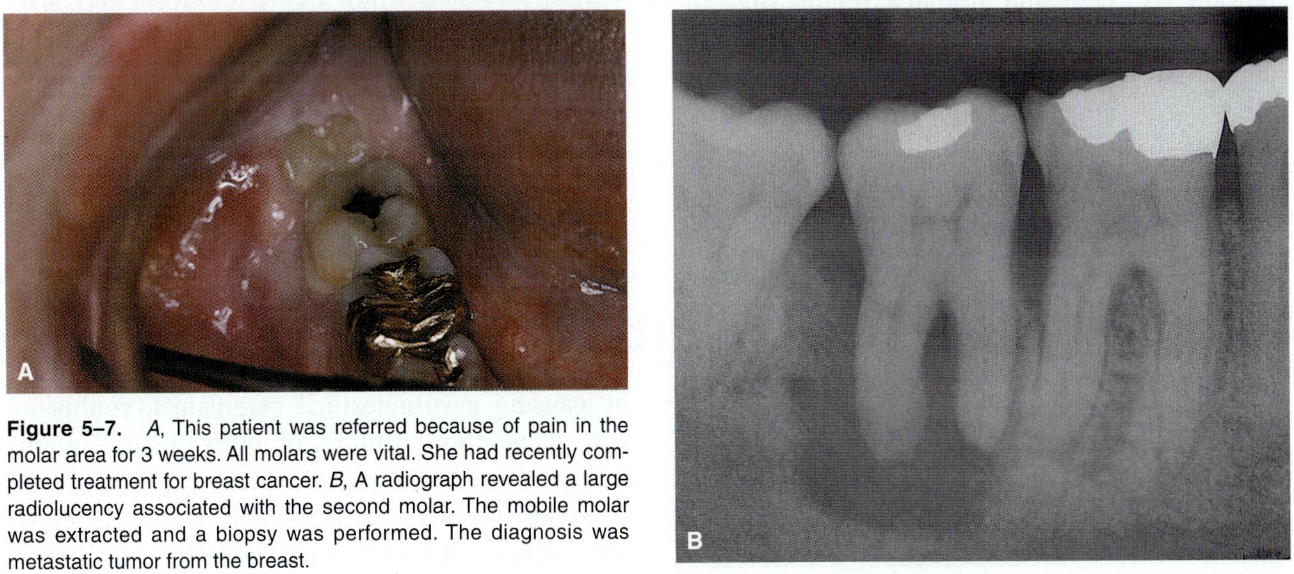

Figure 5–7. *A*, This patient was referred because of pain in the molar area for 3 weeks. All molars were vital. She had recently completed treatment for breast cancer. *B*, A radiograph revealed a large radiolucency associated with the second molar. The mobile molar was extracted and a biopsy was performed. The diagnosis was metastatic tumor from the breast.

Table 5–2. TUMOR NODE METASTASIS STAGING SYSTEM FOR ORAL CARCINOMA

Primary Tumor (T)	
TX	= Primary tumor cannot be assessed
T0	= No evidence of primary tumor
Tis	= Carcinoma in situ
T1	= Tumor 2 cm or less in greatest dimension
T2	= Tumor more than 2 cm but not more than 4 cm in greatest dimension
T3	= Tumor more than 4 cm in greatest dimension
	(Lip) Tumor invades adjacent structures (eg, through cortical bone, into deep [extrinsic] muscle of tongue, maxillary sinus, skin)
T4	= (Oral cavity) Tumor invades adjacent structures (eg, through cortical bone, into deep [extrinsic] muscle of tongue, maxillary sinus, skin)
Regional Lymph Nodes (N)	
NX	= Regional lymph nodes cannot be assessed
N0	= No regional lymph node metastasis
N1	= Metastasis in a single ipsilateral lymph node, 3 cm or less in greatest dimension
N2	= Metastasis in a single ipsilateral lymph node, more than 3 cm but not more than 6 cm in greatest dimension; in multiple ipsilateral lymph nodes, none more than 6 cm in greatest dimension; in bilateral or contralateral lymph nodes, none more than 6 cm in greatest dimension
N2a	= Metastasis in single ipsilateral lymph node more than 3 cm but not more than 6 cm in greatest dimension
N2b	= Metastasis in multiple ipsilateral lymph nodes, none more than 6 cm in greatest dimension
N2c	= Metastasis in bilateral or contralateral lymph nodes, none more than 6 cm in greatest dimension
N3	= Metastasis in a lymph node more than 6 cm in greatest dimension
Distant Metastasis (M)	
MX	= Presence of distant metastasis cannot be assessed
M0	= No distant metastasis
M1	= Distant metastasis

late-stage disease, the overall poor 5-year survival rate of approximately 56% is unfortunately expected (see Table 5–5). The much worse survival rate in blacks again reflects the larger number of advanced lesions at the time of diagnosis. Therefore, delay in diagnosis appears to represent the most valid explanation for the dismal therapeutic results. This delay underscores the necessity for more effective public and professional education regarding signs, symptoms, and early diagnosis. In addition to stage and primary tumor site, the patient's functional status (Karnofsky performance status) may significantly influence prognosis.[6]

Table 5–3. TUMOR NODE METASTASIS (TNM) CLINICAL STAGE GROUPING

Stage	Tumor Size	Nodal Involvement	Distant Metastasis
Stage 0	Tis	N0	M0
Stage I	T1	N0	M0
Stage II	T2	N0	M0
Stage III	T1	N1	M0
	T2	N1	M0
	T3	N0, N1	M0
Stage IV	T4	N1	M0
	Any T	N2, N3	M0
	Any T	Any N	M1

CAUSE OF DEATH

The most common cause of death resulting from uncontrolled tumor is infection (septicemia or pneumonia). Infection results from two main sources: direct invasion by microorganisms entering through tumor-induced ulcerations and "lowered resistance" owing to anorexia or loss of masticatory function with resultant inability to consume adequate nutrients, causing anemia and weight loss (cachexia). These problems may arise as a result of treatment or mental depression and despair. Some patients die of hemorrhage evoked by tumor-induced erosion of blood vessels. In a study of cause of death in 94 patients with head and neck cancer at the M. D. Anderson Cancer Center, 46% died from infection and 13% from hemorrhage.

Hypercalcemia is unusual in head and neck carcinomas but can occur in advanced cases.[7,8] It indicates a poor prognosis and complicates management by causing gastrointestinal complaints, confusion, and dehydration. Failure of other organ systems from metastases is an infrequent cause of death, although distant spread probably occurs in about 10% of head and neck cancer patients.[2]

Table 5–4. 5-YEAR RELATIVE SURVIVAL RATES FOR THE THREE LEADING ORAL CANCER SITES, UNITED STATES, 1973–1996, COMPARING STUDY INTERVALS BY SEX AND RACE

		5-Year Survival Rate (%)*			
		Men		Women	
Site	Interval	White	Black	White	Black
Tongue	1973–1984	41	25	48	40
	1985–1996	47	27	58	32
Lip	1973–1984	94	–	87	–
	1985–1996	95	–	95	–
Floor of the mouth	1973–1984	52	38	64	41
	1985–1996	52	33	63	59

Adapted from the National Cancer Institute.
*With an adjustment to expected longevity.
Dashes indicate that numbers were too low to enable calculation of a 5-year survival rate.

Patients with head and neck cancer are at high risk of second primary tumors.[9] The excess mortality associated with these second tumors significantly influences survival (see Chapter 1, "Epidemiology"). For example, one study reported in *Lancet* found that 27% of 377 patients treated for floor of the mouth carcinoma developed second malignancies; two-thirds of these second cancers were in the respiratory and upper digestive tracts, whereas the others were in the mouth. These tumors were reported to have developed at a constant rate of 3.6% per year and led to an excess mortality of 5.2% per year.[9]

CHEMOPREVENTION

For patients with stage I or II oral and pharyngeal carcinomas, there is a 2 to 5% per-year risk of developing a second, new, primary aerodigestive tract tumor. New strategies are now focusing on preventing these new primary cancers from becoming established.

The term chemoprevention was first used by Sporn to indicate the pharmacologic inhibition of carcinogenesis or its reversal in the premalignant stage. It is believed that epithelial carcinogenesis evolves through three stages: induction, promotion, and progression, as has been noted in animal models. Through both epidemiologic and animal studies, natural and synthetic substances have been found that can interfere with the epithelial carcinogenic process during either the promotion or the progression phase.

Most of the research conducted in the prevention of upper aerodigestive tract tumors has focused on the use of retinoids or carotenoids.[10,11] The term retinoid refers to vitamin A–derived substances, either natural or synthetic, that are involved in normal epithelial growth and differentiation. Data from epidemiologic, in vitro, and animal studies support the role of retinoids in the prevention of epithelial carcinogenesis. The initial studies using either vitamin A or vitamin A analogues were conducted in patients with leukoplakia (see Chapter 3, "Leukoplakia and Erythroplasia").

In the 1980s, Hong and colleagues[12] conducted the first double-blind, randomized trial comparing 13-*cis* retinoic acid (13-CRA) at 1 to 2 mg/kg/day versus a placebo in patients with leukoplakia. The clinical response rate in this trial was 67%, com-

Table 5–5. ORAL AND PHARYNGEAL CANCER, UNITED STATES, 1992–1997: STAGE AT DIAGNOSIS AND RELATIVE 5-YEAR SURVIVAL RATES BY RACE

	Incidence by Race (%)	
Variable	White	Black
Stage at diagnosis		
Localized (stages I and II)	38	18
5-year survival rate by stage		
Localized	82	72
Regional metastasis	45	29
Distant metastasis	21	18
All cases	58	34

Adapted from the National Cancer Institute.

pared with 10% in the placebo group ($p = .002$), but, more importantly, histologic assessment showed a reversal of dysplasia in 54% of the retinoid group versus 10% of the placebo group ($p = .01$). Nevertheless, toxicity, particularly mucocutaneous, and triglyceride elevation were significant. Also, there was a 50% relapse rate within 3 to 4 months after the end of retinoid therapy.

In a follow-up study, patients initially receiving 13-CRA at 1.5 mg/kg/day for 3 months were then randomized to either low-dose 13-CRA at 0.5 mg/kg/day or beta carotene at 30 mg per day for a 9-month period. Response rates from the induction phase were similar to those of the previous study, but there were significant differences in the randomized arms: 8% of patients on low-dose 13-CRA had progressive disease versus 52% in the beta carotene arm ($p = .001$).

The results using beta carotene alone for oral leukoplakia have been conflicting. Although its lack of toxicity makes beta carotene an attractive chemopreventive agent, results have been disappointing as to its effectiveness. The encouraging results obtained using 13-CRA for premalignant lesions led to its use in the adjuvant setting for patients who had been rendered free of their oral and pharyngeal carcinomas after local therapy. Hong and colleagues, in a double-blind, randomized study, administered 13-CRA at 50 to 100 mg/m^2 daily for 1 year with a 3-year follow-up.[12] They noted a significantly reduced incidence of second primary tumor development in the CRA arm versus the placebo group (4% versus 24%; $p = .005$). Mucocutaneous dryness and hypertriglyceridemia were adverse side effects. A larger, confirmatory randomized trial is now being conducted by the Radiation Therapy Oncology Group (RTOG) for patients with early stage I and II carcinomas to define further the role of the retinoids as chemopreventive agents. In this trial, a less toxic dose of 13-CRA (30 mg/day for 3 years) is compared with placebo in a double-blind fashion.

Based on prior data suggesting limited efficacy for 13-CRA in moderate or severe dysplasia of the oral cavity, a phase II pilot study combining 13-CRA with α-tocopherol (vitamin E) and interferon-α was conducted in patients with moderate to severe dysplasia of the oral cavity and larynx. Of 36 patients entered in this study, evaluation was noted for clinical and histologic response in 30 patients at 6 months and 21 patients at 12 months of therapy. There was clearly a difference in favor of the laryngeal lesions, with 9 of 19 patients (47%) demonstrating complete histologic reversal of dysplasia versus only 1 of 11 patients (9%) with a histologic complete response in the oral cavity ($p = .05$). The most commonly seen side effects were mucocutaneous (ie, dry skin, cheilitis), but arthralgias, myalgias, and fatigue were commonly seen, and 36% of the patients had grade III reactions. The authors concluded that the combination of 13-CRA, α-tocopherol, and interferon-α is active for laryngeal dysplasia, and confirmatory trials are in progress.

The future of chemoprevention for upper digestive tract lesions seems to parallel that for invasive cancers in that new targets that are up-regulated in squamous cell dysplasia need to be identified and exploited. To that end, two new markers, cyclooxygenase 2 (COX-2) and epidermal growth factor receptor (EGFR) and its accompanying tyrosine kinase, have been recently noted to play a role in squamous cell carcinogenesis and are up-regulated in dysplastic tissue.[13,14] These new targets were recently the focus of an ongoing trial using COX-2 inhibitors and inhibitors for EGFR (C225, Iressa, OSI774). More importantly, new targets will have to be elucidated by molecular probing, the reversal of which may be more important than histologic reversal of dysplasia.

MODERN MOLECULAR ANALYSIS OF ORAL CANCER

Like all cancers, oral cancer represents an accumulation of molecular lesions in genes that encode for proteins that control cell cycle, cell survival, cell motility, and angiogenesis. These complex changes give the tumor cells an independent growth advantage, leading to the ability to invade and metastasize to distant sites.[15]

These alterations in the genotype and phenotype of cancer cells have lent themselves to analysis using molecular methods. These tools are directed at studying changes in the genome, genetic expression and protein alterations that are common in both neoplastic and preneoplastic states. This section reviews methods that are used to analyze tumor deoxyribonucleic acid (DNA), ribonucleic acid (RNA), and protein and show how these alterations, once characterized, can be used to profile oral cancer and precancer and their potential for screening, prediction of progression, and prognostic studies.

That cancer is a genetic disease underpins the fundamental need to analyze DNA in tumor specimens. Oral cancer is characterized by complex karyotypes as the result of gene amplifications, reduplications, translocations, and deletions.[16] Many methods have been developed to study DNA in tumor cells, including chromosome karyotyping, Southern blot hybridization, in situ hybridization methods, flow cytometry, and polymerase chain reaction (PCR)-based analyses. Each has specific applications and limitations and also depends on the source tissues for analysis. The least sensitive assays involve karyotyping, in which metaphase analysis can identify gross chromosomal alterations. By contrast, PCR is an extremely sensitive method that can detect single nucleotide alterations in a variety of tissues from differing sources.

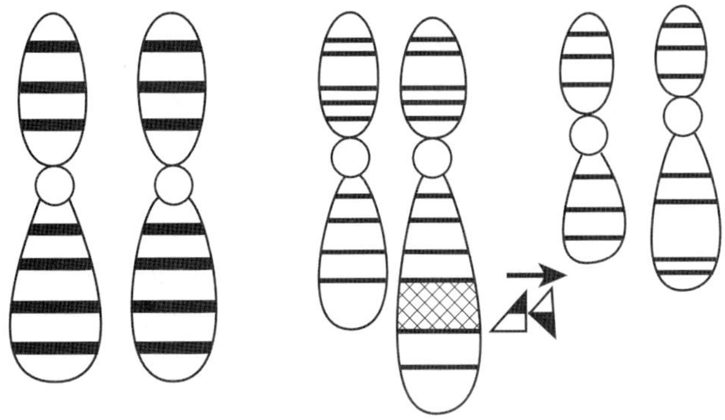

Figure 5–8. Metaphase analysis of chromosomes from tumor cells involves growing the cells in culture and then arresting them in metaphase. The chromosomes are stained using the Giemsa method, which permits detection of chromosome loss, gain, or translocation from one chromosome (*solid arrow*) to another (*open arrow*).

Cytogenetic Studies

Cytogenetic studies involve the analysis of chromosomal abnormalities in tumor cells. The most common approach is chromosomal karyotyping using tumors or cell lines that are grown in culture and arrested in metaphase. The cells are then spread on a microscope slide, treated with a Giemsa stain, and then analyzed microscopically to identify areas of chromosomal gain, loss, or translocation (Figure 5–8). Using this method, most oral SCCs show a complex karyotype with frequent regions of chromosome gain and loss. Consistent and reproducible cytogenetic abnormalities have been identified, including loss of chromosomes 3p, 5q, 8p, 9p, 18q, and 21q. Loss of a region on chromosome 18q has been associated with poor outcome in many head and neck SCCs. Breakpoints associated with chromosomes 1p22, 3p21, 8p11, and 14q have been associated with more radiation-sensitive oral SCCs.[16]

Although metaphase analysis of tumors is useful to detect regions of gross chromosome loss, gain, or translocation, the method is relatively crude owing to the low resolution of analysis. A refinement of this analysis is the use of fluorescence-labeled probes to detect chromosomal alterations in both metaphase and interphase cells. A DNA probe, labeled with a fluorochrome, specific for a chromosome segment or a whole chromosome, is used. Fluorescence in situ hybridization (FISH) can be used to order genes and DNA segments on chromosomes to a resolution of 2 to 3 Mb. Based on the amount of fluorescence, FISH can be used to identify regions of gene amplification or loss. Although better than metaphase spreads, the resolution is still not high. An important advantage of FISH is its application to cells in interphase; thus, it can be applied to fixed tissues in which the cells cannot be cultured in vitro. FISH has proven useful for determining gene amplification by multiple gene copies and numerical changes in chromosomes. Here FISH is usually combined with confocal microscopy, a computer-assisted imaging method to examine thin serial sections of whole cells in interphase. Chromosome deletions, translocations, and breakpoints can also be detected using FISH. In head and neck SCCs, precancer amplification of the *cyclin D1* gene and loss of component exons of the *p16* gene have all been reported using FISH.

When the cytogenetic abnormality is unknown, a suitable probe for FISH cannot be selected. Comparative genomic hybridization (CGH) permits the development of a detailed map of chromosomal differences between normal and tumor cells by detecting increases (amplifications) or decreases (deletions) of segments of DNA (Figure 5–9). The technique involves labeling tumor DNA with biotin, which is detected with fluorescein, and labeling normal DNA with digoxigenin, which is detected with rhodamine. DNA samples from both normal and tumor cells are then hybridized together onto a metaphase spread of unlabeled normal chromosomes. Regions of gain or loss of DNA such as deletions, duplications, or amplifications are seen as changes in the relative ratios of red and green. Thus, areas of amplification are represented by green and areas of loss by red. Subtle changes in color may not be discernible by the naked eye, thus requiring sophisticated image analysis software for quantification of these gene regions.[17]

A major disadvantage of CGH is its relative insensitivity because only chromosomal changes larger than 5 Mb can be detected. However, the technique is useful for identifying relatively small chromosome translocations that cannot be detected by traditional Giemsa staining of metaphase spreads (karyotyping) and for identifying novel gene amplification or loss in tumors. Balanced rearrangements such as inversions and translocations cannot be detected by CGH. Regions of chromosomal alterations in oral SCCs using CGH have included chromosomes 3p, 5p, 11q13, and 19q in addition to other regions of gain and loss identified by traditional metaphase karyotyping.

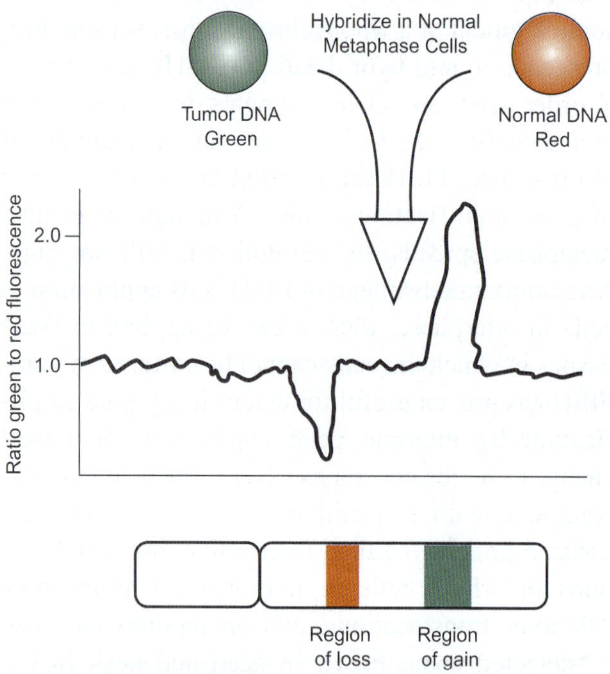

Figure 5–9. Comparative genomic hybridization is an in situ method that can be used to detect regions of gene loss or gain. Tumor deoxyribonucleic acid (DNA) is labeled to produce green fluorescence and normal DNA is labeled to produce red fluorescence. Both tumor and normal DNA are then hybridized onto normal metaphase chromosomal spreads. Amplified regions of DNA are detected when the ratio of green to red fluorescence is greater than 1, resulting in green fluorescence. Regions of chromosomal loss are detected when the green-to-red ratio is less than 1, resulting in red fluorescence.

Both traditional metaphase analysis and FISH have consistently shown cytogenetic alterations at the 11q13 locus in many head and neck SCCs. This locus contains the *cyclin D1, BCL-1, fibroblast growth factor*s *3* and *4 (FGF3, FGF4), (INT2)*, and *EMS1* genes. Amplification of the *cyclin D1* gene has been found in head and neck SCCs with a frequency ranging from 17 to 55%.[18] In some tumors, this change has been associated with a decreased survival rate, increased recurrence rate, and more frequent metachronous tumors. *Cyclin D1* gene amplification has been correlated with greater local tumor invasion, lymph node metastases, and high stage at presentation.

Oral precancerous lesions have also been studied using FISH to determine amplification levels of the *cyclin D1* gene. Here amplification is a frequent event in both low-grade and high-grade oral epithelial dysplasias, suggesting that *cyclin D1* gene amplification is an early event in oral carcinogenesis.

Polymerase Chain Reaction

PCR has proven to be an important tool in the detection of chromosome gain or loss in many human cancers. PCR typically begins with the isolation of DNA (genomic DNA) from a fresh tissue specimen or from tissue in a paraffin block. If RNA is the object of analysis, it must first be converted to complementary DNA (cDNA) through reverse transcription. Heating DNA separates the complementary double strands into single-stranded forms intended to act as a template dictating the nucleotide sequence in vitro. Two short oligonucleotide primers are designed to anneal (bind) to the template and flank a region of interest. A thermostable DNA polymerase, isolated from *Thermophilus aquaticus*, known as Taq polymerase, catalyzes the sequential addition of the four nucleotides (deoxynucleotide triphosphates [dNTPs]) to the primers. Cooling the solution permits the primers to bind to the template DNA, and then the Taq polymerase catalyzes the addition of dNTPs to the template between the primers. Salts and buffers permit the Taq polymerase to catalyze the reaction. This process is then repeated, and with each cycle, there is an exponential increase in the quantity of DNA such that after n cycles the amount increases by 2^n. A typical PCR application involves 30 to 40 cycles; therefore, after 35 cycles, 3.44×10^{10} (2^{35}) copies of the template DNA have been made.[17]

Further refinement for the detection of gene loss has been made using the PCR amplification of highly polymorphic microsatellite markers. These di- and trinucleotide repeat sequences (ie, CGCGCGCG) litter the genome, and by comparison of neoplastic cells to normal cells from the same individual, regions of gene loss suggesting the presence of putative tumor suppressor genes can be identified. The underlying principle of this method, termed allelic imbalance analysis, is that all tumor suppressor genes to become inactive require the loss of one copy on one chromosome and mutation of the other copy on the other chromosome. This method has been used to show frequent deletion of a region on chromosome 17p in oral precancers and cancers. This region corresponds with loss of one allele of the *p53* gene (see below). A region on chromosome 9p21–22 is also frequently lost in many oral precancers and SCCs and contains the *p16* tumor suppressor gene. Other regions frequently lost or altered in oral precancers and SCCs include chromosomes 3p, 4q, 11q, and 13q. Recently, it has been shown that the patterns and frequency of allelic imbalance are statistically associated with a higher risk of transformation of oral precancer to SCC.[19]

DNA Sequencing Methods

Smaller genetic alterations common in oral SCC and precancer include single nucleotide substitutions, deletions, and insertions. Because a mutational event is required for inactivation of most tumor suppressor genes, the goal of many tumor studies is the determination of its DNA sequence. Sequencing methods have been employed for several decades, but improvements in technology have reduced testing time to several hours and permitted characterization of genes composed of up to hundreds or thousands of nucleotides. Today most manual and automated sequencing methods are based on the generation of complementary single-stranded DNA using DNA polymerase. Here four mixtures are prepared, each containing DNA polymerase and all the dNTPs (deoxyadenosine triphosphate [dATP], deoxycytidine triphosphate [dCTP], deoxythymidine triphosphate [dTTP], and deoxyguanosine triphosphate [dGTP]). One of the nucleotide precursors is labeled with a radioactive or fluorescent marker in each mixture. In addition, each of the four reaction mixtures contains a limiting amount of one dideoxynucleotide (dideoxyadenosine triphosphate [ddATP], dideoxycytidine triphosphate [ddCTP], dideoxythymidine triphosphate [ddTTP], or dideoxyguanosine triphosphate [ddGTP]), which, when incorporated into the DNA, causes premature chain termination. Therefore, in the reaction tube containing the ddGTP, nucleotides will be added to the complementary strand until a ddGTP is added. When this occurs, chain elongation ceases as ddGTP (or ddCTP, ddATP, or ddTTP, depending on the reaction tube) lacks the 3′-hydroxyl group required for subsequent nucleotide addition. Thus, the reaction tube mixture containing the ddGTP will generate multiple strands of DNA of various lengths, all terminating at positions where ddGTP has been incorporated. Similarly, the other three tubes will all contain DNA fragments of various lengths, terminating at positions where the respective dideoxynucleotide has been added. The contents of each of the four tubes are individually separated via gel electrophoresis, with each band produced corresponding to the size of the terminated DNA fragments. Because smaller fragments travel faster in the gel, those fragments that were terminated early by addition of the dideoxynucleotide will migrate farthest in the gel.[17]

In the past, DNA sequencing was performed using laborious and time-consuming manual techniques. Today this process is often automated by using fluorescence-labeled nucleotides read by a laser during passage through an electrophoresis seqencing gel. The fastest methods available involve sequencing analysis by capillary electrophoresis whereby parallel tiny fiber-optic glass tubes contain a special polyacrylamide sieving medium for separation of fluorescence-labeled DNA fragments generated by the sequencing reaction.

DNA sequencing methods have been used to characterize mutational events in both oral precancer and cancer. The *p53* tumor suppressor gene plays a critical role in the normal regulation of cellular growth and proliferation. The gene encodes a nuclear phosphoprotein that acts as a sequence-specific transcription factor and is involved in cell-cycle regulation and cellular responses to DNA damage. The *p53* tumor suppressor gene encodes an oligomeric nuclear phosphoprotein that is important in regulating cell proliferation. There is now a well-established link between cell-cycle arrest at G1/S following exposure to ionizing radiation and *p53* induction. Mutations in the *p53* gene are the most commonly reported genetic abnormality in human cancers, including carcinomas arising in the oral cavity, with reported prevalence from 30 to 60%. In addition, *p53* alterations are frequently identified in precancerous lesions, with the reported prevalence varying from 10 to 50%.[20] The timing of this change in the development of oral cancer has yet to be clearly established within this setting, with some reporting *p53* alterations as an early event in the development of oral cancer and others suggesting that it is a late finding.

Gene Expression (Messenger RNA) Analysis

Alterations at the gene level are often reflected in abnormalities in messenger RNA (mRNA) expression, either up or down. In oral SCCs and precancers, changes in the relative expression of specific mRNA species are common and can be used to profile specific cell populations. Traditional methods to study RNA include Northern hybridization, ribonuclease protection assay, and nuclear run-on methods. These methods are typically suitable for the laboratory research setting where abundant, high-quality RNA is available for analysis or where cells are grown in culture and dynamic changes in the amount of RNA can be measured. Another important method to determine the amount of RNA in cells is based on PCR. So-called quantitative PCR is based on the continuous monitoring of the amount of product at the end of each cycle. One of the most popular ways to do this is based on the 5′s to 3′-endonuclease activity of Taq DNA polymerase to detect target sequences during PCR. Included in the PCR mixture is a short oligonucleotide probe designed to hybridize within the target sequence but not to be extended in the 3′ direction. When the probe is hybridized to the target, no signal is produced owing to the presence of a quencher molecule that suppresses the fluorescence of a reporter molecule on the probe. During PCR, the probe hybridizes to the target DNA, and Taq polymerase cleaves the probe into shorter fragments, thereby releasing the quencher from the reporter molecule. The amount of fluorescence generated is therefore directly proportional to the amount of PCR product generated. By measuring the amount of PCR product produced at the end of each single cycle, PCR growth curves can be plotted and measurements taken from the exponentially expanding region of the reaction.[21]

Another important advance in the quantitative study of mRNA expression has been the development of microarray technology, commonly referred to as "gene chips." Using microarrays, the expression levels of hundreds to thousands of genes can be determined at the same time, providing a unique profile of increased or decreased gene expression in tissues.

DNA microarray technology relies on the hybridization of a "probe" to multiple defined genomic DNAs, cDNAs, expressed sequence tags, or oligonucleotides that have been "printed" onto specific locations of a solid phase or "chip." The probe is usually cDNA fragments produced by reverse transcription of tumor mRNA and then labeled with a fluorescent marker. The probe and the spotted cDNAs are hybridized, resulting in varying red/green and yellow fluorescent emissions. These emissions are then scanned by a reader consisting of argon lasers and a scanning fluorescence confocal microscope. The use of computer image analysis permits quantification of the intensity of thousands of different genes on the array, which can then be compared to the expression in normal tissues.

Because this is evolving technology, the scope of applications has yet to be defined. Some of the types of studies that have used microarray technology include gene expression studies in tumors versus normal tissues, genotyping of mutations in tumors, functional analyses of genes expressed in yeast, and gene mapping to identify loci of disease susceptibility genes. Molecular expression profiles have been examined in forms of lymphoma and melanoma, with findings suggesting alternative taxonomy based on molecular differences in the expression of novel genes. In oral SCCs, microarray studies have identified complex patterns of gene expression consisting of increases and decreases in the expression of specific markers. Recently, gene profiling has been used to distinguish tumors with a poor prognosis from those associated with a more favorable outcome. Therefore, this suggests that, in the future, microarray analysis may become part of the diagnostic workup of patients with oral cancer and precancer.

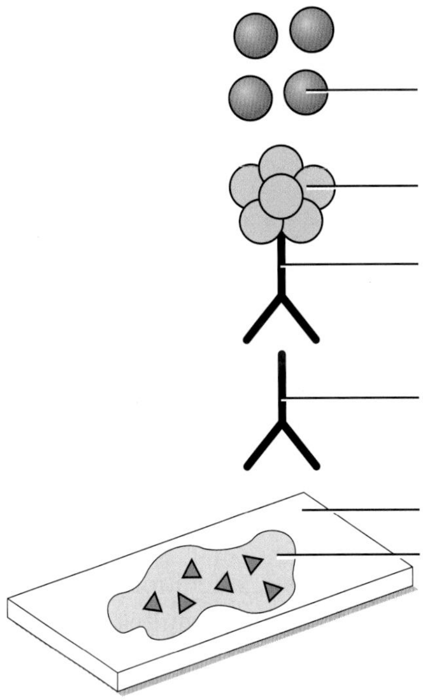

Figure 5–10. Immunohistochemistry involves the localization of a target antigen in tissue sections using conjugated antibodies. In this example, a primary antibody is used to localize the target antigen, which is then detected using a secondary antibody-enzyme conjugate. The enzyme is used to catalyze the precipitation of a chromogen, producing a color where the primary antibody is located. Differing numbers of antibodies can be used to increase or decrease the sensitivity of the assay.

Immunohistochemistry

The ultimate effector molecule of a cell is a protein. Thus, genetic alterations and changes in the expression of different RNA species in normal, premalignant, and malignant oral epithelial cells are ultimately reflected in changes in protein expression. There are many ways to analyze proteins in cells, including Southern blotting, two-dimensional gel electrophoresis, and flow cytometry. These are all suitable for laboratory study in which the cells of interest can be grown and manipulated prior to analysis. For the analysis of oral precancer and cancer, the most important method for the study of proteins in vivo has been using immunohistochemistry (Figure 5–10).[22] This method involves using a polyclonal or monoclonal antibody to a specified epitope (protein of interest) and applying it to a tissue section. The bound antigen-antibody complex can then be visualized using a series of labeled secondary antibodies and enzyme-activated chromogens. Immunohistochemistry has proven invaluable in the quantification and localization of overexpressed proteins in oral precancer and cancer. For example, this method can be used to detect p53 protein in tissue sections. Mutant p53 protein has a relatively long half-life, unlike the wild type, and thus can be more readily detected by immunohistochemistry (Figure 5–11). Other mechanisms of stabilization of the p53 protein are recognized, for example, by binding to viral proteins or cellular proteins.

The accumulation of altered p53 protein appears to be a common step in the development of many human cancers and has been reported frequently in cancers of the breast, colon, and lung. In the oral cavity, there is much variability in the reported prevalence of altered p53 protein expression in oral carcinomas, ranging from 20 to 50% of cell lines and tumor tissues.[20] Part of this variability may be attributable to differences in the method of p53 protein detection. It is recognized that with antigen retrieval methods, both wild-type and mutant p53 protein can be detected by immunohistochemistry. Abnormal expression of p53 protein has also been reported in 10 to 50% of oral epithe-

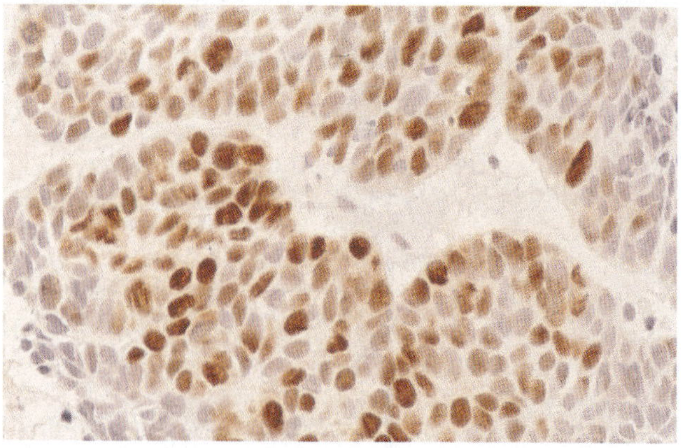

Figure 5–11. Immunohistochemical demonstration of p53 protein expression (brown staining) in nuclei of an oral squamous cell carcinoma (ABC × 400).

lial dysplasias.[20] Furthermore, alterations of p53 are thought to be an early event in multistage carcinogenesis of oral epithelium.

The development of oral precancer and cancer is a complicated process involving changes in the genome and expression of cellular proteins. Modern molecular analysis has identified many alterations in these tissues and paved the way for advances in the detection and treatment of the disease.

REFERENCES

1. de Braud F, Heilbrun LK, Ahmed K, et al. Metastatic squamous cell carcinoma of an unknown primary localized to the neck: advantages of an aggressive treatment. Cancer 1989;64:510.
2. Merino OR, Lindberg RD, Fletcher GH. An analysis of distant metastases from squamous cell carcinoma of the upper respiratory and digestive tracts. Cancer 1977;40:145–51.
3. Silverman S Jr. Demographics and occurrence of oral and pharyngeal cancers. The outcomes, the trends, the challenge. J Am Dent Assoc 2001;1312:7S–11S.
4. Anneroth G, Hansen LS, Silverman S Jr. Malignancy grading in oral squamous carcinoma. I. Squamous cell carcinoma of the tongue and floor of mouth: histologic grading in the clinical evaluation. J Oral Pathol 1986;15:162–8.
5. Moore C, Flynn MB, Greenberg RA. Evaluation of size in prognosis of oral cancer. Cancer 1986;58:158–62.
6. Mor V, Laliberte L, Morriss JN, et al. The Karnofsky Performance Status Scale: an examination of its reliability and validity in a research setting. Cancer 1984;53:2002–7.
7. Brodaus AE, Mangin M, Ikeda K, et al. Humoral hypercalcemia of cancer. Identification of a novel parathyroid hormone-like peptide. N Engl J Med 1988;319:556–63.
8. Won C, Decker DA, Drelichman A, et al. Hypercalcemia in head and neck carcinoma. Incidence and prognosis. Cancer 1983;52:2261–3.
9. Tepperman BS, Fitzpatrick PJ. Second respiratory and upper digestive tract cancers after oral cancer. Lancet 1981;ii: 547–9.
10. Lippman SM, Batsakis JG, Toth BB, et al. Comparison of low-dose isotretinoin with beta carotene to prevent oral carcinogenesis. N Engl J Med 1993;328:15–20.
11. Papadimitrakopoulou VA, Clayman GL, Shin DM, et al. Biochemoprevention for dysplastic lesions of the upper aerodigestive tract. Arch Otolaryngol Head Neck Surg 1999;125:1083–9.
12. Hong WK, Endicott J, Itri LM, et al. 13-cis-retinoic acid in the treatment of oral leukoplakia. N Engl J Med 1986; 315:1501–5.
13. Mestre JR, Chan G, Zhang F, et al. Inhibition of cyclooxygenase-2 expression. An approach to preventing head and neck cancer. Ann N Y Acad Sci 1999;889:62–71.
14. Srinivasan M, Jewell SD. Evaluation of TGF-alpha and EGFR expression in oral leukoplakia and oral submucous fibrosis by quantitative immunohistochemistry. Oncology 2001;61: 284–92.
15. Califano J, van der Reit P, Westra W, et al. Genetic progression model for head and neck cancer: implications for field cancerization. Cancer Res 1996;56:2488–92.
16. Carey TE, Van Dyke DL, Worsham MJ. Nonrandom chromosome aberrations and clonal populations in head and neck cancer. Anticancer Res 1993;13:2561–7.
17. Jordan RC, Daniels TE, Greenspan JS, Regezi JA. Advanced diagnostic methods in oral and maxillofacial pathology. Part I: molecular methods. Oral Surg Oral Med Oral Pathol Oral Radiol Endod 2001;92:650–69.
18. Rousseau A, Lim MS, Lin Z, Jordan RC. Frequent cyclin D1 gene amplification and protein overexpression in oral epithelial dysplasias. Oral Oncol 2001;37:268–75.
19. Rosin MP, Cheng X, Poh C, et al. Use of allelic loss to predict malignant risk for low-grade oral epithelial dysplasia. Clin Cancer Res 2000;6:357–62.
20. Shahnavaz SA, Regezi JA, Bradley G, et al. P53 gene mutations in sequential oral epithelial dysplasias and squamous cell carcinomas. J Pathol 2000;190:417–22.
21. Ginzinger DG. Gene quantification using real-time quantitative PCR. An emerging technology hits the mainstream. Exp Hematol 2002;30:503–12.
22. Jordan RC, Daniels TE, Greenspan JS, Regezi JA. Advanced diagnostic methods in oral and maxillofacial pathology. Part II: immunohistochemical and immunofluorescent methods. Oral Surg Oral Med Oral Pathol Oral Radiol Endod 2002;93:56–74.

6

Treatment

MARK I. SINGER, MD, FACS (Surgical Management)
JEANNE M. QUIVEY, MD (Radiation Therapy)
THEODORE L. PHILLIPS, MD (Radiation Therapy)
ALAN M. KRAMER, MD (Chemotherapy)
SOL SILVERMAN JR., MA, DDS

Long-term survival and functional results of treatment depend on the stage of the tumor, histology, and treatment plan. The treatment plan is developed at pretreatment conferences (tumor boards) by multidisciplinary consultants and subsequent patient/family concurrence. Additional important outcome factors include the patient's nutritional status, general health, tobacco use, alcohol intake, and anticipated compliance with the rigors of therapy.

Curative treatment modalities include surgery and radiation or a combination. Chemotherapy is used with these modalities to enhance cure rates and to preserve function, which has led increasingly to organ preservation strategies. When survival is in doubt, the use of these approaches, with pain control, is considered for palliation and quality of life.

SURGICAL MANAGEMENT OF MALIGNANCY OF THE ORAL CAVITY

Effective treatment requires the cooperative efforts of surgeons, radiation oncologists, dental practitioners, and rehabilitation specialists. The side effects of treatment are permanent and diminish oral function. Treatment planning is based on careful cancer staging (see Chapter 5, "Spread of Tumor, Staging, and Survival"), which allows for prognostication and facilitates the reporting of outcomes. Physical examination, open biopsy, or fine-needle aspiration biopsy and radiologic imaging studies that include computed tomography (CT), magnetic resonance imaging (MRI), and positron emission tomography (PET) are used to classify and stage the disease.

Most of the major functional disabilities following treatment are related to the volume of the disease, extent of mandible loss, reduction of tongue mobility, loss of dentition, xerostomia, diminished mastication, and anesthesia of the oral cavity. The treatment plan considers an adequate resection of tumor and surrounding normal tissue and the addition of the lymphatic drainage. This requires operative exposure of the disease, control of the vasculature, and identification of the innervation to the tongue, floor of the mouth, and teeth critical to long-term disease control. Metastases to the regional lymphatics occur commonly, about 25% of the time in stage I disease, and they must be encompassed in the treatment field, either with surgery or radiotherapy.

The first levels of lymph nodes that are involved by metastasis are either the submental group or the submandibular group (Figure 6–1). The nodes of the submandibular region cluster anterior or posterior to the facial vein. Additional lymphatics may exit the oral cavity to communicate with the deep jugular system between the digastric muscle and the omohyoid muscle. Metastatic squamous cell carcinoma from the oral cavity is predictable by its metastatic pattern from superior to inferior. Cancer of the lips and anterior floor of the mouth may metastasize early to the submandibular region, whereas more posterior primary lesions will extend deeply to the region of the jugular lymph nodes. As tumor growth

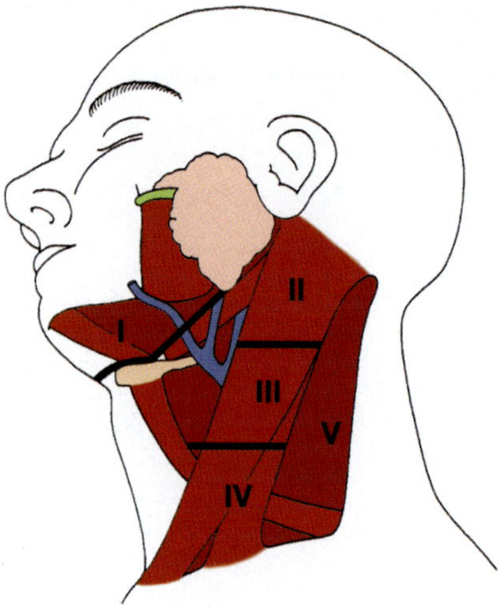

Figure 6–1. Cervical lymph nodes and topical level classification.

continues, middle and lower lymph node groups will become affected (Figure 6–2).

PHYSIOLOGIC CONSIDERATIONS AND TREATMENT PLANNING

The oral cavity should be viewed as a complex structure made up of muscles, surrounded by the jaws, driven by the tongue, lubricated by the salivary glands, defined by the teeth, and containing exquisite sensory innervation. The mouth is central to the intake of nutrition and depends on the effective coordination of mastication, bolus transport, and management of liquids. In addition, the human quality of vocalization, articulated as speech, depends on the structures of the oral cavity. The alteration of these structures by disease and treatment affects the patient's quality of life, functioning, and ability to interact socially. Surgical defects from the treatment of cancer are well described, and techniques have been developed for rehabilitation (see Chapter 8, "Restoration of Palate, Tongue, Mandible, and Facial Defects").

TREATMENT SPECTRUM

Surgical resection and radiation therapy are the main methods for treatment. The selection of one or the other or a combination of both is determined by the tumor's location, size, and proximity to the jaws; the patient's clinical status; and the experience of the treatment team. Staging is critical (see Chapter 5). Stage I cancer usually responds equally well to either, but morbidity may be greater with one or the other when considering the complications owing to the proximity to bone, teeth, and other intraoral structures (see Chapter 7, "Complications of Treatment"). The more advanced stages usually require a combination of modalities, sometimes including chemotherapy (see the end of this chapter).

In addition to the treatment of the primary tumor, the cervical lymphatics commonly require treatment. The clinically negative neck (no evidence of lymph node involvement) may be treated electively by radiation or modified neck dissection. Undetected or occult

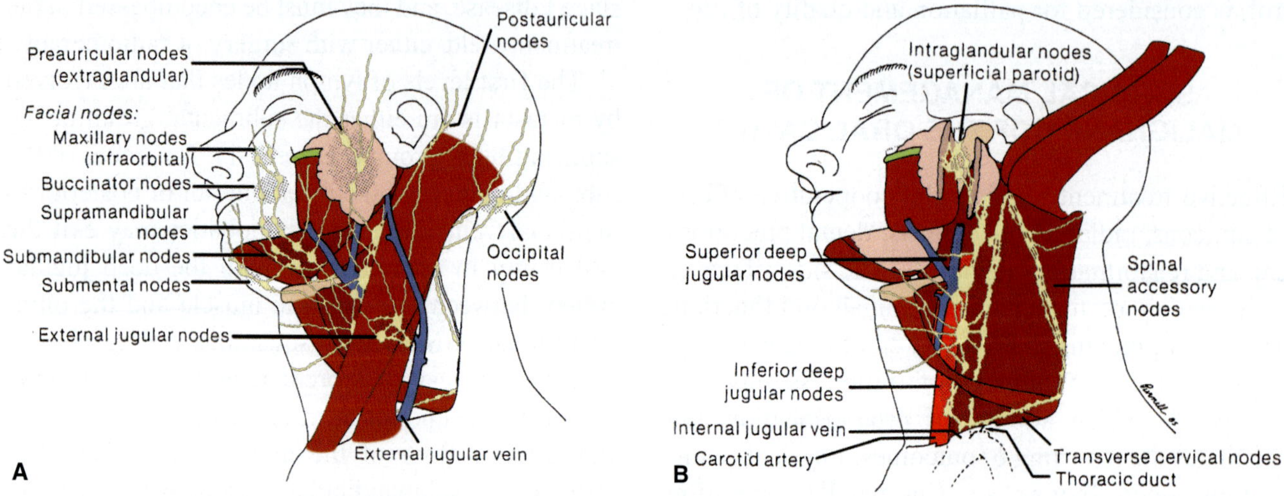

Figure 6–2. Cervical nodal drainage patterns. *A*, Superficial cervical and facial nodes. *B*, Deep cervical drainage patterns. Note that the sternocleidomastoid muscle is reflected.

metastatic disease occurs in 20 to 50% of cases. When the statistical risk of cervical metastasis exceeds 20%, management of the neck is indicated. Of course, experience is coupled with staging and grading of the tumor. Prophylactic irradiation of the clinically negative neck is as effective as modified neck dissection.

SURGICAL CONSIDERATIONS

Local surgical excision may be used for malignancies that extend to 2 cm and can be removed by the transoral approach (Figure 6–3). Greater extension posteriorly or deeply requires a transcervical approach. When the mandible is involved, radiocurability is unlikely, and resection of the primary tumor with proximal mandible and neck dissection is required (Figures 6–4 and 6–5). Radiologic imaging studies for early mandibular involvement are not very sensitive. Encroachment on the mandible requires a bone margin without segmental sacrifice, whereas when a margin is not possible because of deeper invasion, segmental resection is required.

When the mandibular structure is affected, dental rehabilitation is very difficult, and a continuous dialogue with dental practitioners is needed. The anterior arch of the mandible is critical to function, and when it is sacrificed, reconstruction with either a prosthetic implant or bone graft may be used with subsequent lengthy rehabilitation (see Figure 6–4). Osseointegration of implants for dental prostheses is a major advance for this patient population provided that the bone has not been irradiated. The maxilla is easier to manage from the dental standpoint and is more often sacrificed for effective cancer margins (Figure 6–6). The maxilla is usually replaced by a prosthodontic obturator device, with good results.

MANAGEMENT OF THE NECK

Elective neck dissection is recommended for control of micrometastases before they grow and become clinically evident. It is generally indicated following radiation failure and/or stage III and IV disease. The classic radical neck dissection is an en bloc resection of the lymphatics of the lateral neck. It encompasses the internal jugular vein, submandibular gland and triangle, sternocleidomastoid muscle, and the eleventh cranial nerve (see Figure 6–5). A number of modifications have been proposed that preserve one or more of the named structures. Preservation of the eleventh nerve is the most important to reduce the operative morbidity of the paralyzed trapezius muscle and resultant painful shoulder.

The selection of the type of dissection is controversial. Equivalent results are often seen in modified neck dissection versus radical neck dissection in the negative neck when patients undergo adjunctive postoperative radiation therapy. Palpable neck disease is probably better managed with radical neck dissection; however, a definitive, prospective, randomized trial remains to be completed to resolve this important issue.

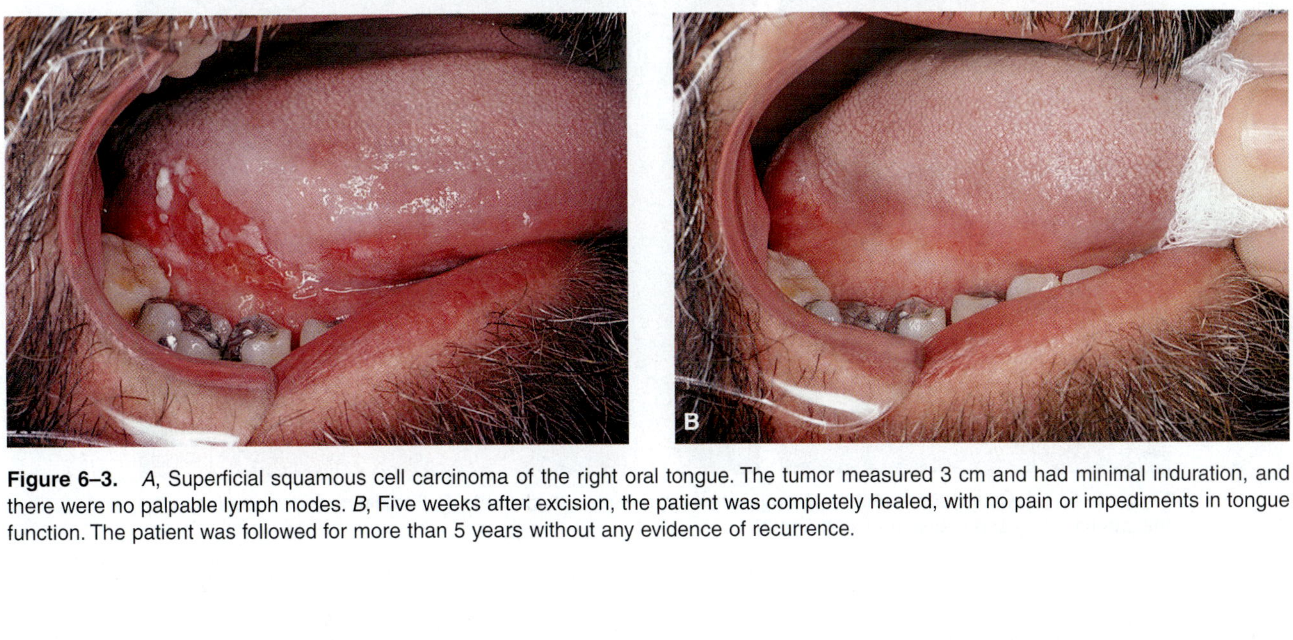

Figure 6–3. *A*, Superficial squamous cell carcinoma of the right oral tongue. The tumor measured 3 cm and had minimal induration, and there were no palpable lymph nodes. *B*, Five weeks after excision, the patient was completely healed, with no pain or impediments in tongue function. The patient was followed for more than 5 years without any evidence of recurrence.

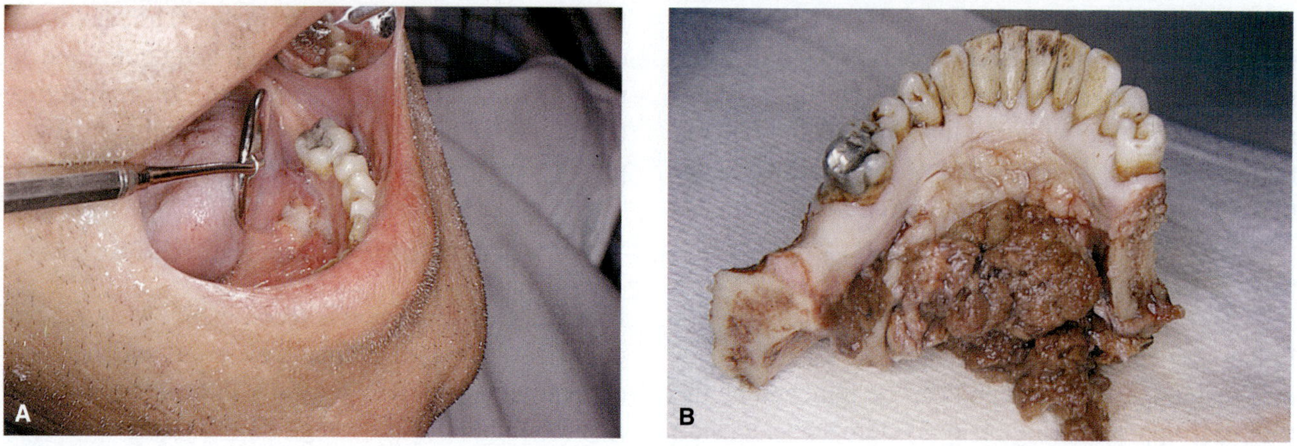

Figure 6–4. *A*, A deeply infiltrating squamous cell carcinoma involving the entire anterior floor of the mouth and mandible. *B*, Treatment involved composite resection followed by radiation. Reconstruction was critical to function, appearance, and quality of life.

Combining surgery and radiation is widely advocated for advanced-stage disease to improve survival and decrease the likelihood of locoregional recurrence. Chemotherapy has been added for advanced disease, with increasingly promising results. Preoperative irradiation is effective in reducing local failure, but significant surgical complications have led to a change to postoperative radiation therapy, which is, in theory, equally effective. Traditionally, a 2 cm region of normal tissue around the malignancy is the surgical goal in either case.

The combined treatment of oral cavity cancer requires a number of considerations. Dental evaluation and care are important before starting treatment. Antibiotics are needed both before surgery as prophylaxis and during healing. When the primary oral site and contents of the neck dissection are removed in continuity, after radiation therapy, coverage of the carotid artery is necessary to prevent fatal hemorrhage. This is managed by a muscle flap.

RECONSTRUCTION

Although cure rates have not changed much during the past two decades, better function and appearance have been made possible by advances in reconstruc-

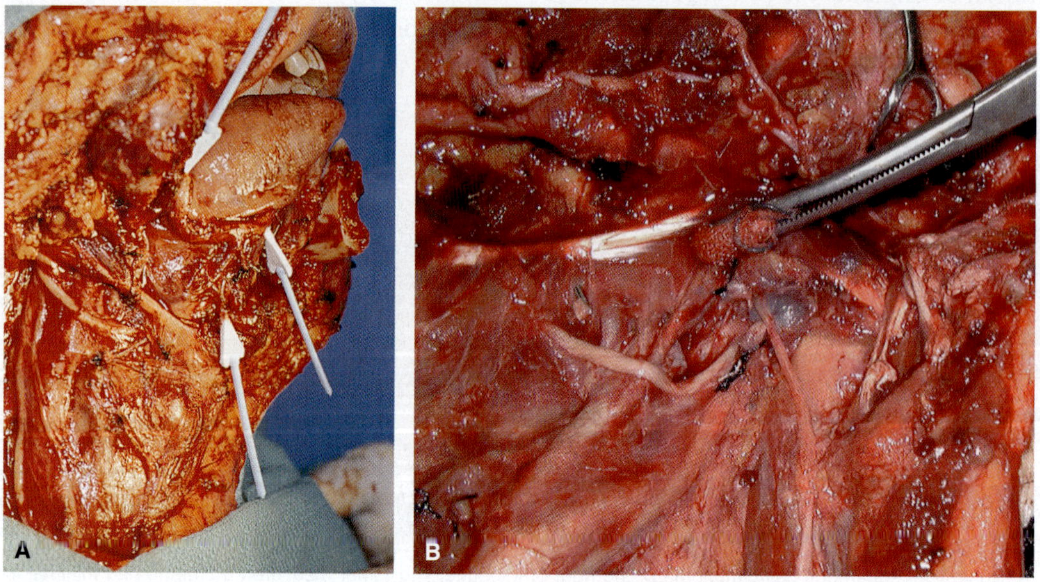

Figure 6–5. *A*, Composite resection of tongue, mandible, and neck contents. *B*, Radical neck dissection sparing the carotid artery and cranial nerves X and XII.

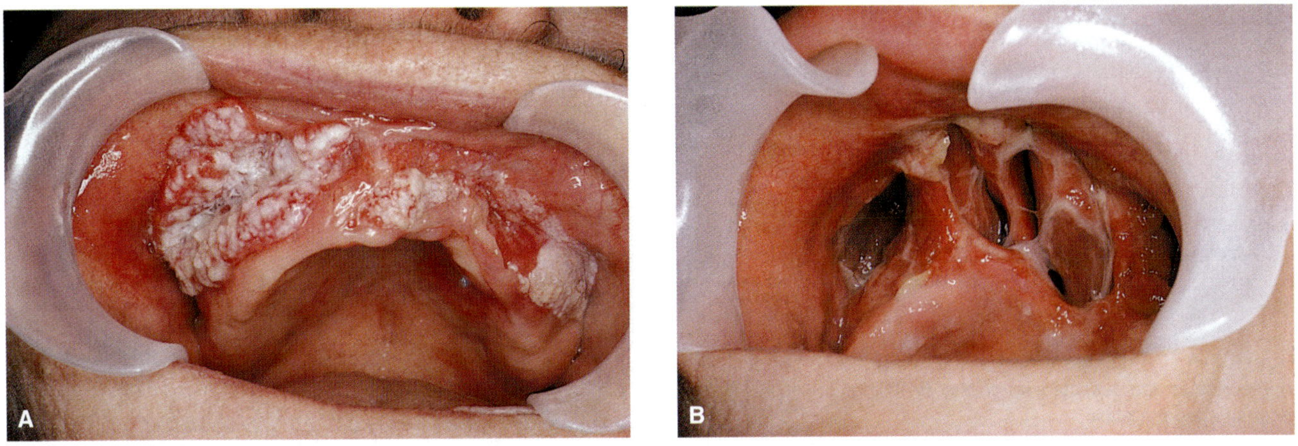

Figure 6–6. *A*, Squamous cell carcinoma involving anterior maxillary gingiva and bone. *B*, Postsurgical maxillary tissues 1 month following surgery. A maxillary prosthesis replaced the defect, leading to good function. The tumor has now been controlled for more than 10 years.

tive surgical techniques. The earliest methods for reconstruction used primary closure or tongue flaps to reconstruct the oral cavity. In addition, split-thickness skin grafts have been used regularly in simple cases for rapid wound resurfacing. The 15-year period from 1965 to 1980 saw regional pedicle flaps widely used. The first reliable head and neck flap was the deltopectoral flap, followed by the breakthrough development of the myocutaneous flaps, which include the pectoralis major, trapezius, and sternocleidomastoid flaps. The deltopectoral flap provides a relatively reliable skin lining in one to two stages, whereas the pectoralis major myocutaneous flap is a one-stage procedure, with the muscle carrier providing effective carotid artery protection (Figure 6–7).

These pedicle flaps provide safety for the patient when the surgeon operates in the postirradiated field and a satisfactory oral cavity reconstruction outcome. The flaps are done primarily with the resections and decrease the need for multiple operative revisions. With the shift to postoperative radiation therapy, the flaps are hardy and protect the mandibular remnants and reconstruction from the major complications of osteoradionecrosis.

Reconstruction of the mandible after segmental resection is more complicated.[1,2] The procedure is variably known as the "commando" or the composite resection, and when the anterior arch is resected, it is sometimes called the "Andy Gump" defect (see Figure 6–4). It involves removal of the primary tumor and the mandible and a neck dissection in continuity. Formerly, surgeons used free bone grafts, usually the rib or iliac crest, or prosthetics of either titanium or acrylic, and currently use free tissue microvascular transfer of the fibula, iliac crest, or radius (Figure 6–8).

The newer techniques use bone and soft tissue, which are revascularized when transferred to the neck. The procedure is reliable (the graft failure rate usually does not exceed 5%) and provides excellent cosmetic appearance and good function. When the bone grafts receive osseointegrated implants, a denture can be applied and can contribute to the return of near-normal mastication (see Chapter 8). Most of the soft tissue reconstructions, that is, pectoral or fibular skin, are insensate and immobile, decreasing the acuity of intraoral proprioception and the effi-

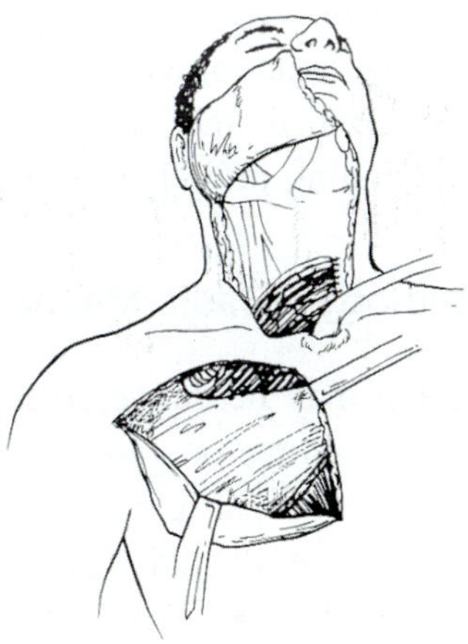

Figure 6–7. Diagram of a pectoralis major myocutaneous flap.

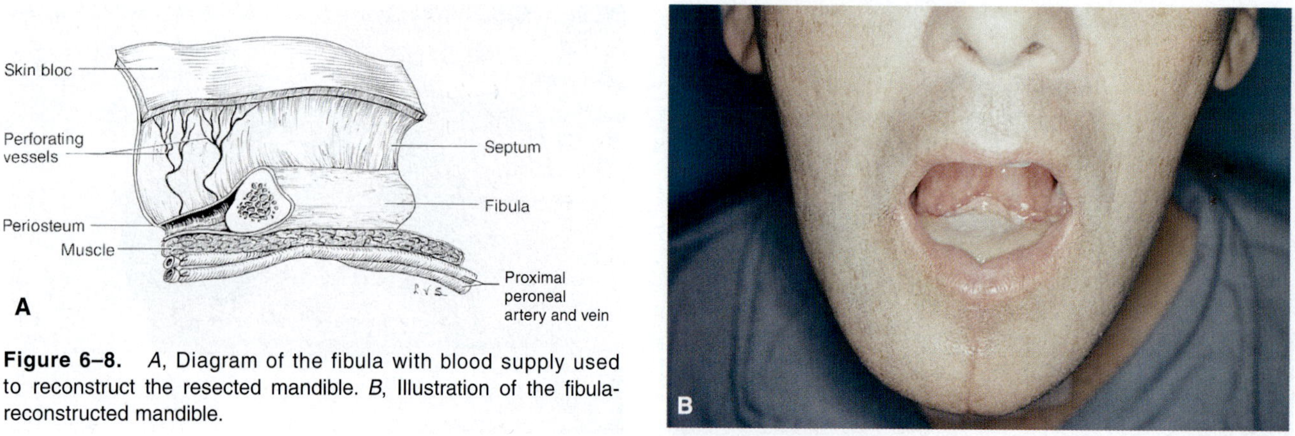

Figure 6–8. *A*, Diagram of the fibula with blood supply used to reconstruct the resected mandible. *B*, Illustration of the fibula-reconstructed mandible.

ciency of oral phases of swallowing. Current clinical research is directed to micro–free flap reconstruction of the oral cavity and microreinnervation of the oral cavity flaps with the remnants of the inferior alveolar nerve, lingual nerves, and, in some cases, glossopharyngeal nerve.

RADIATION THERAPY

Choice of Treatment

In selecting between radiation therapy and surgery or a combination of radiation with surgery for the treatment of oral cancer, it is necessary to understand the basic mechanisms by which radiation acts on tumors and normal tissues. The major factors influencing the choice of treatment are the following: (1) the relative cure that can be obtained with radiation compared with surgery or another modality, (2) the relative morbidity associated with radiation treatment versus surgery, (3) the cosmetic and functional result of radiation versus surgery, and (4) improved local control and survival that can be achieved by combining radiotherapy and surgery.

Radiobiology—Basic Mechanisms

Ionizing radiation may be delivered in the form of external beams of x-rays or gamma rays, external beams of electrons or particles (neutrons or protons), or internally implanted sources of beta or gamma rays.[3] Radiation kills cells by primary and secondary interactions with the cells making up the tissues. In general, the photons of x-rays or gamma rays dislodge electrons from the atoms of the tissue. These charged particles cause ionization along their tracks, which results in chemical changes in the water in the cell and in the critical macromolecules of the cell, primarily the deoxyribonucleic acid (DNA). The major site of action of ionizing radiation on mammalian cells is in the nucleus, where it causes breakage of chromosomes and disruptions or misrepair of the DNA molecule.

Although many of the changes can be repaired, certain chromosomal and DNA breakages are not repaired normally and result in the inability of the cell to undergo more than a few subsequent divisions. In some types of cells, such as mature lymphocytes and tumors with wild-type *p53*, radiation has a direct effect on the function of the nucleus and causes programmed cell death (apoptosis). In most cases, the damage is to the DNA and chromosomes, and cell death results after several divisions. It should be noted that cells need not actually die to be mitotically "dead." For instance, they may divide once or twice but then remain in a postmitotic state and form giant cells that are no longer capable of causing tissue or tumor regeneration.

There is a constant relationship between the radiation dose and the fraction of cells that will survive, which can be expressed in the form of a survival curve. These curves are presented in terms of the logarithm of survival versus the dose and, in most instances, bend downward after a finite initial upward slope. This exponential-type survival makes it necessary to use increasing doses of radiation as the number of cells in any given tumor increase to achieve complete tumor cell sterilization. Variation exists in the shape of the survival curve for various types of tumors and between tumor and normal tissue cells. Although these variations are relatively small after high doses, survival at a dose of 20 cGy, a common clinical dose, can vary from 20 to 80%, depending on tumor histology and subtype. This may explain some of the differences in sensitivity of tumors to radiotherapy. The cellular repair and kinetic growth changes that take place during fractionated radiotherapy can become as important as the shape of the individual cell survival curve.[4,5]

Differential Effects on Tumor and Normal Tissue

The events that cause cell death occur in both normal tissue and tumor. The differential ability of ionizing radiation to sterilize a tumor without unacceptable damage to normal tissue is attributable to five major biologic differences between tumor and normal tissue:

1. In general, the number of normal clonogenic cells present in the surrounding tissue is far greater than in the tumor. Thus, after complete sterilization of all clonogenic cells in the tumor, there will be surviving surrounding epithelial cells and underlying vasculoconnective tissue cells that can repopulate the area formerly occupied by the tumor. The fraction of cells surviving after irradiation depends on the dose: the higher the dose, the smaller the fraction surviving and, conversely, the larger the tumor, the greater the dose required to ensure sterilization of its cells.
2. Repair takes place in cells after radiation damage. This process is usually considered to be an intracellular repair of damage to the major nuclear components and is known as sublethal damage repair. Although this occurs in both tumor and normal tissue, it appears to be depressed in the portions of tumors that have poor vascularity and are hypoxic. In addition, repair is depressed in certain tumor types, such as lymphoma. It may occur to a greater extent in slowly dividing normal tissues than in most tumors. Thus, when radiation is given in multiple doses, there can be more repair of damage in the normal tissue than in many but not all tumors.
3. Repopulation or proliferation of cells can occur after irradiation in both tumor and normal tissue if viable clonogenic cells remain. Mitosis will be delayed on the average of 1 minute per centigray. Normal tissues seem able to respond to the radiation injury with more rapid cell proliferation. This homeostatic biologic mechanism does not appear to be available to tumors. However, tumors may, in some cases, speed up their proliferation when they become smaller and better vascularized if all of their cells have not been killed.
4. Oxygenation plays an important role in radiation sensitivity. Cells are three times more resistant when hypoxic. Although the centers of many tumors are hypoxic, making them more resistant to radiation, it is now known that some areas of tumors reoxygenate during treatment. This process can occur in a few hours to a few days. What otherwise would be resistant portions of tumors thus become more sensitive during a course of fractionated radiation therapy lasting days or weeks. Reoxygenation seems to occur because of fluctuations in blood flow in tumor capillaries and tumor shrinkage.
5. Cell position in the cell cycle (resting, DNA synthesis, mitosis) can cause variations as great as a factor of three in cell sensitivity to radiation. If tumor cells are in a vulnerable position in their cycle, whereas normal tissue cells are in a more resistant phase, a better differential between tumor and normal tissue damage may result. The use of halogenated pyrimidine sensitizers that are incorporated into DNA takes advantage of the fact that, for some tumors, more cells are in the S phase of the cycle than in some surrounding normal tissues (brain, soft tissue).

New Approaches

Many experimental approaches are being employed to increase the tumor cell kill and decrease damage to normal tissues during radiotherapy. One approach is the use of neutrons that deposit their energy in dense patterns.[6] These high linear energy transfer (LET) radiations differ from conventional x-rays in that the damage they cause is less likely to be repaired and is less influenced by the concentration of oxygen. These differences may yield greater tumor control for a given level of normal tissue damage in those cases in which repair of tumor cells is unusually great or when hypoxia persists throughout treatment. Several trials have shown that high LET treatment is more effective than low LET radiation in salivary gland tumors. No advantage has been proven in other head and neck cancers.

A second approach to increasing the cell kill of hypoxic tumor cells is the use of radiosensitizers. Some of these chemicals have the ability to sensitize hypoxic cells to radiation in much the same way that oxygen does, but because they are inert and not metabolized by the tissue, they can reach the hypoxic centers of tumors. The best analogue yet developed, etanidazole, has been tested in patients with head and neck cancer without evident benefit in survival or local control.

A third method under clinical investigation is the use of radioprotective compounds that selectively decrease the radiation injury to normal tissue. Current studies are focusing on Ethyol (amifostine) for reduction in salivary gland injury.[7] To date, most studies have been small because of theoretical concerns that the tumor might also be protected. However, some investigators report improved morbidity with no apparent impact on tumor control.

Hyperthermia, the induction of temperatures in the range of 42°C to 45°C, is being applied to the treatment of oral cancer in conjunction with radiotherapy.[8] Either external applicators using ultrasound or microwaves or interstitial needles heated by microwave antennas, local current fields, or ferromagnetic seeds can be used to induce elevated temperatures for 15 to 60 minutes and, with special needles, continuously for several days. When this is combined with radiation, the effect can be doubled or the necessary radiation dose reduced. A randomized trial has shown improved control of neck disease with combined radiotherapy and hyperthermia. The most striking responses have been in melanomas and in readily accessible neck nodal masses.

Cytotoxic chemotherapy is often used in combination with radiation.[9] Although many trials have explored the use of induction or preirradiation chemotherapy with some tumor responses, particularly in oropharyngeal cancers, only chemotherapy concurrent with radiation has been shown to improve local control and decrease the incidence of distant metastatic disease. Although the combination can increase local tumor response, it has not yet been proven to increase survival in oral cancer. Meta-analysis of a number of head and neck cancer trials using radiation and chemotherapy combinations does seem to suggest a small survival benefit, particularly with the use of concurrent chemotherapy, particularly with cisplatinum.[10]

Standard radiation fractionation schedules for head and neck cancers employ a single daily treatment, 5 days a week, for approximately 6 1/2 to 7 1/2 weeks. Altered fractionation patterns have the potential as well to improve results in oral cancer.[4] They can be either hyperfractionated (an increased number of fractions with a lower dose per fraction) or hypofractionated (a decreased number of fractions with a higher dose per fraction), and the overall treatment time might also be compressed (accelerated) so that a larger number of treatments are given either two or three times each day and the overall treatment time can be 3 to 6 1/2 weeks. Squamous cell cancers have been found to have widely varying potential doubling times. Those with long doubling times do well with standard fractionation (200 cGy per day, 5 days a week). Those with short doubling times have poorer local control with radiotherapy and, in at least one study of accelerated hyperfractionation (120 cGy twice daily), do better than with conventional patterns. Three different patterns of accelerated treatment, all of which shorten the total time taken to deliver the treatment, were compared with standard fractionation in a large Radiation Therapy Oncology Group (RTOG) study for head and neck cancer. This study shows a clear benefit with two of the accelerated hyperfractionation treatment schedules: treatment twice daily (120 cGy) for the whole course of therapy and a concomitant boost technique that uses 180 cGy daily up to 3,240 cGy and then twice daily for the final 12 days of therapy, with the second fraction of 150 cGy directed to the gross tumor only. Because of patient convenience, the latter treatment schedule has been adopted by many centers to treat locally advanced (T3 and T4 versus stage III and IV) lesions.

Finally, sophisticated radiation treatment planning systems are being applied to many head and neck tumors, including those in the oral cavity and oropharynx. This is called intensity-modulated radiation therapy (IMRT), which allows more optimal dose delivery (Figure 6–9). The radiation oncologist uses the information from CT and MRI scans to identify targets for high-dose deposition (the site of the gross tumor volume [GTV]) and intermediate-dose deposition (the clinical target volume [CTV], which includes areas at high risk for microscopic spread, such as tissue immediately adjacent to the GTV, and clinically uninvolved lymph nodes). The critical adjacent structures including the spinal cord, mandible, and salivary glands are also identified, and the computer planning system uses sophisticated algorithms to deliver a low radiation dose to these structures. There are pilot studies of IMRT for oropharyngeal cancers that are currently ongoing. Because this technique allows a dose gradient between tumor target and adjacent normal tissues, it is possible to use a higher daily dose for the GTV than the CTV or normal tissues. It is hoped that these techniques will allow a higher cure rate with lower long-term complications such as poor salivary function, dental caries, and mandibular osteoradionecrosis.

Thus, we see that although radiation damages both tumor and normal tissue, a number of factors influence tumor response, and a fractionated, multiple-dose course of radiation therapy can effect complete sterilization of the tumor with adequate survival of normal tissue. Some basic principles are evident. The smaller the number of clono-

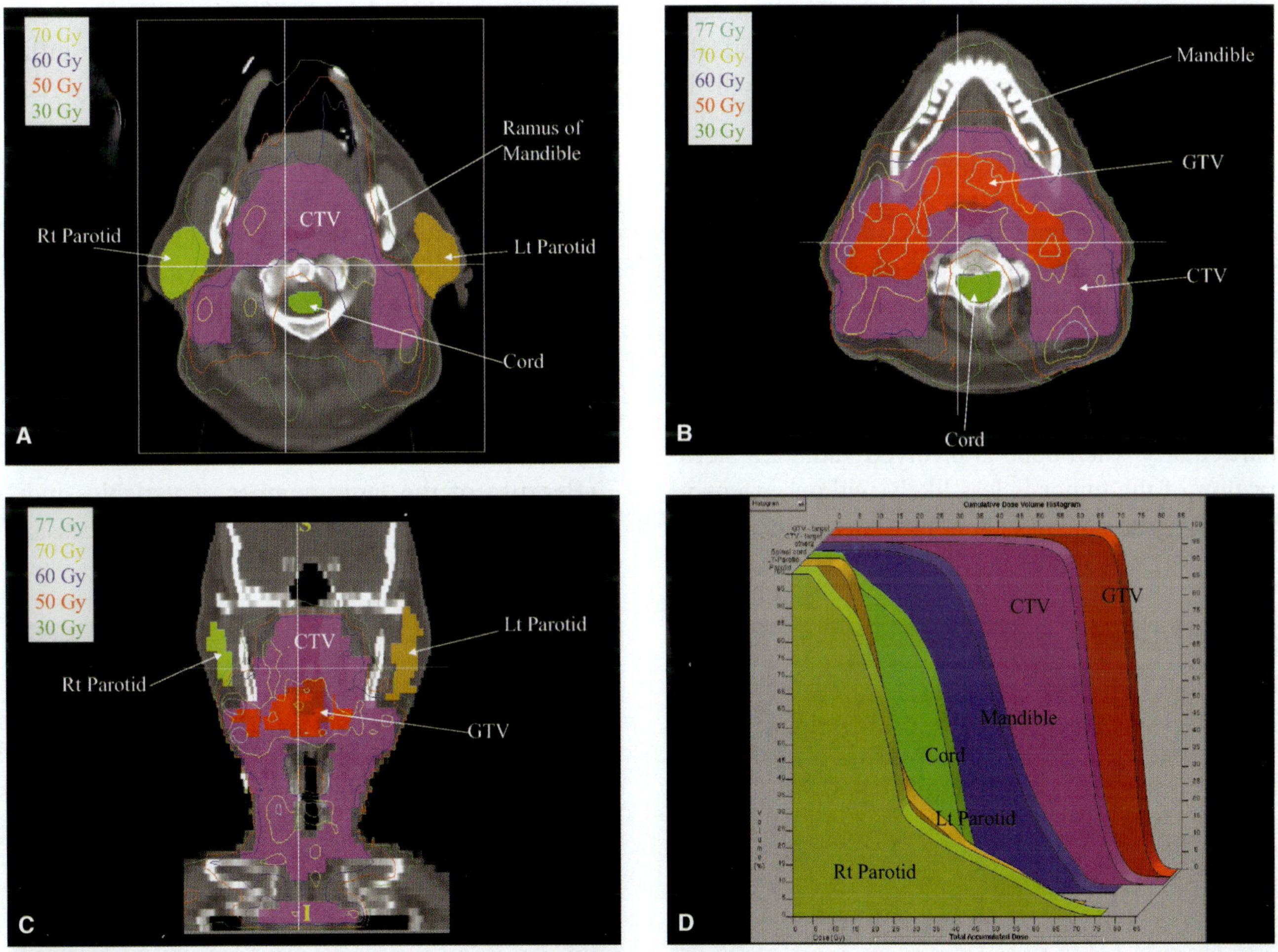

Figure 6–9. Intensity-modulated radiation therapy plan for the treatment of a carcinoma of the base of the tongue (T2N1). *A*, Axial view through the level of the parotid glands with the clinical target volume (CTV) in purple and the dose contours superimposed. *B*, Axial view through the level of the gross tumor volume (GTV) in red and the dose contours as labeled. *C*, Coronal view with the dose contours superimposed on the CTV and GTV and parotids in color wash. *D*, Dose volume histogram displaying the cumulative dose to the tumor targets and to the normal tissues, including the mandible, spinal cord, and parotids.

genic tumor cells present, the greater the probability of radiation sterilization and/or the lower the dose required for a given probability of sterilization. Certain tumor cell types, such as lymphomas, will have greater radiosensitivity and radiocurability. Large necrotic tumors with anoxic foci, particularly those deeply invading bone or muscle in which reoxygenation may not occur, will be more resistant to radiation. Damage to normal tissue depends on dose as well, and the incidence of complications will increase, with larger tumors requiring higher doses.

Selection of Patients for Radiation Therapy

Based on the foregoing principles, the selection of patients for radiation therapy for cancer of the oral cavity can be approached rationally. Those lesions that are small (under 3 cm and superficial, ideally exophytic, and without necrotic areas) will be amenable to radiation sterilization (Figures 6–10 to 6–12). The choice of radiation therapy versus surgery for such early, superficial lesions will depend on the functional and cosmetic results of the two modalities. If a regional excision can be accomplished without much morbidity, this would often be the treatment of choice because there would be no residual radiation injury.

For lesions that are large and deeply invasive, and particularly when bone is involved, radiation sterilization of the tumor is less likely without extensive normal tissue damage; therefore, surgery or a combination of irradiation and surgery is usually required. When the lesion is potentially extremely radiosensitive (according to histology), as in various lymphomas, radiotherapy would be the treatment of choice over surgery.

If the location and clinical behavior of a lesion indicate significant lymphatic permeation, then radiotherapy is often advantageous, either alone or in combination with surgery, because a greater volume of the potentially involved lymphatic structures can be covered. For example, in carcinomas of the tongue or the floor of the mouth, bilateral irradiation of the neck can prevent the development of lymph node metastases in a neck that shows no clinical signs of involvement. In addition, prophylactic treatment of the lower neck and supraclavicular areas when the upper neck is involved can prevent the involvement of lymph nodes in this region.

The patient's medical condition has some influence on the selection of the treatment modality. A 5- to 8-week course of radiotherapy is debilitating, particularly of the oral cavity region, when mucositis and decreased taste and salivary function make it difficult to maintain weight and nutrition. Thus, poor general condition is a contraindication for radiotherapy, although this modality may be selected for patients in whom radical surgery and lengthy anesthesia are absolutely prohibited. The availability of equipment and expertise are certainly other factors in treatment selection.

Because of the large number of variables indicated in the selection of treatment, it is necessary

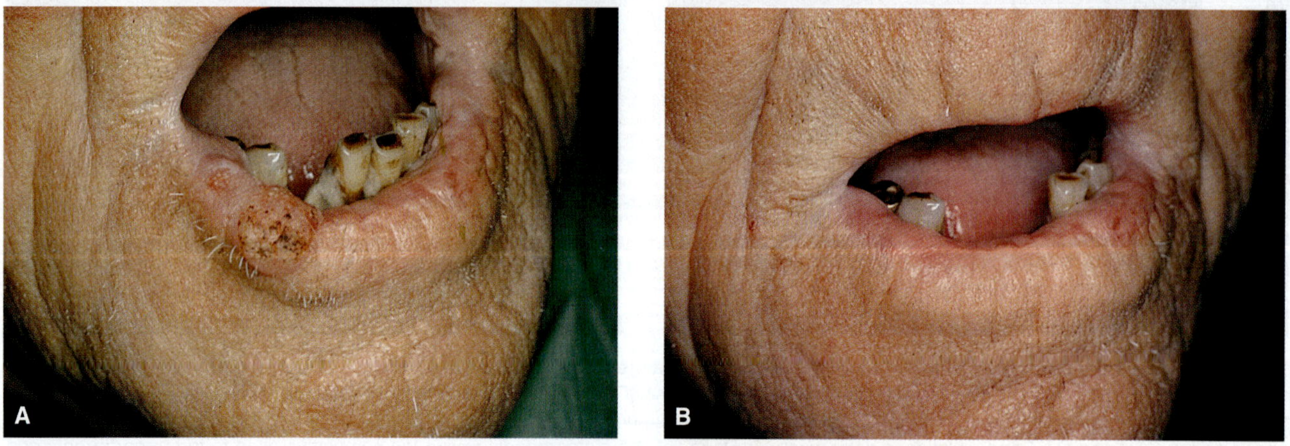

Figure 6–10. *A*, Squamous cell carcinoma of the lower lip. *B*, One month postradiotherapy.

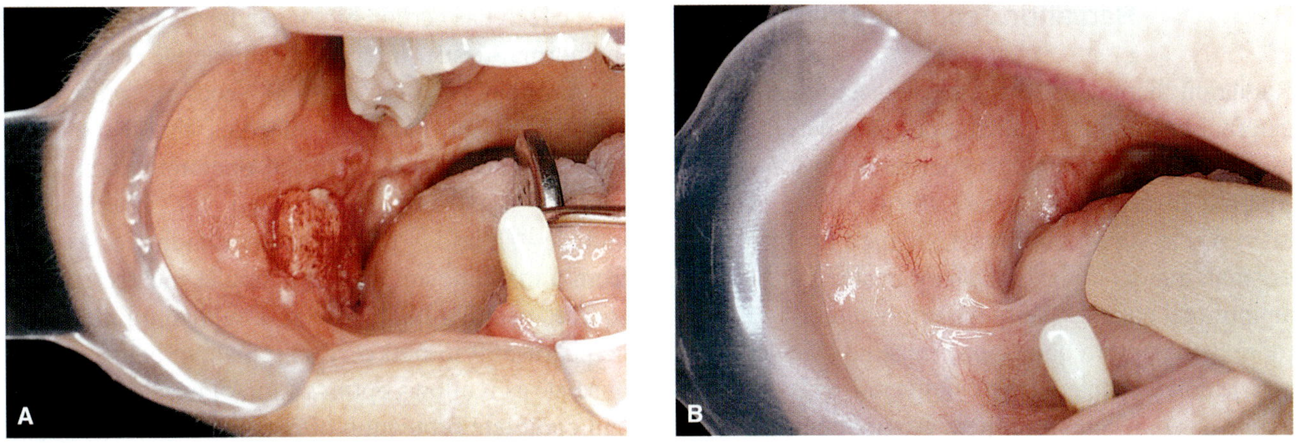

Figure 6–11. *A*, Squamous cell carcinoma of the posterior buccal mucosa. *B*, Complete response following 6,500 cGy. Note the radiation-induced telangiectasia and fibrosis. The patient is asymptomatic.

that a team approach be used in the management of oral lesions. The dentist, head and neck surgeon, radiation oncologist, radiologist, pathologist, medical oncologist, and social worker/nurse should see and evaluate the patient jointly, preferably in a tumor board setting with the patient available for examination. The decision on treatment will be individualized for the exact histologic nature, extent, and depth of invasion of the lesion and the social and physical conditions of the patient.

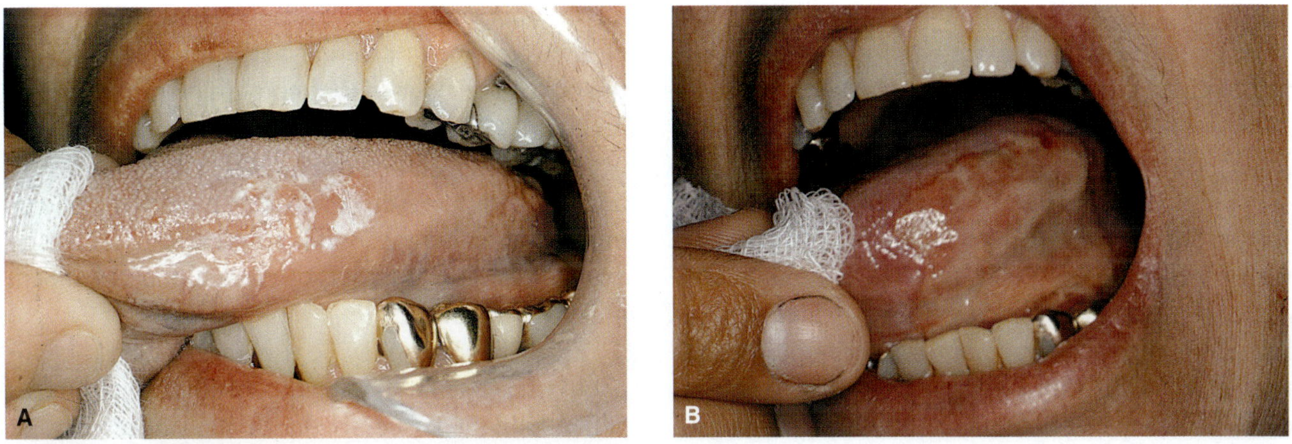

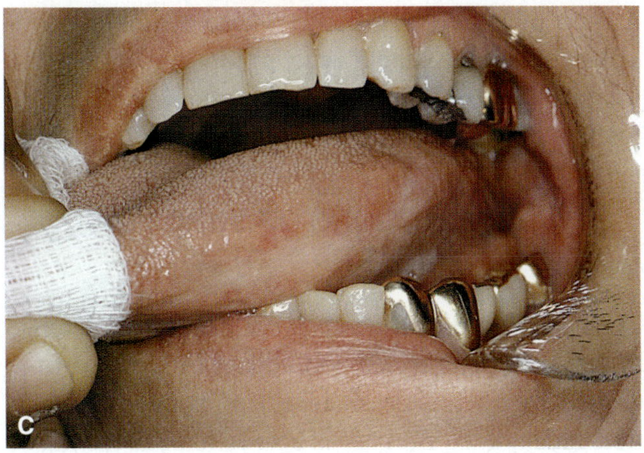

Figure 6–12. *A*, Squamous cell carcinoma (T1N0) presenting as leukoplakia of the tongue. *B*, Management was by interstitial therapy (radium needle implant). Note the mucositis induced at the end of 1 week (calculated dose of 6,500 cGy). *C*, After 1 month, there was no evidence of tumor or loss of function, and the patient was asymptomatic.

Radiation Techniques

Radiation therapy for oral cancer is administered by external beam, interstitial sources, and peroral cones or applicators. Low-energy external beam sources are referred to as orthovoltage (100 to 300 kilovolt x-rays). These superficial x-rays are used for lip lesions or small tumors in the oral cavity treated by means of an intraoral cone. Because the orthovoltage x-rays are more damaging to bone, bone must be shielded. Peroral irradiation may also be delivered with electrons using special small cones or applicators. This approach is useful alone or combined with external beam x-rays for lesions under 3 cm in diameter.

Megavoltage beams from cobalt 60 or linear accelerators of 4 million electron volts (MeV) or higher are used for external beam treatment. Today the cobalt and 4 MeV machines with an 80 cm source axis distance (SAD) have been mainly replaced by linear accelerators producing 6 and 15 or 18 MeV bremsstrahlung x-rays and electrons from 6 to 20 MeV with a SAD of 100 cm. These high-energy photons allow multiple-beam treatment, often with wedges, shaping blocks, and compensating filters to protect uninvolved tissues. Complex treatment plans with these beams often allow delivery of a higher dose to the tumor volume than to the surrounding normal tissues. Automated multileaf collimators are replacing the poured blocks, making multiple fields simple to set up automatically. Three-dimensional imaging allows three-dimensional conformal planning of the therapy, further sparing normal tissues, particularly salivary glands. IMRT techniques provide even more precision and sophistication of treatment planning and optimal beam delivery. However, these techniques can also create greater dose inhomogeneity in the target volume, leading to high-dose "hot spots" while sparing the salivary tissue. Thus, the acute reaction during treatment may be more intense, whereas, in the long term, the salivary function is recovered if the mean dose to the parotid is kept to 250 cGy.

Interstitial implant treatment (brachytherapy) is used commonly for delivery of a high dose to a limited volume (Figure 6–13).[11] Implants deliver the radiation in the immediate vicinity of the implanted isotope and also deliver it at a relatively low dose rate, which has certain biologic advantages in sparing the normal tissue. Interstitial radioactive sources can be placed directly as wires or seeds or, preferably, afterloaded into tubes or needles that have been inserted into the tumor in the operating room. The sources most commonly used for afterloading include ^{192}Ir and ^{125}I. Remote afterloading of iridium from a machine employing a single, intense iridium source, using a high dose rate with multiple treatments of 300 to 600 cGy, is replacing hand loading of seeds as it allows optimization of dose distribution and complete protection of personnel from radiation exposure. The single source can be programmed to traverse up to 18 separate catheters or needles.

When using radiotherapy alone to treat T1 and T2 tumors of the oral tongue, interstitial therapy is essential (see Figure 6–12). Control rates of 80 to 90% are achieved, whereas with external beam alone, the rate is only 30%. Peroral cone therapy with low-energy x-rays or electrons can approach the results of brachytherapy. For floor of the mouth cancers, external beam irradiation controls 80% of T1 lesions and brachytherapy about 90%. It is clearly superior to external beam irradiation for T2 tumors of the floor of the mouth. The problem with brachytherapy for these sites is bone necrosis because of the close proximity of the sources to bone. For this reason, many centers have replaced most brachytherapy with surgical excision and external beam irradiation or peroral cone treatment plus external beam.

Electron beams may be used rather than x-ray or photon beams. They have the advantage of limited penetration in tissue so that a high dose may be given to superficial lesions, with only minimal irradiation of underlying tissue. These beams are usually generated by linear accelerators and are used to treat neck nodes overlying the spinal cord after cord tolerance is approached with photons.

COMBINATIONS OF SURGERY AND IRRADIATION

The need for doses exceeding normal tissue tolerance in larger squamous cell and adenocarcinomas of the oral cavity often necessitates a combination of radiation and surgery. Surgery is able to remove the major

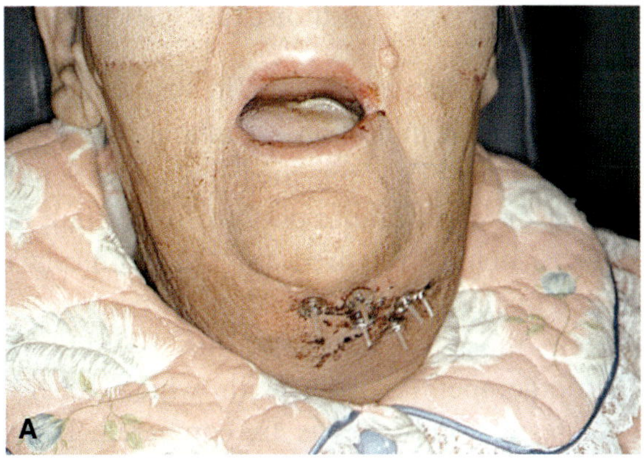

Figure 6–13. *A*, This patient had an ^{192}Ir implant for a squamous cell carcinoma of the floor of the mouth. *B* and *C*, Radiographs of the seeds in place.

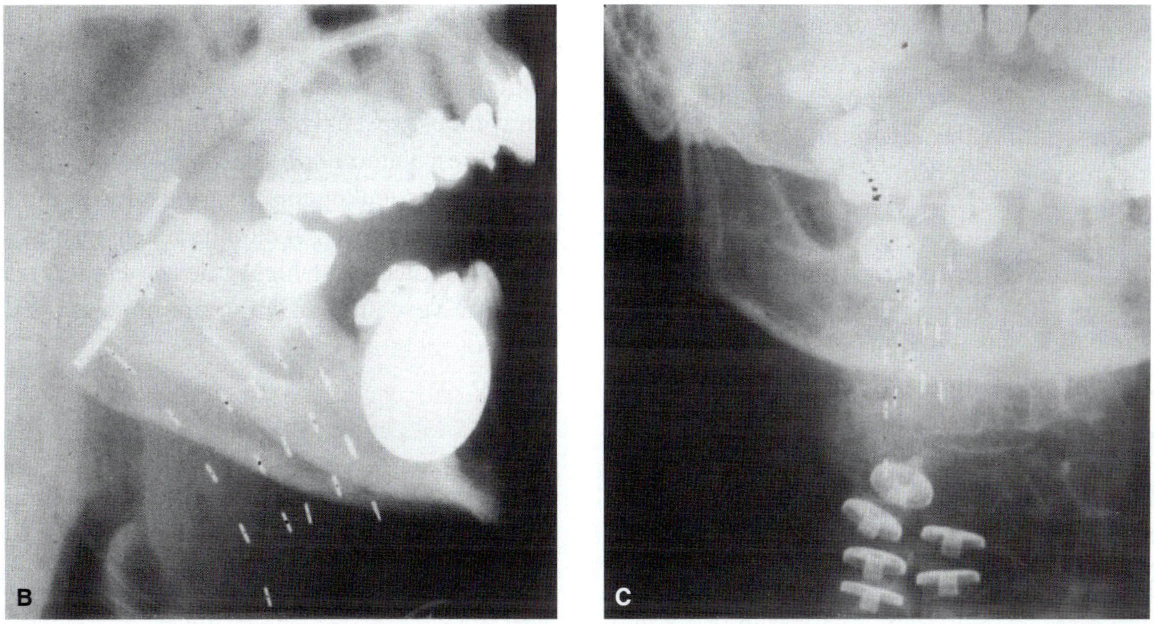

bulk of the tumor, including the potentially resistant central portion, and radiation is then able to sterilize the microscopic routes of spread in the lymphatics and tissue planes not resected in the standard excisional procedures. Combinations of radiation and surgery are used in at least half of all oral cancers.

Radiation can be administered preoperatively for squamous cell lesions to reduce the size of the tumor, sterilize the microscopic involvement of lymphatics and lymph nodes, and increase the margins of normal tissue resected. If the tissues are irradiated using proper fractionation and tissue compensation techniques, perioperative and postoperative complications are significantly reduced.

Postoperative irradiation is used more extensively. Advantages include the delivery of higher radiation doses, sterilization of both the surgical field and those lymphatic draining regions not removed by surgery, and the improvement in the surgeon's ability to judge margins.

ROLE OF CHEMOTHERAPY IN ORAL AND PHARYNGEAL CANCER

Unfortunately, patients with stage III or IV oral and pharyngeal carcinomas have a 60% chance of having a locoregional recurrence and a 20 to 40% risk of developing distant metastases. Chemotherapy is largely palliative in patients with recurrent or metastatic disease.[12,13] In patients with previously untreated locally advanced disease, chemotherapy has been combined with radiotherapy and/or surgery in attempts to increase locoregional control, decrease distant metastasis, and improve survival.[14,15]

CHEMOTHERAPY FOR METASTATIC DISEASE

Patients who have relapsed after extensive surgery and/or radiotherapy are often debilitated with substantial weight loss and pain, contributing to an overall marginal performance status. Before recommending systemic chemotherapy, one must take into consideration the toxicity, response, and cost. Unfortunately, for this group of patients, toxicity remains a problem, and no standard agent or combination can be recommended at the present time. It is reasonable to consider the use of chemotherapy for palliation in patients with adequate physiologic functions to manage/tolerate the toxicities induced by these agents (ie, for those with an adequate performance status).

Single Agents

Six drugs have been extensively tested as single agents in patients with recurrent or metastatic head and neck cancer. They are (1) methotrexate, (2) bleomycin, (3) cisplatin and its analogue carboplatin, and (4) 5-fluorouracil (5-FU) and the taxanes, (5) paclitaxel and (6) docetaxel. Recently, several new classes of drugs have been investigated, with some promise. In describing the various agents, the term "response rate" is used. Both "partial" and "complete" responses are usually temporary and are not synonymous with cure.

Methotrexate

Methotrexate, an antimetabolite, exerts its cytotoxic effect through inhibition of the enzyme dihydrofolate reductase. This enzyme is responsible for maintaining the intracellular pool of folates in a reduced state, which is required for the synthesis of the purine nucleotides.

For most oncologists, this is the standard chemotherapeutic agent with which other single agents and combinations are compared. The overall response rate using methotrexate as a single agent is approximately 31%, with predominantly partial responses seen and few complete responses noted (Figure 6–14). The initial dose of 40 mg/m^2 is given intravenously weekly on an outpatient basis and is usually escalated until toxicity is noted (most often mucositis or leukopenia). Various doses and schedules have been used, including leucovorin as a bone marrow protector at higher doses. Pooled response rates are very similar with both moderate and high doses of methotrexate.

Bleomycin

Bleomycin is a mixture of glycopeptides in the class of antibiotic neoplastic agents that affect the cell cycle in the G_2 and mitotic phases. It has been one of the more frequently used agents for head and neck cancer and has a single-agent response rate of approximately 21%. The dose-limiting toxicity of bleomycin is its cumulative impairment of pul-

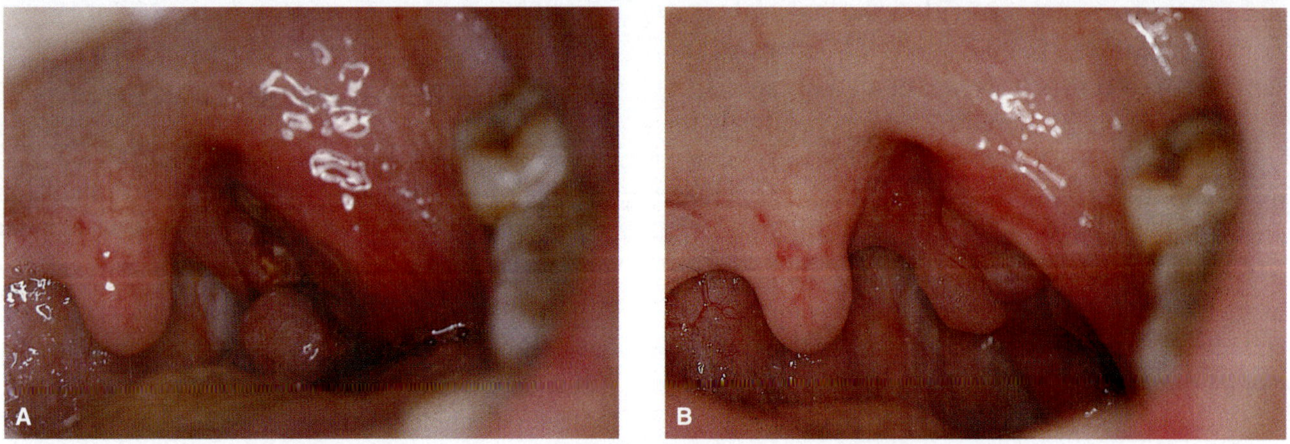

Figure 6–14. *A*, Recurrent squamous cell carcinoma of the left tonsillar fossa. *B*, Postchemotherapy control (complete response) following three cycles of methotrexate. There was a recurrence after 4 months.

monary function, making it difficult to administer after several courses. Bleomycin has equal activity when administered either as a bolus or by continuous infusion. However, the toxicity may be less with continuous infusion. The single-course dosage frequently used is 10 to 15 mg/m^2 daily for 3 to 4 days every 3 to 4 weeks.

Cisplatin

Cisplatin is a heavy metal compound. It is believed to exert its activity by causing DNA cross-linking. This agent has been extensively evaluated in patients with recurrent head and neck squamous cell carcinomas. As a single agent, the response rate is in the range of 28%.

Cisplatin has been given on a weekly basis every 3 weeks as an intravenous bolus or by continuous infusion. All schedules have shown similar response rates. The issue of dose intensity has also been addressed, with dose-related toxicity being a limiting factor, particularly renal toxicity and neurotoxicity. The typical dose used has been between 80 and 100 mg/m^2, with no clear advantage seen when higher doses are used. Currently, cisplatin is usually given every 3 to 4 weeks, with pre- and post-therapy hydration plus mannitol infusion to protect renal function.

5-Fluorouracil

5-FU is one of the most frequently used chemotherapeutic agents for head and neck cancer. It is usually used in combination with cisplatin. 5-FU, a pyrimidine antimetabolite, is converted intracellularly to fluorodeoxyuridine monophosphate, a potent inhibitor of thymidylate synthase (which inhibits DNA synthesis). 5-FU also forms fluorouridine triphosphate, which interferes with the function of ribonucleic acid. As a single agent, it has a response rate of approximately 15%. Recently, it has been observed that 5-FU can be potentiated when used in conjunction with leucovorin, which is the reduced form of folate. Leucovorin stabilizes the 5-FU and thymidylate synthase ternary complex. When 5-FU is administered as a bolus daily for 5 days, the dose-limiting side effect is predominantly bone marrow suppression. If the schedule is altered to a continuous venous infusion over 24 hours daily for 4 to 5 days, the limiting toxicities are mucositis, diarrhea, and skin erythema. The continuous infusion schedule, which reduces myelosuppression, improves 5-FU activity in head and neck squamous cell carcinomas. The dosage most frequently used has been 800 to 1,000 mg/m^2 by continuous infusion for 72 to 96 hours.

Other single agents, not as widely used but with reported activity in the range of 15 to 36% in head and neck squamous cell carcinomas, include carboplatin, an analogue of cisplatin, with a dose-limiting toxicity of myelosuppression, specifically thrombocytopenia; cyclophosphamide and its analogue, ifosfamide; and hydroxyurea. Other general classes of drugs with limited single-agent activity include the anthracyclines (doxorubicin), Vinca alkaloids, mitomycin, and nitrosoureas.

Taxanes

The taxanes (paclitaxel, also known as Taxol, and docetaxel, also known as Taxotere) are a class of agents known to stabilize microtubular formation and disrupt cells during the mitosis phase of the cell cycle. The Eastern Cooperative Oncology Group (ECOG) performed a multicenter phase II study of paclitaxel at a dose of 250 mg/m^2 over 24 hours every 3 weeks with granulocyte colony-stimulating factor support. A 40% major response rate was achieved in 28 evaluable patients. Median survival was 9.2 months, which compared favorably with the 5- to 6-month median survival achieved by cisplatin-based chemotherapy.

The taxanes, when given as a short infusion, have unique toxicity profiles: myelosuppression in the form of neutropenia occurs by day 8 and is usually resolved by day 10. Myalgias usually occur 36 to 48 hours after administration of paclitaxel and are dose limiting; cumulative toxicity is usually in the form of peripheral neuropathy. Toxicities from docetaxel include peripheral edema and/or pleural effusions. Premedication with corticosteroids helps reduce fluid retention secondary to docetaxel and is essential for decreasing the rare allergic reactions from paclitaxel.

Promising New Agents

Promising new agents are gemcitabine (an antimetabolite that blocks division during DNA synthesis) and topotecan (an inhibitor of topoisomerase I involved in DNA replication). In phase II trials, activity was noted in the range of 13% (7 of 54) and 29% (5 of 17) for patients receiving gemcitabine and topotecan, respectively.

Although not yet approved by the US Food and Drug Administration, a new class of therapies referred to as Targeted Therapies holds promise because it represents the next generation of therapeutic development for both solid tumor and hematologic malignancies. Epidermal growth factor receptor (EGFR) is expressed in approximately 70% of patients with squamous cell carcinoma of the head and neck. These new agents have been developed and are being tested in phase II trials to determine overall efficacy and tolerability. C225 is a monoclonal antibody that binds with EGFR on the membrane of the cell. In phase I trials, dose-limiting toxicities are skin rash and allergic symptomatology. ZD-1839 (Iressa) and OSI-774 (Tarceva) are both tyrosine kinase (TK) inhibitors of EGFR. Both are small molecules that inhibit TK inside the cell. Both have the advantage of being oral agents and have minimal toxicity, mostly in the form of a skin rash or diarrhea.

Choice of Chemotherapeutic Agents

In the 1970s, many chemotherapy trials used a combination of agents such as cisplatin, bleomycin, and methotrexate. In the 1980s, cisplatin and 5-FU combined (as a bolus and by continuous intravenous infusion for 96 hours) produced an objective response rate of 78% and a complete response rate of 29% in patients with recurrent and metastatic disease. However, these good response rates were not reproducible. To improve the response rates of cisplatin and 5-FU combinations, trials substituted carboplatin for cisplatin, modulated 5-FU with leucovorin, and dose escalated the cisplatin. Unfortunately, no overall improvements have been observed. An intergroup (ECOG and South Western Oncology Group [SWOG]) conducted a phase III, randomized trial looking at the efficacy and toxicity of the combination of cisplatin and 5-FU compared with cisplatin and paclitaxel (Taxol) for patients with recurrence of metastatic head and neck cancer. The results indicated that both had equal efficacy, with an overall response rate of 22% for cisplatin and 5-FU versus 29% for cisplatin and paclitaxel ($p = 0.4$), but there were fewer toxicities associated with cisplatin and paclitaxel.

Eleven randomized trials have compared single agents, such as cisplatin, 5-FU, and methotrexate, with combination chemotherapy, including cisplatin and 5-FU, for recurrent and/or metastatic head and neck cancer. Combination chemotherapy has not improved disease-free or overall survival. In addition, combination chemotherapy has increased toxicity when compared with single agents. One possible advantage of combination chemotherapy (ie, cisplatin and 5-FU or cisplatin and paclitaxel) is a higher complete response rate, but only in the range of 10 to 15%. Achieving a complete response could translate into a moderate disease-free interval but must be weighed against the expense of the increased toxicities noted with combinations.[16,17]

PRIMARY CHEMOTHERAPY

Primary chemotherapy refers to the use of chemotherapy before local therapy, concurrently with radiation, or after local treatment has been completed. The rationale for using chemotherapy prior to local treatment is to improve patient performance status, obtain tumor shrinkage, and eradicate micrometastases to prevent regional and distant metastases.

Induction (Neoadjuvant)

In the 1970s, cisplatin and bleomycin were combined for two cycles prior to local treatment. This combination used as induction chemotherapy yielded an overall objective response rate of 71%, with a complete response rate of 20%. Subsequently, investigators combined cisplatin and infusional 5-FU for three cycles prior to local treatment and reported an 88% overall response rate, with 54% of the patients achieving a complete response.

More than 21 randomized trials using multiagent induction chemotherapy (most with cisplatin-based regimens) prior to local treatment have been conducted. None has shown that induction chemotherapy has significantly improved survival. Critiques of these studies have included the following complaints: (1) relatively inactive regimens used, (2) variations in local and regional therapies, (3) heterogeneous study populations, and (4) poor patient compliance.

The role of induction chemotherapy as it relates to oral cavity cancer remains uncertain and should be considered experimental.

Concurrent Chemoradiation Therapy

There is enhanced activity when chemotherapy is given either concurrently or by a rapidly alternating sequence with radiotherapy. Local control is improved and may benefit patients with extensive locoregional disease who are not candidates for surgery. The theoretical mechanisms of synergy are as follows: (1) inhibition of repair of radiotherapy-induced DNA damage, (2) decrease in tumor cell repopulation during a course of fractionated radiotherapy, (3) eradication of tumor cell clones that have resistance to one modality of treatment, (4) possible cell-cycle synchronization, (5) increase in tumor reoxygenation and radiosensitivity, and (6) sterilization of micrometastases outside the radiation field.

Concurrent chemoradiotherapy has generally employed only single agents with radiotherapy. At least nine phase II randomized trials of concurrent chemoradiotherapy involving single-agent bleomycin have been reported, with only one showing a significant improvement in disease-free survival and another showing improvements in both disease-free and overall survival.

Four phase III trials using single-agent 5-FU with radiotherapy have shown decreased disease-free survival in three studies, and overall survival advantages were noted only in two studies; dose-limiting mucositis makes this approach less attractive. Multiagent chemotherapy combined with radiotherapy increases mucositis, causing interruptions of radiotherapy. In an effort to lower the toxicity of this approach and to make it feasible to deliver all treatment as planned, a rapidly alternating schedule has been adopted. Several randomized trials using concomitant multiagent chemotherapy resulted in observations of some improvements in disease-free and overall survival compared with radiation alone.

In the largest trial, 157 patients with unresectable stage III or IV squamous cell carcinomas of the oral cavity, pharynx, or larynx were randomized as follows: (1) four courses of cisplatin, 20 mg/m^2, and 5-FU, 200 mg/m^2, given daily as an intravenous bolus for 5 consecutive days during weeks 1, 4, 7, and 10, plus radiotherapy (three courses of 200 cGy, each given in fractions of 20 cGy per day during weeks 2, 3, 5, 6, 8, and 9), and (2) radiotherapy only, 700 cGy total dose given in 20 cGy fractions. Combined treatment was associated with a statistically significant increase in the frequency of complete response (43% versus 22%; p = .037). An estimated 5-year progression-free survival was improved in the combined treatment group (21% versus 9%; p = .008), as well as an overall 5-year survival (24% versus 10%; p = .01). The incidence and severity of mucositis were nearly identical in both treatment arms.

More recently, the Intergroup conducted a randomized phase II trial for patients with stage III and IV unresectable squamous cell carcinoma of the head or neck comparing standard single fractionation radiotherapy to concurrent cisplatin, 100 mg/m^2 for three cycles (days 1, 22, and 43) with concurrent radiotherapy versus the combination of cisplatin/5-FU times three cycles and concurrent radiotherapy, both given in a split-course fashion.[16] Survival favored the chemotherapy/radiotherapy arms, and there was no advantage to having used combination chemotherapy with radiotherapy versus single-agent cisplatin with radiotherapy.

In summary, both single-agent and multiagent concomitant chemoradiotherapy have been shown to improve disease-free and/or overall survival. Because of substantial toxicity using this combined approach, no particular agent(s) have become the new standard approach.

Adjuvant Chemotherapy

Chemotherapy has been employed after standard surgery and/or radiotherapy in an effort to eradicate micrometastases. This approach has not led to improved locoregional control or survival. Problems associated with this approach relate to the patient's poor tolerance of combination chemotherapy and an overall poor compliance.

REFERENCES

1. Cheung SW, Anthony JP, Singer MI. Restoration of anterior mandible with the free fibula osseocutaneous flap. Laryngoscope 1994;104:105–13.
2. Greene D, Sussman S, Singer MI. Segmental reconstruction of the radiated mandible. Laryngoscope 1997;107:1018–23.
3. Hsu I-C, Phillips TL. Oral cavity cancer. In: Leibel SA, Phillips TL, editors. Textbook of radiation oncology. Philadelphia: WB Saunders; 1998. p. 457–77.
4. Fu KK, Pajak TF, Trotti A, et al. A Radiation Therapy Oncology Group (RTOG) phase III randomized study to compare hyperfractionation and two variants of accelerated fractionation to standard fractionation radiotherapy for head and neck squamous cell carcinomas: first report of RTOG 9003. Int J Radiat Oncol Biol Phys 2000;48:7–16.
5. Laramore GE. The use of neutrons in cancer therapy: a historical perspective through the modern era. Semin Oncol 1997;24:672–85.
6. Douglas JG, Laramore GE, Austin-Seymour M, et al. Treatment of locally advanced adenoid cystic carcinoma of the head and neck with neutron radiotherapy. Int J Radiat Oncol Biol Phys 2000;46:551–7.
7. Wasserman T, Mackowiak JI, Brizel DM, et al. Effect of amifostine on patient assessed clinical benefit in irradiated head and neck cancer. Int J Radiat Oncol Biol Phys 2000;48:1035–9.
8. Overgaard J, Gonzalez Gonzalez D, Hulshof MC, et al. Hyperthermia as an adjuvant to radiation therapy of recurrent or metastatic malignant melanoma. A multicentre randomized trial by the European Society for Hyperthermic Oncology. Int J Hyperthermia 1996;12:3–20.
9. Pignon JP, Bourhis J, Domenge C, Designe L. Chemotherapy added to locoregional treatment for head and neck squamous-cell carcinoma: three meta-analyses of updated individual data. MACH-NC Collaborative Group. Meta-Analysis of Chemotherapy on Head and Neck Cancer. Lancet 2000;355:949–55.
10. Schuchter LM, Hensley ML, Meropol NJ, Winer EP. 2002 update of recommendations for the use of chemotherapy and radiotherapy protectants: clinical practice guidelines of the American Society of Clinical Oncology. J Clin Oncol 2002;20:2895–903.
11. Puthawala A, Nisar Syed AM, Gamie S, et al. Interstitial low-dose-rate brachytherapy as a salvage treatment for recurrent head-and-neck cancers: long-term results. Int J Radiat Oncol Biol Phys 2001;5:354–62.
12. Krakoff IH. Systemic treatment of cancer. CA Cancer J Clin 1996;46:134–41.
13. Kramer AM. The role of chemotherapy in head and neck malignancy. Oral Maxillofac Surg Clin North Am 1993;5:303–17.
14. Merlano M, Vitale V, Rosso R, et al. Treatment of advanced squamous cell carcinoma of the head and neck with alternating chemotherapy and radiotherapy. N Engl J Med 1992;327:1115–21.
15. Vokes EE, Weichselbaum RR. Measurable impact: multimodality therapy of head and neck cancer. Int J Radiat Oncol Biol Phys 1993;27:481–2.
16. Adelstein DJ, Adams GL, Li Y. A phase III comparison of standard radiation therapy (RT) versus RT plus concurrent cisplatin (DDP) versus split-course RT plus concurrent DDP and 5-fluorouracil (5-FU) in patients with unresectable SCCHN: an Intergroup Study [abstract 1624]. Proc Am Soc Clin Oncol 2000;19:411.
17. Murphy B, Li Y, Cella D, et al. Phase III study comparing cisplatin and 5-fluorouracil versus cisplatin and paclitaxel in metastatic/recurrent head and neck cancer [abstract 894]. Proc Am Soc Clin Oncol 2001;20:226.

7

Complications of Treatment

SOL SILVERMAN JR., MA, DDS

Cells die in two ways: first and most commonly, by apoptosis (genetically programmed cell death), and second, by necrosis (destruction associated with injury). Radiation and chemotherapy accelerate apoptosis and cause necrosis. Thus, normal tissue functions are altered by therapy, causing signs and symptoms that often limit and/or complicate treatments aimed at eliminating all malignant cells/tissues. Additionally, margins of normal-appearing cells are removed or treated to reduce the risks of recurrences of neoplasia. Still, these patients are at risk for recurrences and of developing second primary head and neck cancers (see Chapter 1, "Epidemiology," and Chapter 5, "Spread of Tumor, Staging, and Survival").

RADIATION EFFECTS

Ionizing radiation delivered in doses intended to kill cancer cells induces unavoidable changes in the surrounding and adjacent normal tissue, causing compromises in function and host defenses and severe complications.[1–4] The degree of these changes is directly proportional to the volume of tissue irradiated and the total dose given and is inversely proportional to the number of fractions and total time in which this dose is delivered. These radiation changes are the direct result of the killing of normal tissue cells as expressed at the tissue level. It is this radiation damage to normal cells that determines the limiting factor in maximal treatment of many cancers. Various techniques, such as intensity-modulated radiation therapy (IMRT) and intraoperative radiation therapy (IORT), as well as certain drugs, are used in an attempt to spare normal cell functions (see Chapter 6, "Treatment") and mitigate the complications of cancer treatments.

The radiation effects associated with treatment of the oral cavity include acute skin reactions or dermatitis, alterations in pigmentation, loss of hair, and delayed skin and subcutaneous changes, including telangiectasia, fibrosis, and edema. Intraoral changes include acute mucositis (erythema, pseudomembrane-covered ulcerations, and hyperkeratosis). Epithelial ulcerations may become so severe as to require a temporary break in treatment to allow some repair. Unfortunately, interruption of treatment also allows for deoxyribonucleic acid (DNA) repair of radiation-damaged malignant cells. Analgesic, antibiotic, and anti-inflammatory medications can be helpful in treating both signs and symptoms. There is also a risk of post-treatment delayed soft tissue necrosis, which may not occur for months or even years. Damage to the bone and its blood supply can result in osteonecrosis and sequestration or progressive osteonecrosis. Radiation changes in the salivary glands result in abnormal saliva (hyposalivation and biochemical changes), as well as the subjective complaint of dry mouth (xerostomia). The altered saliva secondarily leads to decalcification and caries. Overgrowth of candidal fungi (candidiasis) also is a common sequela. Xerostomia is a very common complaint in patients during and following head and neck irradiation. Radiation also directly damages the taste buds. The principal taste buds occur in the tongue, and when they are in the beam of radiation, there is almost always a resultant loss or alteration of taste (dysgeusia, ageusia) that may be transient or sometimes permanent.

Radiation effects on chromosomes (mutagenesis) may predispose cells to subsequent malignant behavior. However, this is usually a long-term effect, which therefore has not been a significant threat or complication in treating adults with head and neck cancers. The loss of salivary protection (quantity and quality) against carcinogens may increase the risks of epithelial neoplasia, particularly in those patients who continue to smoke.

MUCOCUTANEOUS CHANGES

Unless intraoral or interstitial treatment is used, most patients will develop some erythema and moderate tanning of the skin in the treatment portal (Figure 7–1). Interestingly, radiation energy can not only stimulate melanin production and pigmentation, it can also arrest melanocyte production of melanin, leading to white patches (vitiligo). Hair follicles are quite radiosensitive; therefore, if hair is in the treatment beam, it will cease to grow and will fall out. Although this is often transient, it may be permanent.

The acute oral mucosal reaction (mucositis) is secondary to radiation-induced mitotic death of the basal cells in the oral mucosa.[5] Because these cells require about 2 weeks to mature, there is a delay of about 2 weeks between the beginning of radiation therapy and the appearance of mucositis. Inflammation occurs, causing an associated erythema. Oral microorganisms also probably play a role in mucositis, although prophylactic antibiotics do not seem to be helpful in prevention. If the radiation is delivered at a rate equivalent to the ability of the oral mucosa to regenerate, then only mild mucositis will be seen. When the weekly or daily dosage is increased just slightly, destruction (necrosis) will outpace proliferation, and a rather marked mucositis will develop (Figure 7–2). This occurs at dosages above 180 cGy (1 cGy = 1 rad) per day, 5 days per week. The reason for a higher daily dosage (either as one or two fractions) is the possibility of a greater killing effect on cancer cells. Acute mucositis is not related to late radiation-induced atrophy and telangiectasia of the mucosa (Figure 7–3). This late change often increases

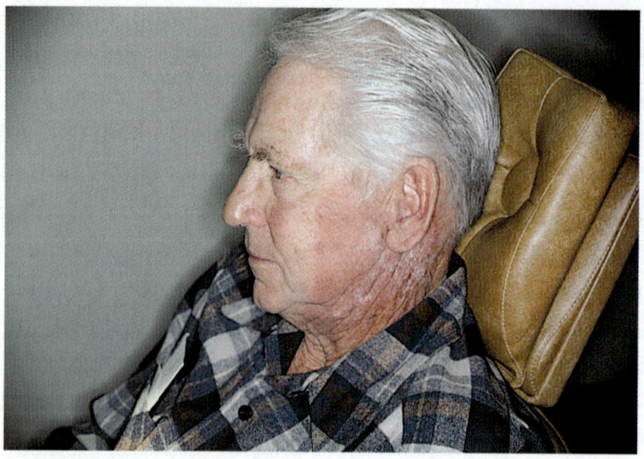

Figure 7–1. This patient had just completed a course of radiotherapy for an oropharyngeal squamous cell carcinoma. Notice skin "burns" outlining the field. The skin reaction slowly resolved with the possibility of a resultant "tanning" or pigmentation and suppressed hair follicles, precluding the need for shaving.

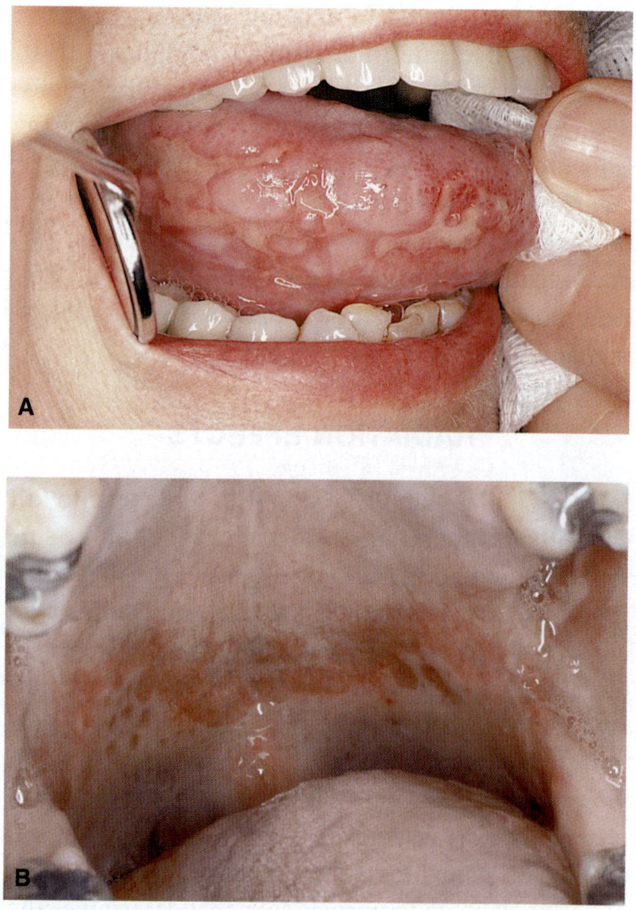

Figure 7–2. *A*, Acute mucositis seen at the fourth week of irradiation (approximately 4,000 cGy). *B*, Acute mucositis of the oropharynx during the fifth week of radiation (approximately 5,000 cGy) for a base of the tongue carcinoma. Analgesics and prednisone systemically controlled the signs and symptoms so that radiation could be continued without interruption. The patient was then able to take in fortified liquids to maintain hydration and minimal nutrition.

the risk of pain and/or necrosis. Mucositis can be so severe as to preclude the intake of even liquids, sometimes forcing interruption of treatment and/or hospitalization. Nasogastric and gastrostomy tubes are used many times to avoid treatment stoppage to allow intake of appropriate nutrients and fluids. Smoking has been associated as a cofactor in worsening acute mucositis reactions.[6]

Management of acute mucositis may sometimes require up to a 3- to 5-day interruption of therapy. Topical anesthetics (viscous lidocaine) may be of some value, but the pain usually requires systemic analgesic drugs, sometimes at the level of morphine.[7,8] However, in many instances, narcotic analgesics are not satisfactorily effective. Because infections may be associated, appropriate diagnosis and antimicrobial agents must be considered for either fungal or bacterial organisms. Viral infections are rarely a complication of radiation-induced mucositis. A short course of systemic prednisone (40 to 80 mg daily for up to 1 week) has been helpful in reducing inflammation and discomfort. There are numerous ongoing multicenter trials seeking to establish the efficacy of agents that will prevent or modify radiation-induced and chemotherapy-associated mucositis.[9] Examples of some of these agents include sialogogues, nonsteroidal anti-inflammatory drugs, and certain prostaglandin analogues. With the increasing use of combined radiation/chemotherapy treatment approaches, the problem of mucositis is increased further.[10]

LOSS OF TASTE

Taste buds, which occur primarily in the circumvallate and fungiform papillae, are very sensitive to radiation.[11] Because of their location in the tongue, they are included in the beam of radiation for most oral cancers. Therefore, patients will develop a partial loss of taste (hypogeusia) or, most usually, complete loss of taste (ageusia) during treatment. The alterations in taste for sweet, sour, bitter, and salt are variable and are caused by damage to the cells in the taste buds and/or their innervating nerve fibers. Often some taste buds are altered, causing confusing perceptions of taste (dysgeusia). The cells comprising taste buds usually will regenerate within 4 months of treatment. However, the degree of long-term impairment of taste is quite variable from patient to patient.

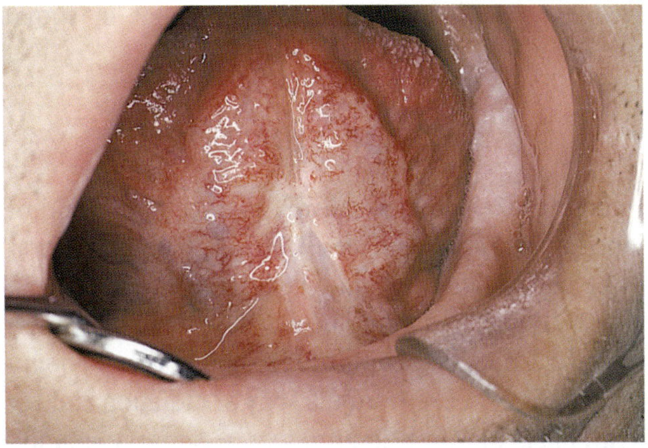

Figure 7–3. This patient had radiotherapy for a carcinoma of the tongue, with resultant tumor control. Note the residual mucosal fibrosis and telangiectasia, which are frequently found in irradiated mucosa.

Dietary consultations regarding recipes with pleasing textures and tastes are essential to improve food intake. However, there are tremendous patient-to-patient differences, which preclude standard recommendations. Failure of taste perception, in addition to pain, dysphagia, hyposalivation, and depression, is associated with the loss of pleasure in eating and thus a loss of appetite. This is compounded by frustrations in food preparation. Weight loss, weakness, malaise, and dehydration often follow. This situation is further complicated when prior surgery has caused problems with mastication and swallowing. Appetite can sometimes be enhanced by megestrol, a hormone, taken in a dosage of 40 mg four times daily, as needed.

Zinc supplements exceeding Dietary Reference Intakes (DRIs) appear to help in some patients (50 to 100 mg elemental zinc daily) to restore or enhance taste.[12,13] This can be prescribed as ZnSO4, 220 mg, taken once or twice daily with food. In addition to improving taste perception in some patients, zinc has occasionally improved saliva production. Although zinc serves as a critical enzyme element in many biochemical reactions, its role in taste and saliva remains unknown. Saliva probably has a modulating effect on the acuity of some tastes (sour, bitter, salt, sweet) through biochemical interactions, as well as providing an ionic environment in signal transduction for taste cells.[14]

SALIVARY FUNCTION

Exposure of the major salivary glands to the field of ionizing radiation induces fibrosis, fatty degeneration, acinar atrophy, and cellular necrosis within glands (Figure 7–4). A critical dose level has not been identified, but complaints of xerostomia usually begin within a few weeks from the start of radiation and for many patients last indefinitely.[15] Salivary gland–sparing techniques (eg, IMRT, cytoprotectants such as amifostine, and prophylactic saliva stimulants such as pilocarpine) have not been predictively effective. The serous acini appear to be more sensitive than the mucinous. Therefore, in addition to diminished glandular secretions, the saliva is thick, sticky, and bothersome to the patient.[16] Some patients are unable to produce more than 1 mL of pooled saliva in 10 minutes and sometimes essentially none.

The duration of this depressed salivary function (hyposalivation) varies from patient to patient. In many patients, there is some regeneration several months after treatment, and the undesirable signs and symptoms of xerostomia (discomfort, difficulty in speech and swallowing) are at least partially reversed. However, recovery of adequate saliva for oral comfort and function may take from 6 to 12 months; in others, the saliva remains inadequate and is the source of major post-treatment complaints. When both parotid glands are exposed to the treatment beam, saliva diminution is most marked, and the prognosis for recovery is the worst. Obviously, the higher the dosage of irradiation, the worse the prognosis for xerostomia and prolonged hyposalivation. Again, IMRT is a function of radiation treatment planning designed to spare salivary glands and preserve function (see Chapter 6). The effectiveness has yet to be completely determined both objectively and subjectively.

Management involves a variety of regimens.[17] Frequent sips of water and water rinses are most commonly used and are essential for partial control of radiation-induced xerostomia. Patients are instructed to carry with them plastic bottles of water for constant use. Sugarless chewing gum and tart candy may be helpful. In some patients, pilocarpine hydrochloride solution (1 mg/mL) or Salagen tablets (5 mg) have been effective in stimulating saliva production.[18–22] Five milligrams, three or four times daily, has been an optimal dosage for most patients. Some patients require up to 30 mg per day, and in others, there is no help at even higher dosages. It is always a balance between the beneficial and adverse effects. The most common side effects include sweating, a "flushed" feeling, and stomach discomfort, but these usually occur only at higher dosages.

Alternative sialogogues are cevimeline (Evoxac, US Food and Drug Administration [FDA] approved

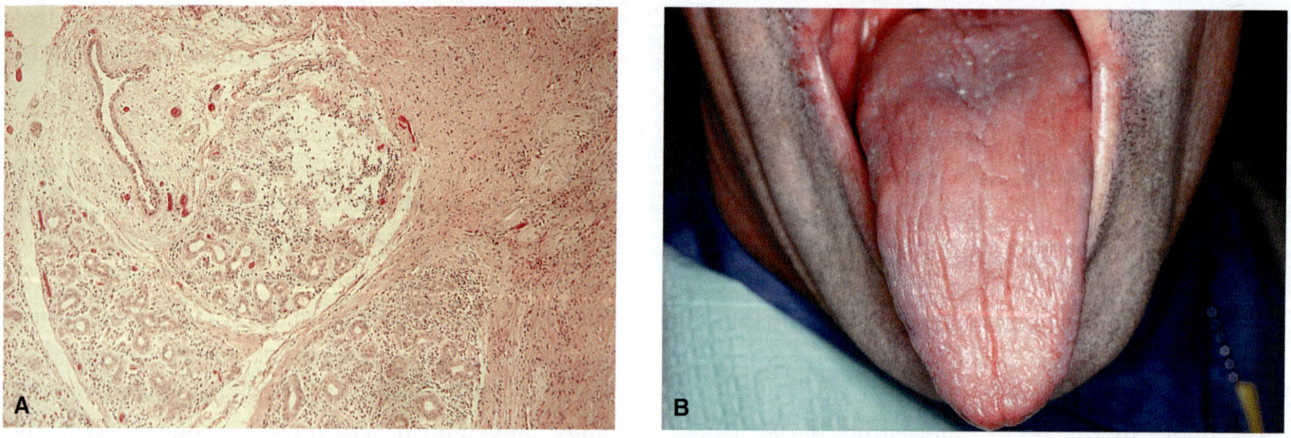

Figure 7–4. *A,* Microscopic view of an irradiated salivary gland. Note the fatty degeneration, inflammatory infiltrate, and absence of acini with relative prominence of remaining ducts. *B,* Hyposalivation and xerostomia are common sequelae and frequently a major complaint from head and neck radiation therapy. The complications include chronic discomfort, difficulties in mastication and swallowing, altered speech, and poor hygiene.

for Sjögren's syndrome), 30 mg three times daily, and bethanechol (Urecholine, FDA approved for improving postsurgical urinary retention), 25 to 50 mg three to four times daily. These drugs are effective for many of the xerostomic irradiated patients suffering from hyposalivation. Prospective comparative controlled studies have not been carried out on these agents. Benefit can usually be determined within a few weeks. Responses are variable, and drug tolerance over time does not seem to be a problem. It is not yet fully apparent that commencing a sialogogue at the time of starting radiation preserves or enhances salivary function, in spite of some reports indicating a positive effect.

In a small, double-blind, controlled study of 12 patients irradiated for head and neck cancer at the Oral Medicine Clinic, University of California at San Francisco (UCSF), pilocarpine administration (15 to 30 mg daily) appeared to be beneficial. All 12 patients had marked xerostomia that had failed to improve even though 6 months had elapsed since radiation treatment. After receiving pilocarpine, 9 of 12 patients improved subjectively, 9 of 12 had increased stimulated parotid flow rates, and 6 of 12 demonstrated improvement in whole saliva volume. While on placebo medication for 3 months, none of the 12 showed objective or subjective benefit. Other studies have reported similar findings.

Synthetic saliva solutions and saliva substitute lubricants have been of limited help in the majority of patients with dry mouth, although some favorable reports have been published.[23] One over-the-counter product (Oral Balance) is helpful for some patients. In patients for whom the salivary complaint is related to "thickness" (excess mucus-type secretions), guaifenesin (Organidin NR) dispensed as a solution or tablets (both to be swallowed) may help as a mucolytic agent (200 to 400 mg three to four times daily).

NUTRITION

Because of painful mucositis, alteration of taste, and degrees of xerostomia, the lack of desire or frank inability to eat is a common—almost universal—complaint in patients receiving external irradiation to the oral cavity. This is particularly the case when the field includes the oropharynx as well as more aggressive therapy in attempts to control tumors. These complications of treatment, in combination with difficulty in mastication and swallowing caused by the tumor and the treatment, will result in weight loss. A marked weight loss tends to produce weakness, inactivity, discouragement, further anorexia, and susceptibility to infection. Therefore, close attention must be given to food intake and weight maintenance during treatment and follow-up (see Chapter 2, "Etiology and Predisposing Factors"). Dietary supplements, menu preparations, and encouragement to eat become important factors. Diets vary, depending on the patient's attitude and effort, previous surgical intervention, saliva and taste status, food texture, and pain.

There is usually little change in the peripheral blood count before, during, or after head and neck treatment, either in response to poorer nutrition or to irradiation. Therefore, anemia, bleeding, or immune deficiencies have not been complications when chemotherapy is not used.

DENTAL CARIES

Patients who have not shown any degree of carious activity for years may develop decalcification, dental decay, and varying degrees of tooth disintegration after irradiation (Figure 7–5).[24] The cervical areas are most typically affected. This condition appears to be attributable to the lack of saliva and to changes in the chemical composition of teeth. One result of radiation xerostomia is a pronounced shift toward a highly acidogenic, highly cariogenic oral microflora. The protective influence of saliva has been demonstrated by the extensive dental destruction found in animals subjected to salivary gland ligation or removal and in patients with xerostomia caused by drugs (eg, diuretics, antidepressants) or disease (eg, Sjögren's syndrome).

Radiation-induced dental effects primarily depend on salivary changes and occur when the glands are included in the field of treatment, not on direct irradiation of the teeth themselves. Direct irradiation of teeth may alter the organic or inor-

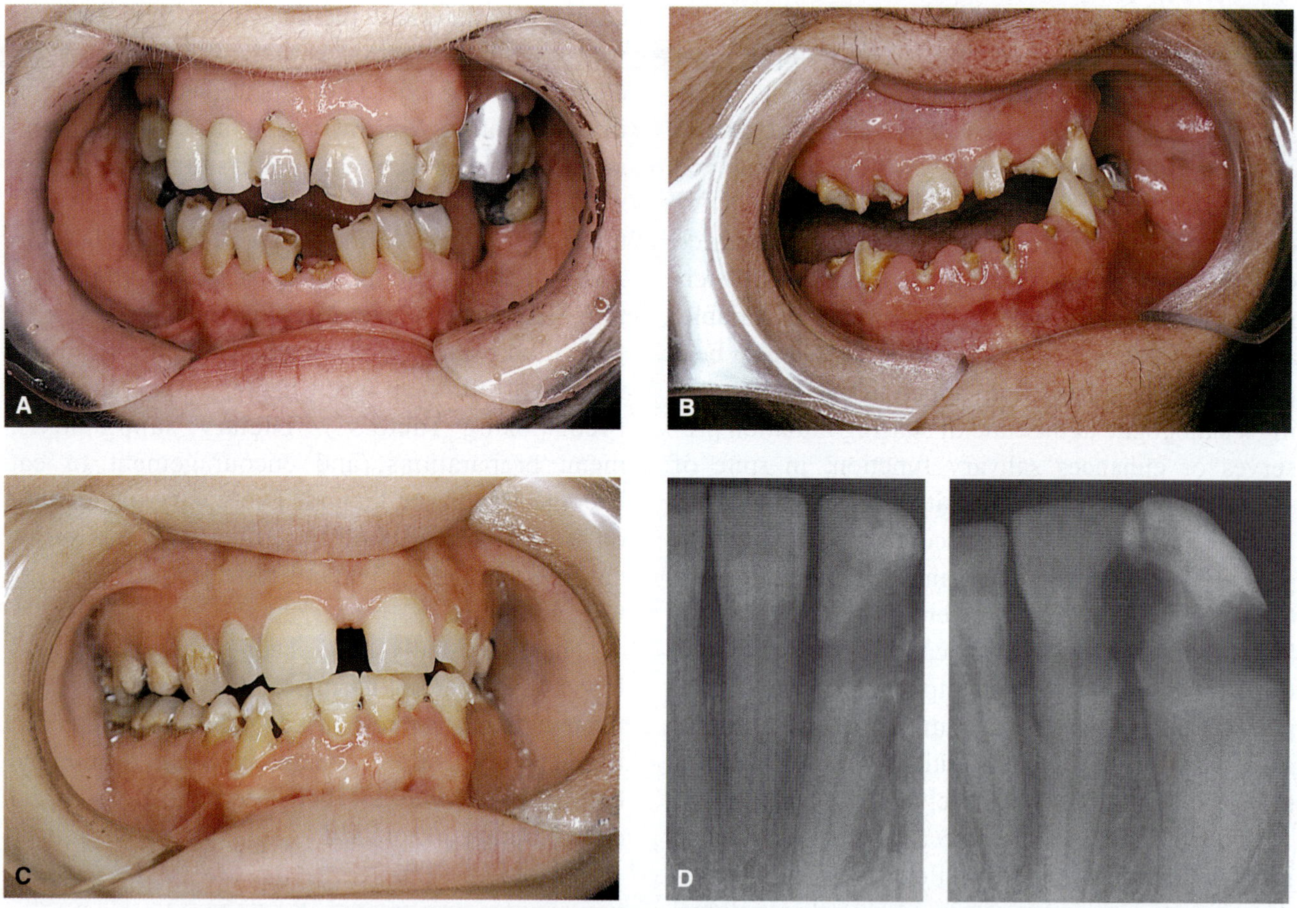

Figure 7–5. *A,* Radiation caries exhibiting commonly found incisal and cervical decalcification. Optimal hygiene, topical fluoride, thorough rinses, and maintenance of mouth moisture minimize this complication of head and neck radiation and xerostomia. *B,* As a result of failure to institute preventive measures or poor patient compliance, dental destruction can cause serious problems with infection, pain, and function. *C,* Note unusual loss of tooth structure in this irradiated patient. *D,* Radiographs of patient in Panel C showing marked dental deterioration.

ganic components in some manner, making them more susceptible to decalcification, but this has not been shown clearly.[25] Remineralization of enamel by salivary substitutes (remineralization solutions and pastes) has been reported. There do not appear to be any clinical or histologic pulpal differences in noncarious human adult teeth, whether they have been in or out of the primary field of radiation. Studies in monkeys have also found no dental pulp damage.

To prevent or at least minimize radiation caries, oral hygiene must be maximal, including intensive home care and frequent office visits for examination and prophylaxis. Mouth rinsing is essential. Antiseptic mouthrinses, such as chlorhexidine, if tolerated, are helpful in eliminating debris and controlling microbial flora. In patients with hypersensitive mucosa, non–alcohol-containing and unflavored mouthrinses are available. Daily topical fluoride applications, as a rinsing solution, a gel delivered by means of a tray, or brushed on as a paste or gel, are all effective.[26,27] Attempts should be made to increase salivary flow either by local or systemic means. Foods and beverages containing sucrose should be avoided as much as possible. If carious lesions develop, removal and restoration should take place immediately. Use of dental radiographs is often indicated to monitor caries activity.[28] In case of pulpal involvement, there are no contraindications for root canal therapy.[29,30]

CANDIDIASIS

Infections of the mouth by *Candida albicans* are commonly seen in irradiated patients (Figure 7–6 and Table 7–1) and are related to the alterations in the saliva.[31,32] Clinically, the signs may be confused with

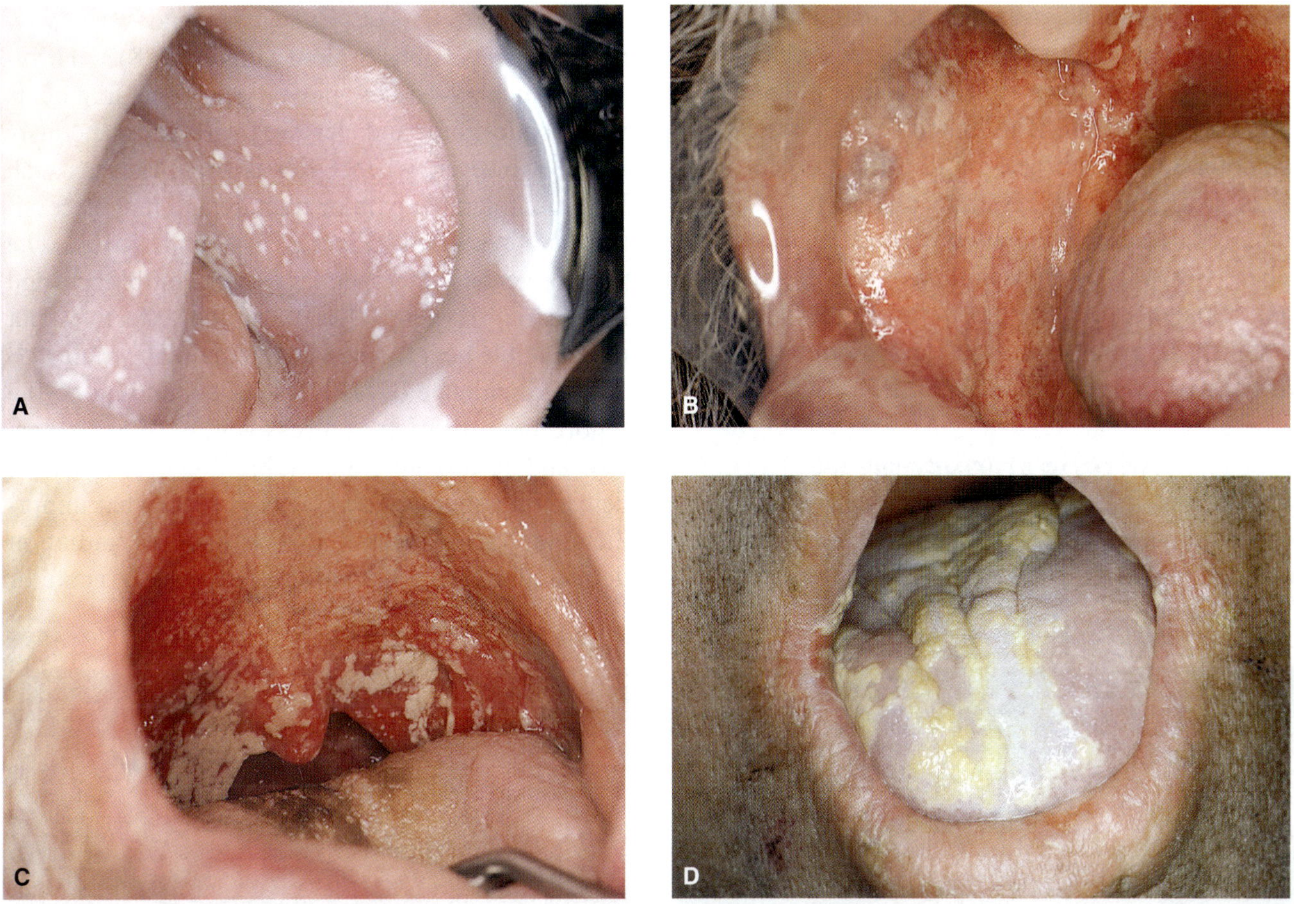

Figure 7–6. *A–D,* Varying appearances of oral candidiasis in irradiated patients with marked hyposalivation/xerostomia.

radiation mucositis or other sources of infection. Candidiasis is usually painful. Management is primarily with the use of antifungal drugs. Systemic administration (200 mg ketoconazole daily with food or fluconazole 100 mg daily) is usually more effective for both response and compliance. Duration of treatment depends on control of signs and recurrences. Obviously, the longer the use, the greater the risk for developing fungal tolerance (resistance). Therefore, limited use as necessary is wise.

Topical administration entails the use of nystatin or clotrimazole troches. Nystatin is used by orally dissolving 100,000 U vaginal troches three to five times daily. Nystatin can also be made up as a mouthwash (100,000 U/mL) to swish and swallow or spit out. Clotrimazole troches (Mycelex) are approved by the FDA as 10 mg troches to be dissolved orally up to five times daily. Alternatively, the clotrimazole 100 or 200 mg vaginal troches are effective when dissolved orally once or twice daily. The use of amphotericin B (1 mL swish and swallow four times daily) can be considered, but the effectiveness has not been well documented. Because of pain from mucositis and dryness, patients may experience difficulty in dissolving tablets topically. Suspensions are another alternative form of treatment, but often this treatment is not as effective as the tablets (possibly because of limited contact time between drug and fungus).

Table 7–1. OCCURRENCE OF ORAL *CANDIDA* IN 109 IRRADIATED ORAL CANCER PATIENTS*

	Candida Culture		
Percent of Patients	Before Therapy	End of Therapy	After Therapy*
41	Negative	Negative	Negative
10	Negative	Negative	Positive
27	Negative	Positive	Positive
22	Positive	Positive	Positive

Data from Silverman et al, 1983 (67 men, 42 women).
*Mean time, 14 months.

These control measures for candidiasis are often used in combination. Antiseptic mouthrinses similar to those used for periodontal/plaque control may be helpful if tolerated (eg, chlorhexidine gluconate or Listerine). In addition, topical (viscous lidocaine) or systemic analgesics may be required. Keeping the mouth moist is essential. There is always the possibility of developing fungal resistance, or the need for higher dosages, when these agents are used for prolonged periods of time.

OSTEORADIONECROSIS

Osteoradionecrosis (ORN) is one of the more serious complications of head and neck irradiation for cancer (Figure 7–7).[33] Bone cells and vascularity may be irreversibly injured (Figure 7–8).[34] Fortunately, in many cases, devitalized bone fragments will sequestrate and lesions will spontaneously heal.[35] However, when ORN is progressive, it can lead to intolerable pain or fracture and may necessitate jaw resection (Figures 7–9 and 7–10). The preventive and therapeutic use of antibiotics and hyperbaric oxygen (HBO) can be effective, but reproducible beneficial results remain uncertain.[36,37]

The incidence of ORN varies depending on the reporting institution, aggressiveness of radiotherapy, and follow-up time (Table 7–2). The risk of developing spontaneous ORN is somewhat unpredictable but is related to the dose of radiation delivered and to bone volume. Obviously, acute or

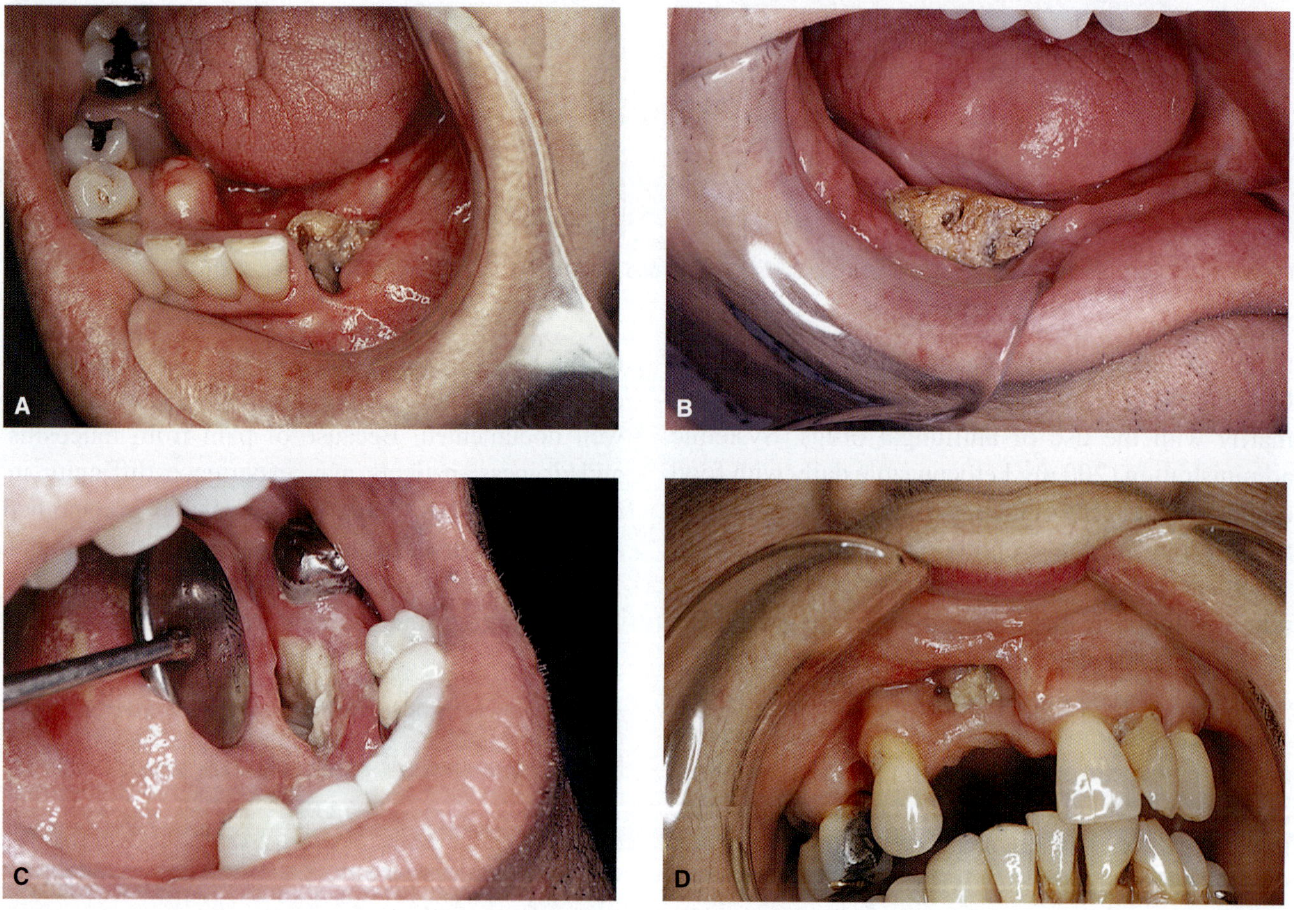

Figure 7–7. Osteoradionecrosis following radiation therapy. *A*, Osteonecrosis following a bicuspid extraction. The mandible had been in the field of radiation for a ventral tongue–floor of the mouth squamous cell carcinoma. After 1 year, the necrotic bone sequestrated. *B*, Spontaneous osteonecrosis 2 years after completion of radiation for a tongue cancer. The patient was not wearing a lower denture. The mandible fractured after 9 months and required a resection. *C*, Spontaneous exposed bone 1 year following radiation for a floor of the mouth carcinoma. Treatment required a surgical resection. *D*, Painful, exposed bone 3 years following radiation for a maxillary sinus malignancy. The necrotic bone sequestrated 4 months after the exposure.

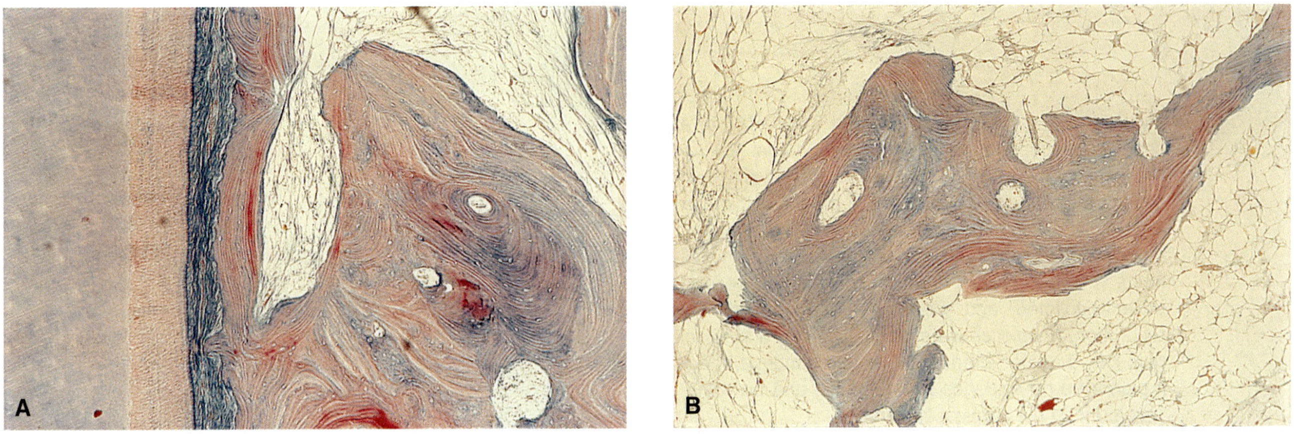

Figure 7–8. Devitalization of bone following radiation therapy. *A,* Note acellularity of periodontal ligament and adjacent alveolar bone. (Left to right, note dentin, cementum, periodontal ligament, lamina dura/trabecular bone). *B,* Trabecular bone and marrow. Note lack of marrow vascularity and fatty degeneration, and absence of trabecular osteoblasts, osteoclasts, and osteocytes.

chronic irritation or trauma to avascular mucosa and bone increases the risk of tissue breakdown and ORN. However, the wearing of dentures does not appear statistically to create a greater risk for ORN (see Chapter 8). The risk seems to be increased in dentulous patients, even more so if the teeth within the treatment field are removed after therapy (see the UCSF study below).[38] Spontaneous bone exposure usually occurs more than 1 year after radiation is completed.

Animal models to study the effects of ionizing radiation on jaw bones have demonstrated changes similar to those observed in human specimens: marrow avascularity and fatty degeneration; reduction of osteocytes, osteoblasts, and osteoclasts; enlarged lacunae; and microfractures.

UCSF Study

To assess the contributory factors in the development of ORN, the records of 100 patients irradiated for head and neck cancer at the UCSF were reviewed retrospectively. The group comprised 60 men and 40 women whose average age was 65 years. At the time of diagnosis, 78 were dentulous and 22 were edentulous. All patients received megavoltage external beam radiotherapy and/or interstitial radium or iridium implants. The maxilla and/or mandible were within the radiation fields. Special care was taken to calculate the bone dose as well as the tumor dose. The dose of external beam radiotherapy was in the range of 5,000 to 7,500 cGy, delivered at 180 cGy per fraction, five daily fractions per week. The total

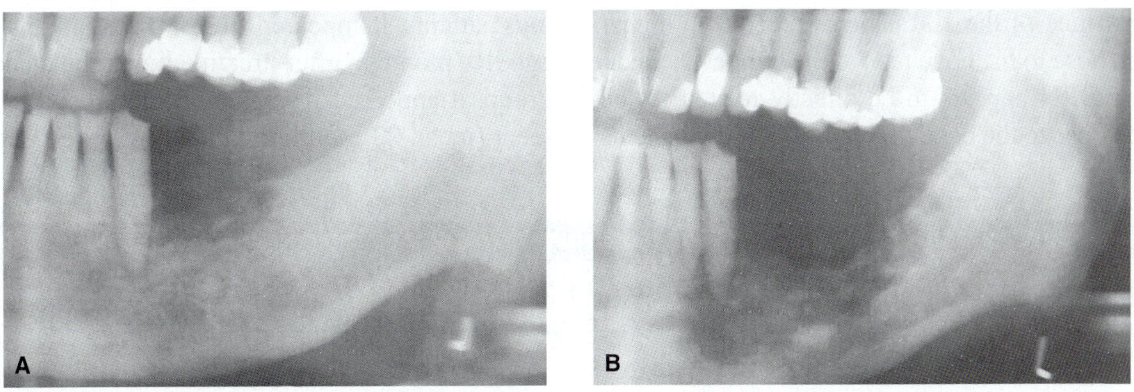

Figure 7–9. This patient was treated with radiotherapy for an anterior floor of the mouth carcinoma. *A,* Almost 2 years later, a painful mandibular osseous lesion became apparent. *B,* One year later, the osteonecrosis progressed, requiring a resection for control.

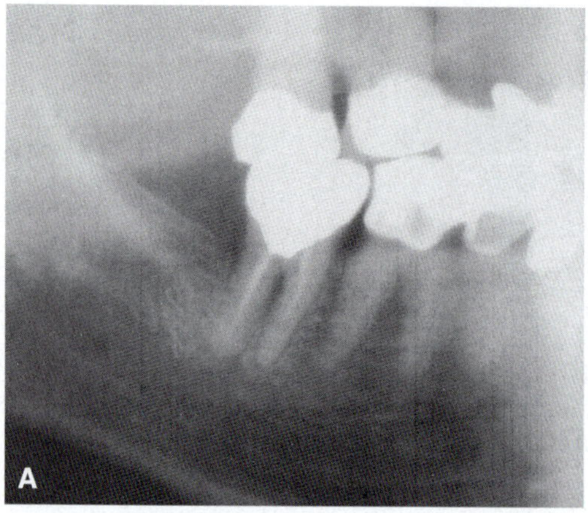

Figure 7–10. This patient received 7,000 cGy for a base of the tongue squamous cell carcinoma. *A*, Preradiation radiograph. *B*, Two years later, the patient developed swelling and pain in the mandibular molar area. Note the bone necrosis. *C*, At 4 years, the osteoradionecrosis continued to increase with frequent bouts of swelling, pain, and suppuration. The second molar exfoliated, and the first molar showed root resorption. Antibiotics were ineffective, and a surgical resection was performed. Magnetic resonance imaging showed no evidence of neoplasia, and no tumor was found in the surgical specimen.

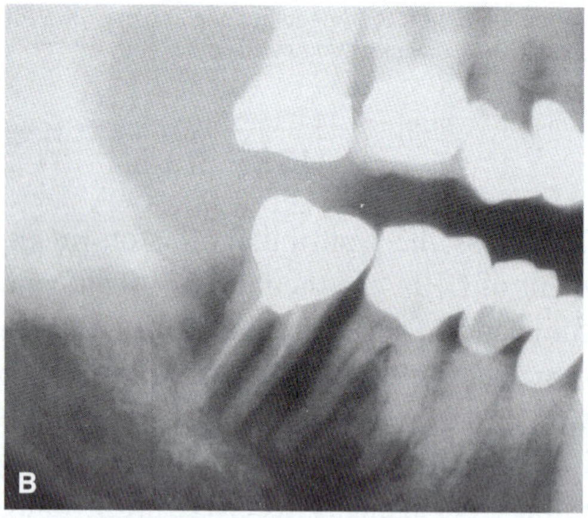

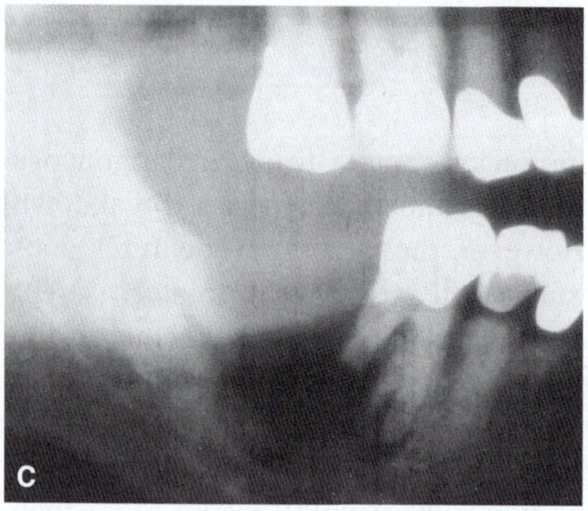

radiation dose included the dose from the external beam and from the interstitial implant.

ORN developed in 22 of these 100 patients. A higher percentage of dentulous patients developed ORN (24%, 19 of 78) than edentulous patients (14%, 3 of 22). All but one necrosis developed in the mandible. There was no correlation between tumor size and the incidence of ORN.

Thirty-nine of the 100 patients received a higher radiation dose to the bone than to the tumor. The incidence of ORN appears to be directly related to the radiation dose to the bone (Table 7–3). Of the patients who received more than 7,500 cGy to the bone, ORN developed in 85% of the dentulous patients and 50% of the edentulous patients. None of the patients who received less than 6,500 cGy developed ORN.

All patients were observed for at least 6 months. The time at which ORN developed was variable. In 15 of the 22 cases, it occurred more than 1 year after radiation treatment was completed. In the edentulous patients, it appeared from 1 to 18 months (average 10 months) after treatment; in the dentulous group, it appeared from 6 to 72 months after treatment (mean 22 months). Follow-up observations of

Table 7–2. REPORTED INCIDENCE OF OSTEONECROSIS IN PATIENTS IRRADIATED FOR HEAD AND NECK CANCER

Source, Year	Hospital	No. of Patients	Years	Dosage (cGy)	Cases of Osteonecrosis
Beumer, 1972	UCSF	278	1961–69	5,000–7,000	10 (4%)
Bedwinek, 1976	MDACC	381	1966–71	6,000–7,500	54 (14%)
Murray, 1980	MDACC	397	1971–75	4,000–> 8,000	77 (19%)
Morrish, 1981	UCSF	100	1971–77	5,000–7,500	22 (22%)

MDACC = M. D. Anderson Cancer Center, Houston, Texas; UCSF = University of California, San Francisco.

Table 7–3. INCIDENCE OF OSTEONECROSIS ACCORDING TO RADIATION DOSE TO BONE

Dose to Bone (cGy)	Incidence of Osteonecrosis	
	Dentulous Patients	Edentulous Patients
< 6,500	0/36 (0%)	0/3 (0%)
6,500–7,500	8/29 (28%)	1/15 (7%)
> 7,500	11/13 (85%)	2/4 (50%)
Total	19/78 (24%)	3/22 (14%)

Data from Morrish RB et al.[38]

those who did not develop ORN ranged from 6 to 76 months (average 24 months).

Table 7–4 shows the incidence of ORN in relation to dental status and extractions. The risk was significantly greater for patients whose teeth were extracted after radiation therapy than for those with extractions before radiation or no extractions at all. Of the 14 dentulous patients who had extractions and developed ORN, the necrosis was associated with dental extraction sites in only 9 and was apparently spontaneous in the remaining 5. All 9 cases of necrosis associated with dental extractions occurred with postradiation extractions.

Certain facts emerge from this study:

1. Patients who were edentulous at the time of diagnosis of cancer had a relatively low risk of ORN.
2. Patients who were dentulous had a greater risk.
3. The increased risk in dentulous patients appeared to be associated with those who had tooth extractions after radiation therapy.
4. Dentulous patients with pretreatment extractions or no extractions appeared to have risks similar to those of the edentulous patients.
5. Spontaneous ORN occurred.
6. The most important risk factor for the development of osteonecrosis appeared to be the radiation dose to the bone, particularly in the mandible.
7. Clinical changes in skin and/or mucosa indicating radiation damage was a risk indicator for ORN.
8. The risk of ORN continued indefinitely following radiation therapy.

The attempt to improve the cure rate in patients with head and neck cancer by means of aggressive radiation therapy, as expected, has led to an increase in complications. For the general principles followed in dental management prior to radiation therapy, see "Treatment Planning" below.

Treatment of ORN

If ORN does not progress clinically or radiographically, the usual management involves periodic observation. Spontaneous sequestration over a period of time often takes place. Analgesic drugs can be taken as needed to control discomfort. The type of analgesic depends on the severity of pain and patient response. If flares of swelling and suppuration occur only occasionally, antibiotics are usually effective. The choice of antibiotic may pose problems (single or combination drugs and dosages), as well as the long-term use with inherent risk of developing microbial tolerance (resistance). If pain and/or flares occur too frequently or present other difficulties for the patient, surgery must be considered. HBO is elective. If it is to be considered, the only possible effectiveness is combining HBO with surgery and antibiotics. HBO involves sequential daily exposure to oxygen under pressure (20 to 30 2-hour daily "dives" at 2 atmospheres oxygen).

Table 7–4. ASSOCIATION BETWEEN DENTAL EXTRACTIONS AND OSTEONECROSIS IN 78 IRRADIATED DENTULOUS PATIENTS

Time of Extractions	Radiation Dose (cGy)		Osteonecrosis	
	Range	Mean	Incidence	Mean Time of Onset after Treatment (mo)
No extractions	6,940–9,280	7,871	5/41 (12%)	29
Before radiotherapy	7,580–9,610	8,500	3/19 (16%)	41
After radiotherapy	6,700–8,100	7,346	11/18 (61%)	20
Total	6,700–9,610	7,666	19/78 (24%)	22

Data from Morrish RB et al.[38] Radiation for dentulous patients without osteonecrosis ranged between 4,950 and 9,700 cGy (mean, 64,50 cGy).

Monochambers and walk-in chambers are available. The basic mechanism is to stimulate angiogenesis (blood vessel proliferation) to promote healing. Vascularized flaps for closure add to the extent, time, and expense of surgery but improve the prognosis for healing. Although no harmful sequelae following HBO have been recorded, the benefits remain unclear. Theoretically, tumor growth could be an issue. The cost, time, and inconvenience remain the main considerations at present. In any event, patients with ORN should be made aware of HBO.

Because higher doses and/or changes in fractionation of radiation increase the risk of necrosis, greater pain, and interference with function, the problem that eventually needs to be addressed is the balance between tumor cure rate and the morbidity associated with more aggressive radiation therapy.

SOFT TISSUE NECROSIS

Soft tissue necrosis may be defined as the occurrence of a mucosal ulcer in irradiated tissue that has no residual cancer (Figures 7–11 and 7–12). The incidence of soft tissue necrosis is related to dose, time, and volume irradiated. The risk is far greater with interstitial implantation and intraoral techniques because of the higher irradiation doses concentrated in a limited field.

In a UCSF study of 278 patients, soft tissue necrosis occurred in 18 cases (6.5%). Eleven of these patients were treated by needle implantation or intraoral cone techniques. The average time of onset was within a year of therapy. Fifteen cases were self-limiting in time periods ranging from 1 to 10 months (average 3 months), but 3 cases required surgical intervention.

Soft tissue necrosis is usually quite painful. Optimal hygiene is required and analgesics are usually helpful, but antibiotics are generally of little help in relieving pain and promoting healing. Because these ulcerations are often at the site of the primary tumor, periodic assessment for recurrence is essential until the necrosis heals.

Dental Treatment Planning

In view of the risk that accompanies high-dose irradiation, special attention to preradiation dental planning is an important function for preventing or minimizing complications stemming from cancer treatment (Figure 7–13). Considerations in the dental management of these patients include the following: (1) anticipated bone dose; (2) pretreatment dental status, dental hygiene, and retention of teeth that will be exposed to high-dose irradiation; (3) extraction techniques; (4) allowance of adequate healing time for teeth extracted before radiotherapy; and (5) patient motivation and capability of compliance with preventive measures.

Because many infections occur months or years after treatment, it is evident that the tissue changes

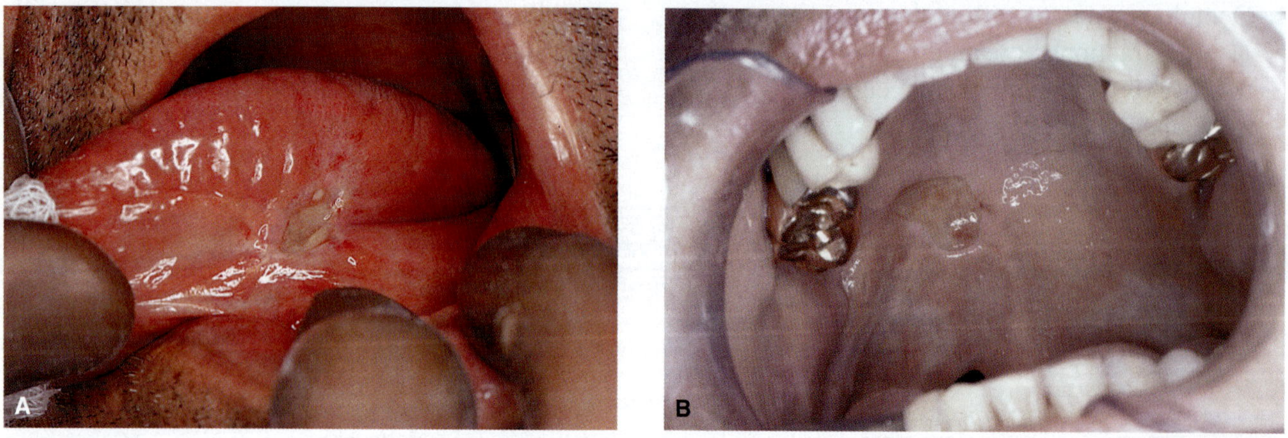

Figure 7–11. *A,* Eight months following brachytherapy for a tongue cancer, this painful necrotic ulcer occurred. After 9 months, the lesion healed. Differentiating necrosis from recurrent tumor sometimes poses a problem. *B,* This immunocompromised liver transplant patient developed a squamous cell carcinoma of the right oropharynx. At 1 year, there was tumor control, but a painful soft tissue necrosis developed. The ulcer healed after 8 months of conservative care.

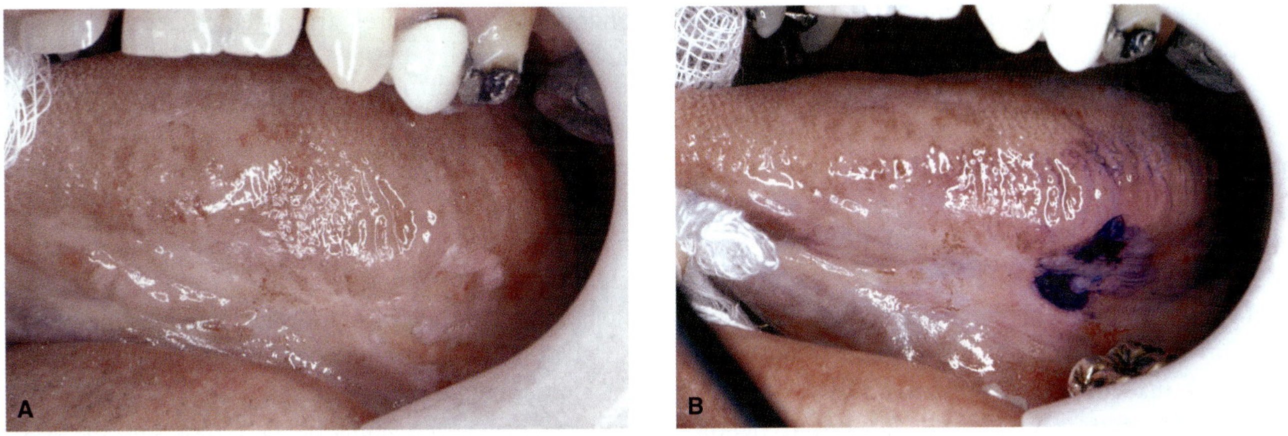

Figure 7–12. This patient was given 6,800 cGy to control a squamous cell carcinoma of the left lateral tongue. Three years following treatment, the patient developed painful ulcerations and mucositis at the previous site of tumor that resembled and were thought to represent a soft tissue necrosis. A biopsy showed recurrent tumor. Note the toluidine blue dye uptake by the tumor.

induced by radiation persist for long periods of time and may be irreversible. Therefore, extreme care must be taken in evaluating the status of the teeth and periodontium before, during, and after treatment, and optimal oral and periodontal hygiene must be maintained because of the lowered biologic potential for healing in response to physical irritation, chemical agents, and microbial organisms. Such attention is critical because of the potentially progressive nature of ORN, which may involve large segments of bone and present a major therapeutic problem, possibly requiring extensive resection.

It is impossible to establish precise formulas for managing preradiation and postradiation dental problems. Extractions are considered primarily for teeth with a poor prognosis owing to such conditions as advanced periodontal disease, extensive caries activity, and periapical lesions. Other considerations are dental sources of chronic soft tissue irritation (trauma) and the degree of patient cooperation in preventive home care and dental office programs. The decision is modified further for each patient on the basis of the individual's prognosis, age, desires, economic aspects, and radiation delivery.

Reported studies and personal experience do not substantiate the practice of extracting all remaining teeth before treatment as a good or reasonable preventive measure. However, teeth with poor prognoses (eg, advanced periodontal disease, pulpal involvement from caries neglect) that require extrac-

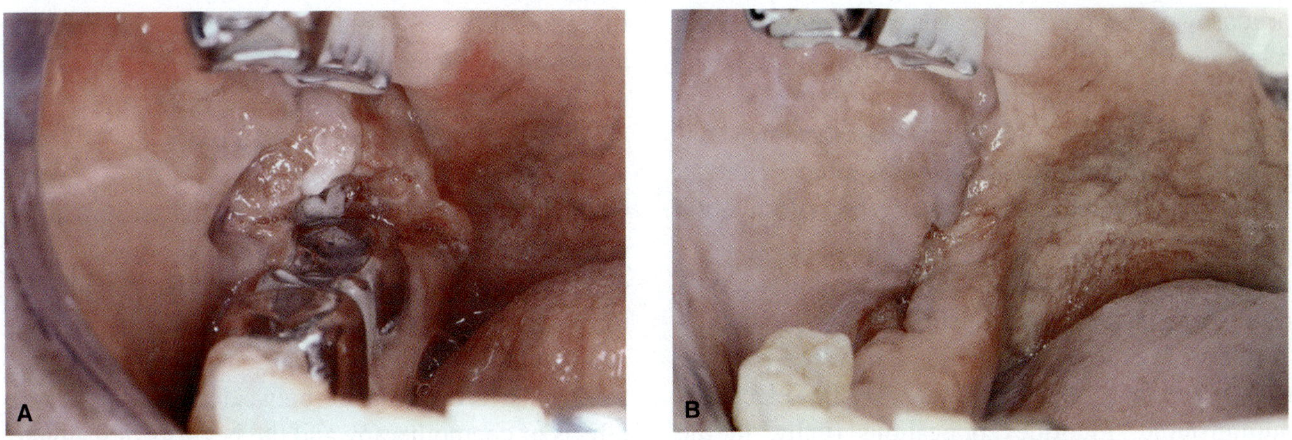

Figure 7–13. This patient was seen for a squamous carcinoma involving the oropharynx and extending to the buccal mucosa. The treatment plan involved primary radiation therapy. *A*, Pretreatment status, requiring molar extractions and commencing the use of a high-potency fluoride dentifrice. Ten days were allowed for postextraction healing. *B*, Five years following treatment, tumor control continued, the patient was asymptomatic, hygiene was good, and there was no evidence of osteoradionecrosis.

tion should have this done before radiation is started to minimize complications/infection during and after therapy. When teeth are extracted either before or after radiation, the alveolar bone must be evenly trimmed and carefully smoothed so that primary tissue closure is possible. This is necessary because suppression of bone cell viability diminishes remodeling, and if a suitable alveolectomy is not performed, the resulting alveolar ridge will be irregular and may increase the risk of subsequent bone exposure and discomfort. A minimum of 1 week to 10 days is arbitrarily allowed for initial healing before radiation is instituted. However, if the situation permits, more time is preferable, up to 14 or even 21 days. Because dosages are fractionated, healing can usually continue before damaging levels of radiation are delivered to a surgical area. Obviously, teeth completely out of the treatment field are not affected similarly. Additionally, the risk of complications is greater for the mandible compared with the maxilla. An explanation is unknown, although it might be related to blood supply.

There is no evidence as to how many teeth should be extracted at one time. Therefore, whether before or after irradiation, all of the teeth indicated for removal are extracted to suit the needs of the surgeon and patient. The use of antibiotics during the healing period is important to control potential infection.

Whenever possible, an attempt is made to retain teeth to support tooth-borne appliances for the tentatively planned rehabilitation of these patients (see Chapter 8). It must be recalled that many teeth, either primarily or secondarily exposed to radiation, remain relatively free of disease and functional for long periods of time. This significantly facilitates rehabilitation. However, tissue-borne prostheses are not contraindicated. In general, mucosa that appears fibrous, telangiectatic, and atrophic (a reflection of radiation damage) is at greater risk for complications.

The periodontium is maintained in optimal condition by periodic routine periodontal procedures.[39] When areas exposed to radiation are treated, extreme care is exercised and antibiotics may be selectively administered. Fluoride applications (daily, in the form of mouthrinses or gels) appear to aid in minimizing tooth decalcification and caries in these patients. There are no unusual contraindications for endodontic procedures for infected teeth that are useful to retain.

Review of the literature and our own experience indicate that carefully controlled studies are necessary before more definitive guidelines can be formulated for managing dental structures that have been or are to be irradiated. This is particularly true because of newer regimens for delivering radiation, as well as combinations with chemotherapy, to attain better responses and survival rates. Until such information is available, each case must be managed individually, based on the patient's needs, the status of the tumor, and the risks known to exist for dental health in irradiated tissues. An overall "one-type" empirical approach for all patients is contraindicated.[35] Additionally, initial patient orientation to mucositis, xerostomia, taste and appetite loss, difficulties with nutritional intake, weight maintenance, and risks associated with continued smoking is critically important to create an understanding of responses to therapy, compliance issues, an acceptable attitude for coping (quality of life), and an optimal outcome.[3]

SURGERY

As indicated, surgical approaches to cancer control include removal of malignant and adjacent normal tissue (margins) in an attempt to remove all cancerous cells. This surgery results in defects that cause problems with appearance and function, which, in turn, can cause severe emotional disturbances. If the margins are inadequate, recurrences follow. Rehabilitation is usually planned at the time of initial treatment (see Chapter 8).

CHEMOTHERAPY

Chemotherapy alone is not an effective treatment for curing oral cancers, although some regimens can enhance radiation and surgery (see Chapter 6). The toxic effects of chemotherapy are usually acute and add to the morbidity of treatment. Therefore, treatment must often balance between the adverse side effects of chemotherapy and the benefits of trying to increase response and survival.

When using cytotoxic chemotherapeutic drugs, it is extremely important to keep patients free from the oral foci of infection and pain to minimize local infection and bacteremia and to enable patients to maintain a nutritious diet. Good oral hygiene (office and home care) is necessary. Nausea is an added and significant problem. The chemotherapeutic agents used to eradicate tumor production also adversely affect normal cells, particularly those that have relatively high turnover rates, such as oral epithelial tissues. The depressant effect of therapy on oral epithelial mitoses can result in thinning and ulceration of the tissues as well as intensify salivary gland and taste dysfunctions. The oral ulcerations may be attributable to direct cellular cytotoxicity from the chemotherapeutic agents, increased susceptibility to microorganisms owing to neutropenia (bone marrow suppression), trauma, or a combination of these factors. Maintaining hydration and adequate nutritional intake are often problems requiring special attention. Feeding tubes (nasogastric, gastrostomy) are frequently the best solution.

It is important to realize that the ability of oral tissues to resist trauma and to repair themselves is significantly compromised, and even irritation from eating and talking can lead to mucosal breakdown. Because continued therapy further induces myelosuppression, leukopenia, and thrombocytopenia, patients grow even more susceptible to infection and bleeding, necessitating special care and precautions. A patient's medical oncologist should be informed of planned dental procedures to confirm if any contraindications exist or if certain precautions/regimens are indicated for oral/dental care (see Chapter 9).

The increased risk of infection is particularly meaningful. The consequences of periodontal and dental infections may be complex and may complicate patient care. Furthermore, the oral cavity can be the site of infections caused by viruses, fungi, and acquired bacterial pathogens. Oral foci of infection can lead to bacteremias, fever, and pain. The reactivation of herpes family viruses such as herpes simplex 1 and varicella zoster can cause significant mucosal breakdown, pain, and hemorrhage and can increase the risk of secondary infection. Fungal infection caused by *Candida* and *Aspergillus* species, in addition to producing local disease, can spread systemically and cause serious infections. Infections can be caused by an overgrowth of bacterial organisms normally found in the oral cavity, as well as by a number of opportunistic pathogenic bacteria, such as *Pseudomonas*, *Klebsiella*, *Serratia*, *Escherichia*, and other gram-negative bacteria. Identification of the source of infection and appropriate selection of antimicrobial agent(s) are critical to effective management.

Children who receive chemotherapy when permanent teeth are developing may suffer a number of abnormalities involving teeth and jaws. These include complete or partial dental agenesis, root malformation, and maldevelopment of jaws.

REFERENCES

1. Cooper JS, Fu K, Marks J, Silverman S Jr. Late effects of radiation therapy in the head and neck region. Int J Radiat Oncol Biol Phys 1995;31:1141–64.
2. Goldstein M, Maxymiw WG, Cummings BJ, Wood RE. The effects of antitumor irradiation on mandibular opening and mobility. A prospective study of 58 patients. Oral Surg Oral Med Oral Pathol Oral Radiol Endod 1999;88:365–73.
3. List MA, Rutherford JL, Stracks J, et al. An exploration of the pretreatment coping strategies of patients with carcinoma of the head and neck. Cancer 2002;95:98–104.
4. Nguyen NP, Sallah S, Karlsson U, Antoine JE. Combined chemotherapy and radiation therapy for head and neck malignancies: quality of life issues. Cancer 2002;94: 1131–41.
5. Dumbrigue HB, Sandow PL, Nguyen K-H, et al. Salivary epidermal growth factor levels decrease in patients receiving radiation therapy to the head and neck. Oral Surg Oral Med Oral Pathol Oral Radiol Endod 2000;89:710–6.
6. Rugg T, Saunders MI, Dische S. Smoking and mucosal reactions to radiotherapy. Br J Radiol 1990;63:554–6.
7. Bruera E, Pereira J, Watanabe S, et al. Opioid rotation in patients with cancer pain. A retrospective comparison of dose ratios between methadone, hydromorphone, and morphine. Cancer 1996;78:852–7.
8. Levy MH. Pharmacologic treatment of cancer pain. N Engl J Med 1996;335:1124–32.
9. Migliorati C, Massumoto C, de Paula Eduardo F, et al. Low-energy laser therapy in oral mucositis. J Oral Laser Applications 2001;1:97–101.
10. Kostler WJ, Hejna M, Wenzel C, Zielinski CC. Oral mucositis complicating chemotherapy and/or radiotherapy: options for prevention and treatment. CA Cancer J Clin 2001;51:290–315.
11. Comeau TB, Epstein JB, Migas C. Taste and smell dysfunction in patients receiving chemotherapy: a review of current knowledge. Support Care Cancer 2001;9:575–80.
12. Ripamonte C, Zecca E, Brunelli C, et al. A randomized, controlled clinical trial to evaluate the effects of zinc sulfate on cancer patients with taste alterations caused by head and neck irradiation. Cancer 1998;82:1938–45.
13. Silverman JE, Weber CW, Silverman S Jr, et al. Zinc supple-

mentation and taste in head and neck cancer patients undergoing radiation therapy. J Oral Med 1983;38:14–6.
14. Spielman AI. Interaction of saliva and taste. J Dent Res 1990; 69:838–43.
15. Torres SR, Peixoto CB, Caldas DM, et al. Relationship between salivary flow rates and *Candida* counts in subjects with xerostomia. Oral Surg Oral Med Oral Pathol Oral Radiol Endod 2002;93:149–54.
16. Makkonen TA, Tenovuo J, Vilja P, et al. Changes in the protein composition of whole saliva during radiotherapy on patients with oral oropharyngeal cancer. Oral Surg Oral Med Oral Pathol 1986;62:270–5.
17. Johnstone PAS, Niemtzow RC, Riffenburgh RH. Acupuncture for xerostomia. Cancer 2002;94:1151–6.
18. Johnson JT, Ferretti GA, Nethery WJ, et al. Oral pilocarpine for post-irradiation xerostomia in patients with head and neck cancer. N Engl J Med 1993;329:390–5.
19. Lockhart PB, Fox PC, Gentry AC, et al. Pilot study of controlled-release pilocarpine in normal subjects. Oral Surg Oral Med Oral Pathol Oral Radiol Endod 1996;82:517–24.
20. Niedermeier W, Matthaeus C, Meyer C, et al. Radiation-induced hyposalivation and its treatment with oral pilocarpine. Oral Surg Oral Med Oral Pathol Oral Radiol Endod 1998;86:541–9.
21. Reikle JW, Hafermann MD, Johnson JT, et al. Oral pilocarpine for radiation-induced xerostomia: integrated efficacy and safety results from two prospective randomized clinical trials. Int J Radiat Oncol Biol Phys 1995;31:661–9.
22. Rode M, Smid L, Budihna M, et al. The influence of pilocarpine and biperiden on pH value and calcium, phosphate, and bicarbonate concentrations in saliva during and after radiotherapy for head and neck cancer. Oral Surg Oral Med Oral Pathol Oral Radiol Endod 2001;92:509–14.
23. Levine MJ, Aguirre A, Hatton MN, et al. Artificial salivas: present and future. J Dent Res 1987;66:693–8.
24. Keene HJ, Fleming TJ. Prevalence of caries-associated microflora after radiotherapy in patients with cancer of the head and neck. Oral Surg Oral Med Oral Pathol 1987; 64:421–6.
25. Kielbassa AM, Munz I, Bruggmoser G, Schulte-Monting J. Effect of demineralization and remineralization on microhardness of irradiated dentin. J Clin Dent 2002;13:104–10.
26. Epstein JB, van der Meij EH, Lunn R, et al. Effects of compliance with fluoride gel application on caries and caries risk in patients after radiation therapy for head and neck cancer. Oral Surg Oral Med Oral Pathol Oral Radiol Endod 1996;82:268–75.
27. Epstein JB, Chin EA, Jacobson JJ, et al. The relationships among fluoride, cariogenic oral flora, and salivary flow rate during radiation therapy. Oral Surg Oral Med Oral Pathol Oral Radiol Endod 1998;86:286–92.
28. Jones GA, Purdy RB, Stoker JW, Palmer JW 4th. Use of dental x-rays on postirradiated patients with head and neck cancer. J Am Dent Assoc 1988;117:599–600.
29. Lilly JP, Cox D, Arcuri M, Krell KV. An evaluation of root canal treatment in patients who have received irradiation to the mandible and maxilla. Oral Surg Oral Med Oral Pathol Oral Radiol Endod 1998;86:224–6.
30. Seto BG, Beumer J III, Kagawa T, et al. Analysis of endodontic therapy in patients irradiated for head and neck cancer. Oral Surg Oral Med Oral Pathol 1985;60:540–5.
31. Ramirez-Amador V, Silverman S Jr, Mayer P, et al. Candidal colonization and oral candidiasis in patients undergoing oral and pharyngeal radiation therapy. Oral Surg Oral Med Oral Pathol Oral Radiol Endod 1997;84:149–53.
32. Rossie KM, Taylor J, Beck FM, et al. Influence of radiation therapy on oral *Candida albicans* colonization: a quantitative assessment. Oral Surg Oral Med Oral Pathol 1987; 64:698–701.
33. Epstein J, van der Meit E, McKenzie M, et al. Postradiation osteonecrosis of the mandible. Oral Surg Oral Med Oral Pathol Oral Radiol Endod 1997;83:657–62.
34. Marx RE, Johnson RP. Studies in the radiobiology of osteoradionecrosis and their clinical significance. Oral Surg Oral Med Oral Pathol 1987;64:379–90.
35. Wong JK, Wood RE, McLean M. Conservative management of osteoradionecrosis. Oral Surg Oral Med Oral Pathol Oral Radiol Endod 1997;84:16–21.
36. Tibbles PM, Edelsberg JS. Hyperbaric-oxygen therapy. N Engl J Med 1996;335:1642–8.
37. van Merkesteyn JPR, Baker DJ, Borgmeijer-Hoelen AMMJ. Hyperbaric oxygen treatment of osteoradionecrosis of the mandible. Oral Surg Oral Med Oral Pathol Oral Radiol Endod 1995;80:12–6.
38. Morrish RB, Chan E, Silverman S Jr, et al. Osteonecrosis in patients irradiated for head and neck carcinoma. Cancer 1981;47:1980–3.
39. Toljanic JA, Siddiqui AA, Patterson GL, Irwin ME. An evaluation of a dentifrice containing salivary peroxidase elements for the control of gingival disease in patients with irradiated head and neck cancer. J Prosthet Dent 1996;76:292–6.
40. Beumer J, Silverman S Jr, Benak S. Hard and soft tissue necroses following radiation therapy for oral cancer. J Pros Dent 1972;27:640–4.
41. Bedwinek J, Shukovsky LJ, Fletcher GH, Daley TE. Osteonecrosis in patients treated with definitive radiotherapy for squamous cell carcinomas of the oral cavity and naso- and oropharynx. Radiology 1976;119:665–7.
42. Murray CG, Herson J, Daly TE, et al. Radiation necrosis of the mandible: A 10-year study. Int J Rad Oncol Biol Phys 1980; 6:543–8.
43. Morrish RB, Chan E, Silverman S Jr, et al. Osteonecrosis in patients irradiated for head and neck carcinoma. Cancer 1981;47:1980–8.

8

Restoration of Palate, Tongue, Mandible, and Facial Defects

JOHN BEUMER III, DDS, MS
IAN M. ZLOTOLOW, DMD
ARUN B. SHARMA, BDS, MSc

Treatment of oral and facial cancers can result in severe oral dysfunction and facial disfigurement, but today it is possible to restore almost all patients to near-normal form and function, enabling them to continue to have useful and productive lives. In the late 1980s, several technical improvements were made—for example, the development of osseointegrated dental implants and free vascularized flaps—but, in recent times, the most significant improvements have been the result of improved collaborations between medical and dental researchers and clinicians. In the leading cancer centers of the world, rehabilitation specialists see and examine the patient prior to their cancer treatment and work with their colleagues in surgical oncology, reconstructive surgery, or radiation oncology to minimize post-treatment morbidities and to develop plans to rehabilitate the patient. Our colleagues in surgery and radiation therapy have begun to realize that minor alterations in their surgical procedures or slight changes in the fields of radiation can have a significant impact on the eventual post-treatment function and appearance of the patient. At present, with a proper multidisciplinary approach to patient care, almost all patients with oral or facial cancer can be very effectively rehabilitated, retaining their ability to speak, swallow, masticate, and control their saliva and enabling them to interact socially with family, friends, and professional colleagues.

Patients with head and neck cancer who require maxillofacial rehabilitation may be arbitrarily classified according to their post-treatment surgical defects and morbidity, which include maxillary, tongue, mandible, and facial defects.

MAXILLARY DEFECTS

Most tumors of the paranasal sinus, palatal epithelium, or minor salivary glands require either a partial or a radical maxillectomy. A radical maxillectomy entails resection of the entire maxilla to the midline, usually with exposure gained by reflection of a lip and cheek flap. A partial maxillectomy is less encompassing and may be performed transorally. The amount of soft palate included in these resections is variable and depends on the site and extensions of the tumor.

Disabilities

Defects of the hard or soft palate produce a variety of problems: hypernasality makes speech unintelligible; mastication efficiency is compromised, particularly for the edentulous patient, because denture-bearing tissue surfaces are lost, and support, stability, and retention of the maxillary prosthesis are compromised; swallowing is awkward because food and liquids may be forced up into the nasal cavity and out the nose; the nasal mucous membranes become desiccated by abnormal exposure to the oral environment; nasal and sinus secretions collect in the defect area; and facial disfigurement can result from a lack of midface bony support or resection of a branch of the facial nerve. In some cases, tumor invasion superiorly requires exenteration of the orbital contents.

Rehabilitation after resection of the hard or soft palate is best accomplished prosthodontically. Customarily, a temporary prosthesis, known as an immediate surgical obturator, is placed at the time of surgery. During the healing period, this prosthesis is relined periodically with temporary denture reliners to compensate for tissue changes secondary to organization and contracture of the tissues adjacent to the defect. When these tissues become well healed and dimensionally stable (usually 3 to 4 months after surgery), the definitive prosthesis is made.

Inadequate retention, stability, and support are the main problems associated with the use of an obturator prosthesis. The remaining teeth, therefore, become extremely valuable in providing support, retention, and stability for these restorations. Unilateral prostheses are particularly difficult because movement of the prosthesis during function may accelerate resorption of alveolar bone and subject abutment teeth to excessive stresses. The purpose of these prostheses is to restore the physical separation between the oral and nasal cavities, thereby restoring speech and swallowing to normal, and to provide support for the lip and cheek.

Treatment

It is essential that the prosthodontist examine and consult with the patient before surgery. The sequence of treatment should be explained to the patient, and diagnostic casts and appropriate radiographs should be obtained. With this information, the prosthodontist is ready to consult with the surgeon about the design and fabrication of the surgical obturator. Modifications in the surgical plan that may improve the prosthetic prognosis without adversely affecting tumor removal should be discussed at this time.

The surgeon can improve the prosthetic prognosis by considering the following modifications[1]:

1. A split-thickness skin graft should be used to line the raw cheek surface of the defect. The skin graft prevents contracture of the cheek flap, provides a keratinized surface to support and stabilize the prosthesis, and forms a scar band at the junction of the skin graft and oral mucosa that can be engaged prosthodontically to improve retention, stability, and support (Figure 8–1).
2. If the surgeon can save some of the palatal mucosa normally included in the palatal resection and reflect this tissue during the bony resection of the palate, it can later be used to cover the medial cut margin of the palatal bone. If this palatal margin of the defect is covered with keratinized mucosa, the prosthesis may engage this surface more completely, thus improving its lateral stability.
3. An attempt should be made to save as much of the maxilla as possible, consistent with tumor control. The more palatal shelf area that remains, the more support will be provided for an obturator prosthesis. Retaining the premaxillary segment is particularly advantageous.

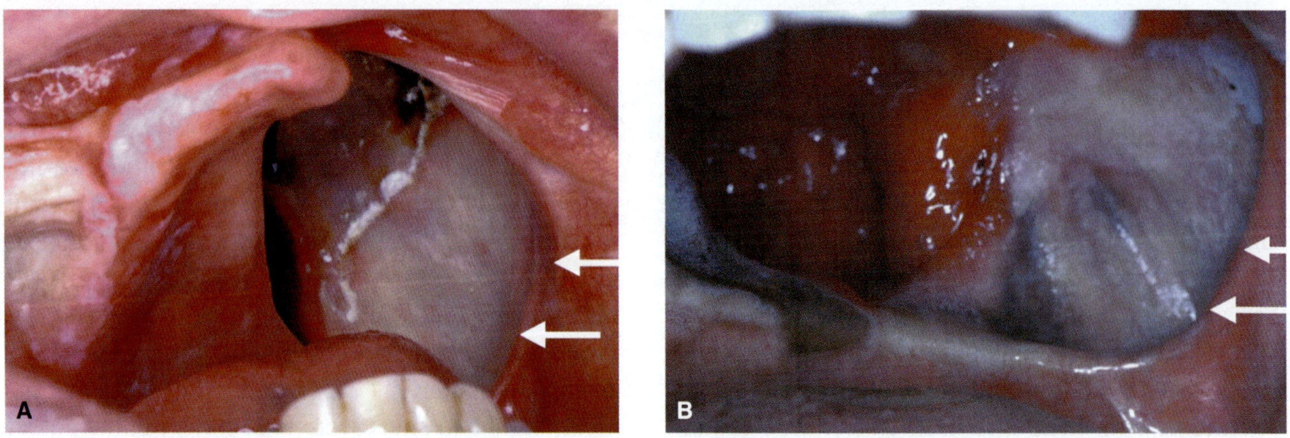

Figure 8–1. A split-thickness skin graft lining the lateral wall of a radical maxillectomy defect greatly enhances the effectiveness of prosthetic rehabilitation. Note undercuts superior to the skin graft mucosal junction (*arrows*).

4. The transalveolar bony resection should be made as far from the tooth adjacent to the proposed defect as feasible. This practice leaves more bone around this tooth, improving its prognosis as a partial denture abutment.
5. If the soft palate does not retain the ability to effect velopharyngeal closure, it should be resected on the side of the tumor. If a posterior, nonfunctioning band of soft palate remains after surgery, it often prevents proper placement of the palatopharyngeal extension of the obturator prosthesis, compromising speech and swallowing (Figure 8–2).
6. In edentulous patients, the placement of osseointegrated implants into appropriate maxillary sites should be considered for patients not scheduled for postoperative radiation. These implants can be used later to facilitate the retention and stability of, and support for, the future obturator prosthesis.

Immediate Surgical Obturator

Immediate or early restoration of a palatal defect with an obturator will greatly simplify the patient's postoperative course. The obturator provides a matrix on which the surgical packing can be placed, minimizes contamination of the wound in the immediate postoperative period, and enables the patient to speak and swallow effectively immediately after surgery.

To fabricate the prosthesis, an irreversible hydrocolloid impression is obtained of the maxillary arch and the anterior portion of the soft palate, and the cast is retrieved. The obturator's size is determined by the surgical boundaries of the resection, as indicated by the surgeon. In the dentulous patient, teeth in the path of the surgical resection are removed from the cast (Figure 8–3). Care should be taken to extend thc surgical obturator posteriorly past the proposed posterior soft palatal resection line to effectively seal off the defect. These prostheses are processed in autopolymerizing methyl methacrylate. They can be altered at surgery by trimming or by adding a temporary denture reliner. The prosthesis is wired to the remaining teeth, alveolar ridge, or other available structures (eg, zygomatic arch, anterior nasal spine) (Figure 8–4).

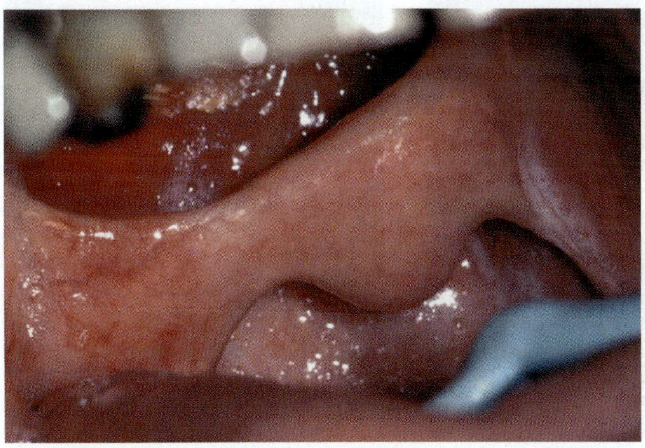

Figure 8–2. This nonfunctional posterior band of soft palate prevents optimal positioning of a pharyngeal obturator extension.

After the surgical packing is removed (6 to 10 days after surgery), the prosthesis is relined with a temporary denture reliner. As healing progresses, the obturator is periodically relined and extended further into the defect, adaptation is improved, and anterior teeth are added as necessary. Three to 5 months after surgery, and after initial wound contracture is essentially complete, the definitive prosthesis is begun. Edentulous patients with maxillary defects often require a longer period of healing because the defect must be engaged more aggressively to maximize stability, support, and retention.

Definitive Obturator Prosthesis

Defects of the hard palate are restored most effectively with a prosthesis. Teeth greatly improve denture retention and stability. Speech, swallowing, mastication, and facial contour can be restored with proper extensions and obturation. The obturator should extend maximally up the lateral wall of the defect (Figure 8–5). This high lateral extension increases retention and lateral stability and provides support for the lip and cheek. The movement of the medial side of the ramus into the distolateral area of the defect must be accounted for during border molding and final impression procedures. The extension superiorly along the medial margin of the defect should not exceed the level of the repositioned palatal mucosa. Further superior extension will impede normal nasal airflow and may result in unnecessary and painful ulceration of the respiratory mucosa lining the nasal septum. In some patients, extension across the nasal surface of the soft palate

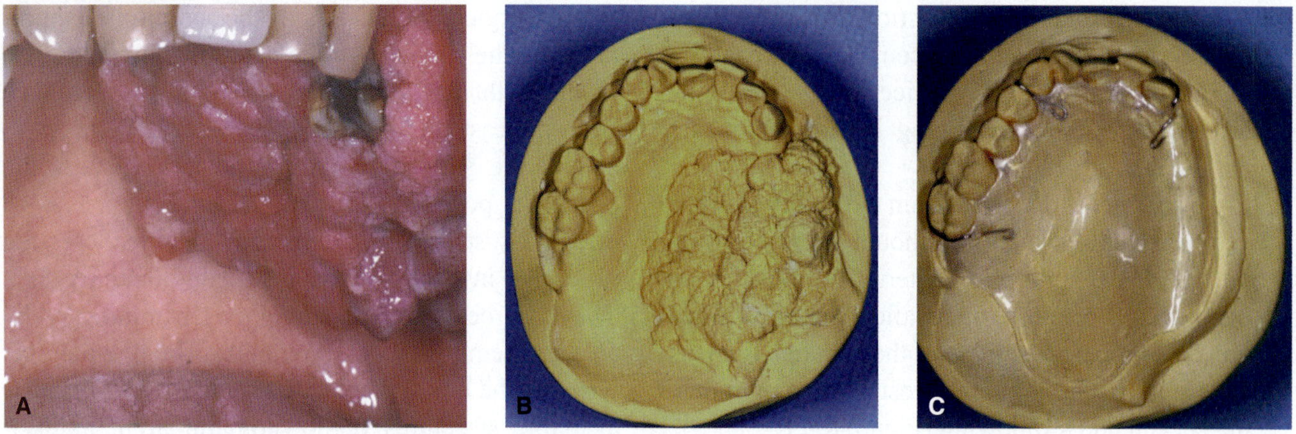

Figure 8–3. *A* and *B*, Tumor-distorted palatal contours. *C*, After the cast is altered to remove teeth and restore palatal contours in the path of the resection, the immediate surgical obturator is completed on the cast.

or into the nasal aperture may be necessary to provide acceptable retention.

Partial denture designs are complicated by (1) multiple axis of rotation, (2) compromised support on the defect side, (3) lack of cross-arch stabilization because of the loss of dentition on the resected side, (4) extended length of the lever arms associated with the obturator prosthesis, and (5) the forces of gravity.

Abutments adjacent to the defect are subject to greater vertical and lateral forces and are more frequently lost than abutments in other positions because the defect offers little support and the long lever arms magnify the loads delivered. If these abutment teeth are to be preserved, it is important that they have positive rests so that occlusal forces can be directed along their long axis. If incisors are adjacent to the defect, it is desirable to fit these teeth with porcelain-fused-to-metal restorations with cingulum rests and to splint them together (Figure 8–6).

The placement of osseointegrated implants dramatically improves the function of the obturator prosthesis, particularly for edentulous patients.[2] The most desirable locations are the premaxillary segment and the maxillary tuberosity. The tissue bars that are secured to the implants have much in common with the concepts of partial denture design for Class I or II distal extension removable partial dentures using the I-bar mesial rest concept. Implants are splinted together, and the bar should be

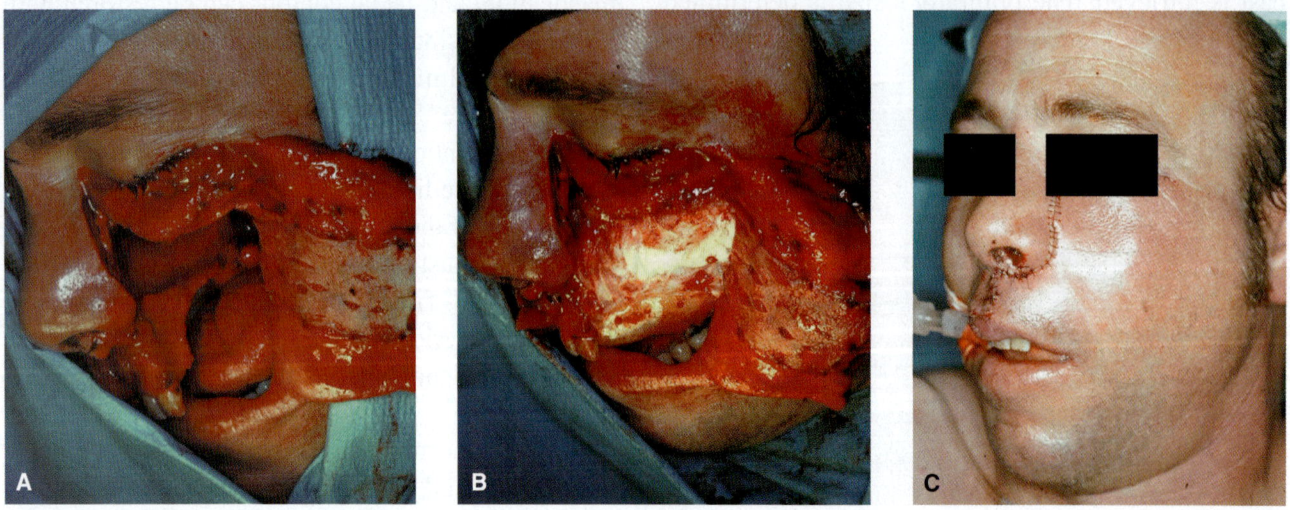

Figure 8–4. *A*, Radical maxillectomy defect. Note that an external skin incision was used for surgical exposure. *B*, A prosthesis serves as a platform for placement of surgical packing. *C*, When the wound is closed, facial contours are nearly normal.

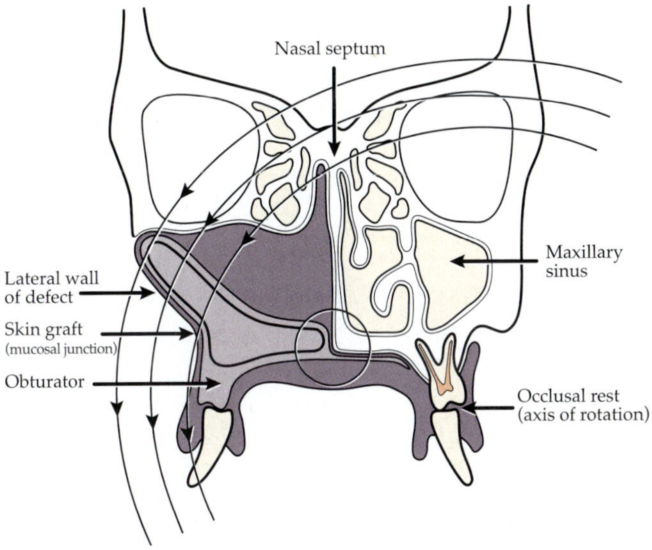

Figure 8–5. A diagrammatic frontal section of a radical maxillectomy with an obturator prosthesis in position. Minimal medial extension enables normal air flow. Maximum lateral extension facilitates retention, stability, and support for the obturator prosthesis.

designed to direct occlusal loads along the long axis of the implants (Figure 8–7). Patients are advised to masticate on the unresected side. Forceful occlusion on the defect side will result in rapid wear of the attachments securing the obturator prosthesis to the retention bar and may also result in bone loss around the implants, particularly the implant adjacent to the defect.

In partially dentulous patients, the basic principles of partial denture design should be followed[3]: (1) major connectors should be rigid; (2) occlusal rests should direct occlusal forces along the long axis of teeth; (3) guide planes should be designed to facilitate stability and bracing; (4) retention should be within the physiologic limits of the periodontal ligament; (5) maximum support and stability should be gained from the residual soft tissue–bearing surfaces, including the defect; and (6) designs must consider the needs of cleansibility (Figure 8–8). When the prosthesis is completed (Figure 8–9), speech and swallowing are restored to normal limits. Most prostheses require relining within the first year because of slow but continuous changes of the tissues on the periphery of the surgical defect.

Definitive Soft Palate Prosthesis

Defects of the soft palate and velopharyngeal complex require different and more complex prosthetic treatment. Palatopharyngeal closure normally occurs when the soft palate elevates and contacts the contracting lateral and posterior pharyngeal walls of the

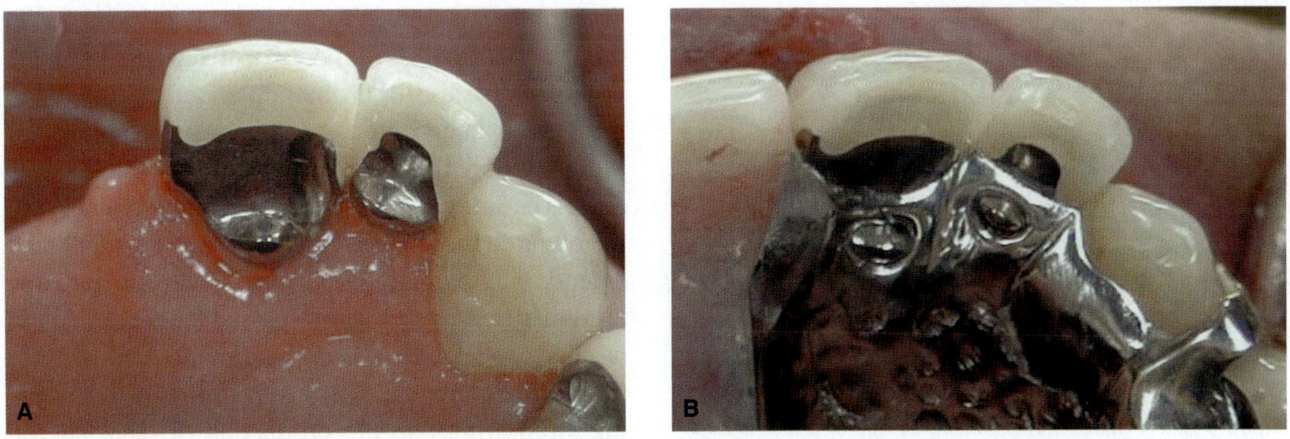

Figure 8–6. Abutments adjacent to the defect are subject to more vertical and lateral forces and are more frequently lost than abutments in other positions. These incisors have been splinted with porcelain-fused-to-metal crowns and provided with cingulum rests.

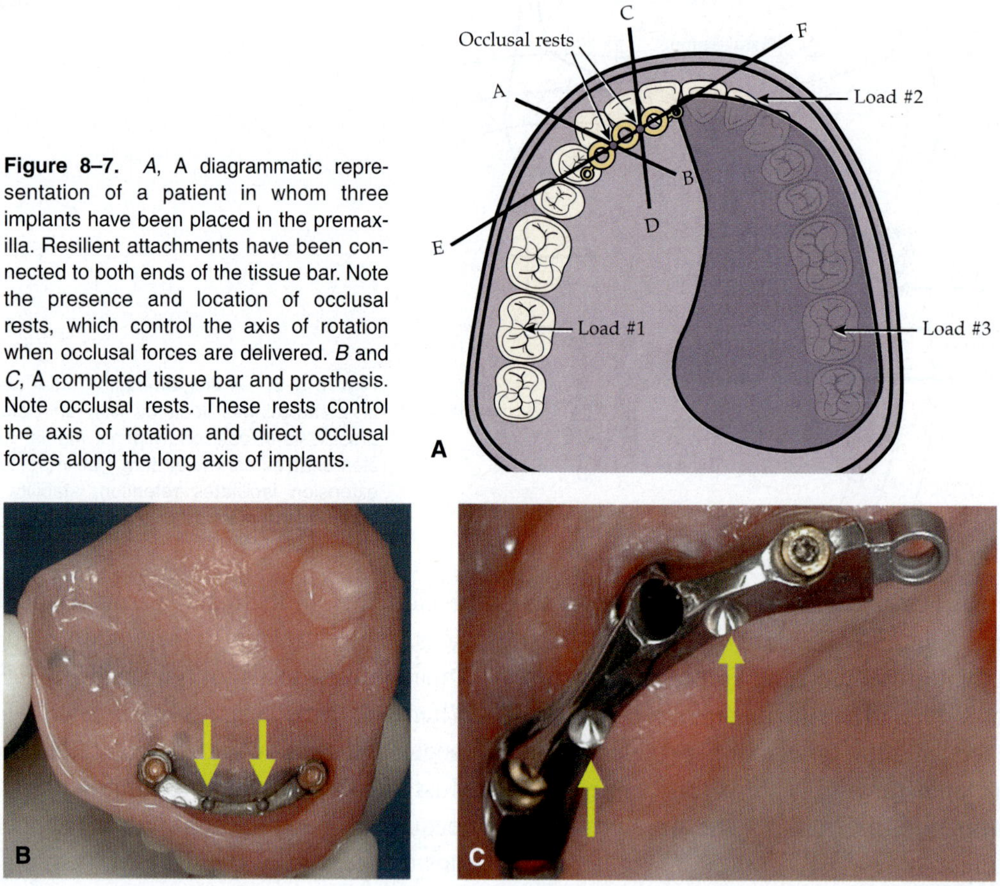

Figure 8–7. *A,* A diagrammatic representation of a patient in whom three implants have been placed in the premaxilla. Resilient attachments have been connected to both ends of the tissue bar. Note the presence and location of occlusal rests, which control the axis of rotation when occlusal forces are delivered. *B* and *C,* A completed tissue bar and prosthesis. Note occlusal rests. These rests control the axis of rotation and direct occlusal forces along the long axis of implants.

nasopharynx. When a portion of the soft palate or lateral pharyngeal wall is excised or when the soft palate is perforated, scarred, or neurologically impaired, complete velopharyngeal closure cannot occur. Speech becomes hypernasal, and normal swallowing is not possible. With a pharyngeal obturator, the patient will be able to re-establish velopharyngeal closure if the residual portion of the velopharyngeal mechanism still exhibits some movement. The obturator must not interfere with breathing, impinge on soft tissues during postural movements, or hamper the tongue during swallowing and speech.

The soft palate obturator remains in a fixed position in the nasopharynx and does not attempt to duplicate normal movements of the soft palate. The inferior surface of the obturator remains level with the hard palate contour, which in most patients is approximately the level of the anterior tubercle of the atlas. The inferior margin of the posterior surface of the obturator contacts Passavant's pad, if present, and extends approximately 10 mm superiorly into the nasopharynx. During breathing and the production of nasal speech sounds, the space around the obturator reflects the potential for muscular contraction. During swallowing and the production of other speech sounds, this sphincteric muscular network moves into contact with the stationary acrylic resin obtura-

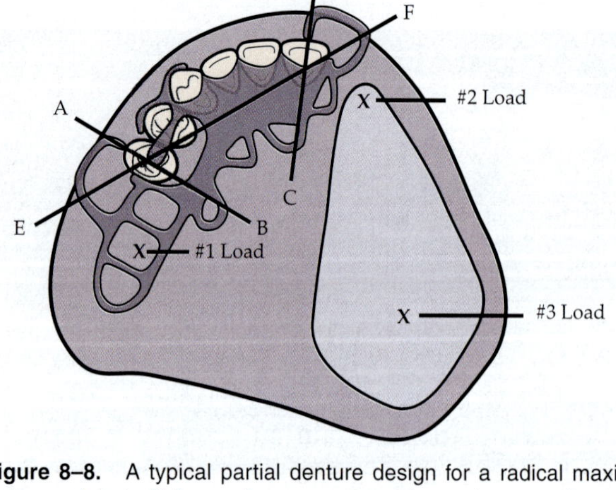

Figure 8–8. A typical partial denture design for a radical maxillectomy defect. Fulcrum lines are dynamic, and once sites of occlusal rests are selected, the axis of rotations depends on the site of load application.

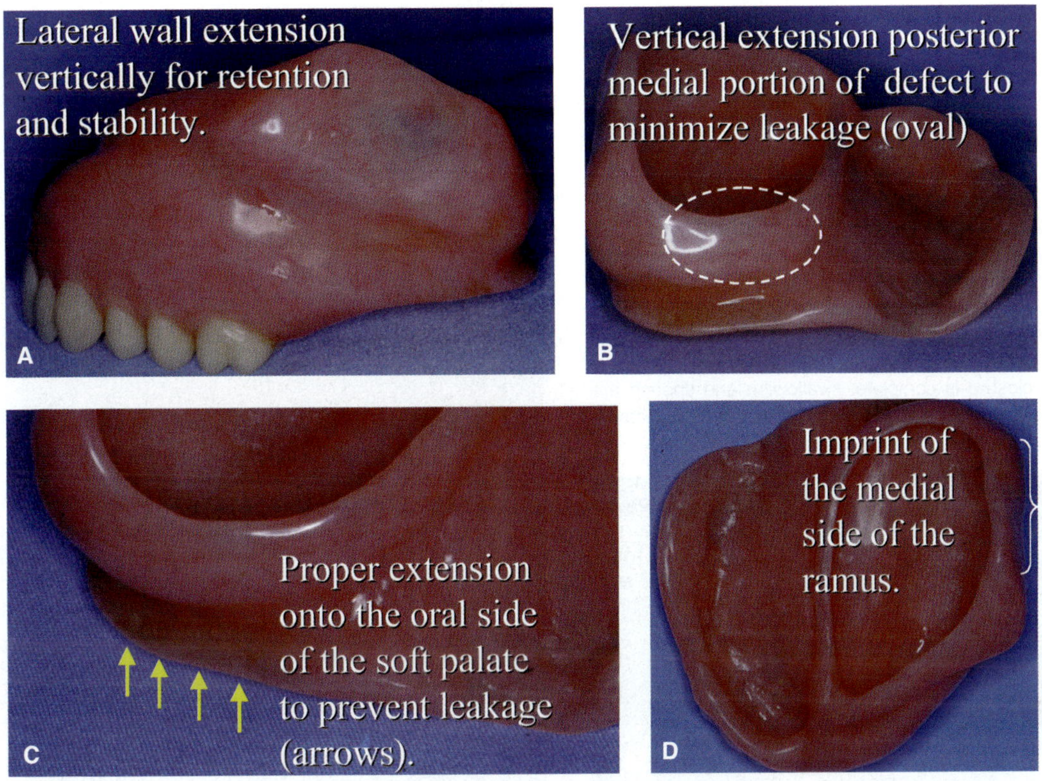

Figure 8–9. *A, B, C, D,* Complete denture with obturator with ideal contours.

tor, establishing velopharyngeal closure (Figure 8–10). A correctly constructed obturator will result in the return of normal speech and swallowing.

TONGUE AND MANDIBLE DEFECTS

Disabilities

Disabilities resulting from tongue and mandibular resections include impaired speech articulation, difficulty swallowing, deviation of the mandible during functional movements, poor control of salivary secretions, and often cosmetic disfigurement.

Advanced tumors of the anterior two-thirds of the tongue and floor of the mouth often require extensive resection of bone and soft tissue. The loss of large portions of the tongue prevents appropriate "valving" and/or interaction with other oral structures. This loss of mobility, combined with the loss of motor and sensory innervation, leads to misarticulation of many speech sounds. Deglutition is less impaired, and most patients learn to swallow fairly efficiently. Tongue function is less affected if the resected portion is restored with either myocutaneous or preferably free flaps. The myocutaneous flap restores bulk, prevents deviation of the mandible, and permits the reconstructed tongue to articulate more effectively with the palatal structures. Myocutaneous flaps, however, can become scarred and immobile. In contrast, tongues reconstructed with vascularized free flaps have the potential of supporting near-normal speech because they are less likely to become heavily scarred and immobile.

If much of the mandible is segmented and removed, the remaining functional mandibular segment will be retruded and deviated toward the surgical side at the vertical dimension of rest. When the jaw is opened, this deviation increases. These factors, combined with impaired tongue function, may prevent effective mastication. The severity and permanence of mandibular deviation vary; some patients attain an acceptable interocclusal relationship without adjunctive therapy, although some frontal plane rotation will be observed (Figure 8–11).

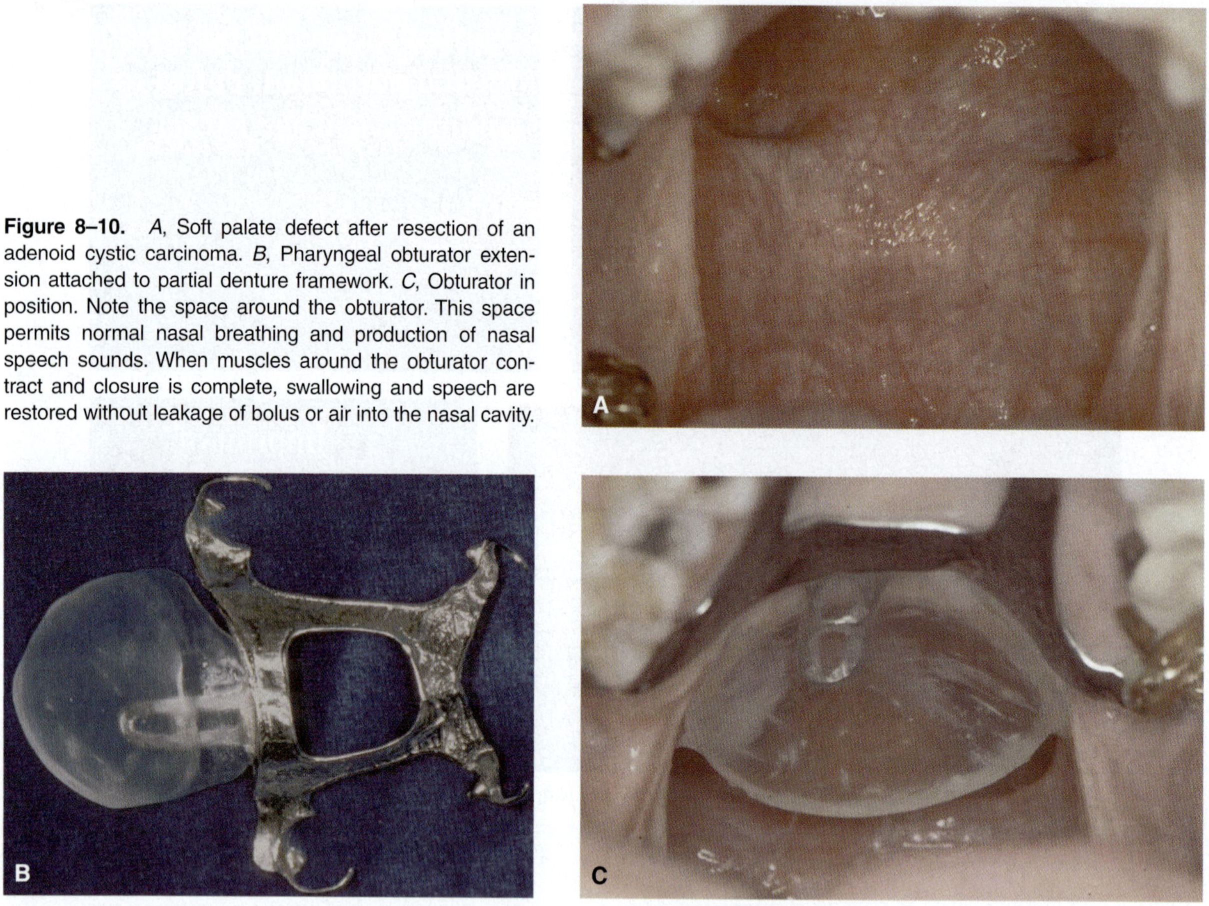

Figure 8–10. *A*, Soft palate defect after resection of an adenoid cystic carcinoma. *B*, Pharyngeal obturator extension attached to partial denture framework. *C*, Obturator in position. Note the space around the obturator. This space permits normal nasal breathing and production of nasal speech sounds. When muscles around the obturator contract and closure is complete, swallowing and speech are restored without leakage of bolus or air into the nasal cavity.

Resections of the tongue and mandible often obliterate portions of the lingual and buccal sulci so that a means of collecting and channeling secretions posteriorly no longer exists. In addition, the motor and sensory innervation of the lower lip on the resected side is often lost, impairing speech, mastication, and control of saliva.

When removal of tumors in the anterior floor of the mouth requires that the mandible be resected anteriorly and when mandibular continuity is not restored, the two remaining posterior fragments are pulled medially by the residual mylohyoid muscles and superiorly by the muscles of mastication. Severe disfigurement and dysfunction result. Free flaps from the fibula can be used immediately to restore the lost hard and soft tissues, and most patients emerge with excellent function and acceptable appearance (Figure 8–12). The nature and degree of the disabilities secondary to impaired tongue function after resection of lesions in the anterior floor of the mouth are proportional to the amount of tissue resected and to the nature of surgical closure. In most cases, motor control is unimpaired, and the functional deficits depend on the degree of tongue mobility.

Surgical Closure and Initial Reconstructive Steps

If the surgical wound is closed primarily (primary closure) by suturing the edges of the wound together, the functional disabilities are compounded. The introduction of the myocutaneous flaps, popularized in the late 1970s, ameliorated some of the disabilities, but it was not until the introduction of vascularized free flaps in the late 1980s that restoration of oral function could be restored to near normal. With proper use of free flaps, tongue bulk can be restored and the mobility of the reconstructed tongue results in acceptable speech, swallowing, and saliva control (Figure 8–13).[4] The

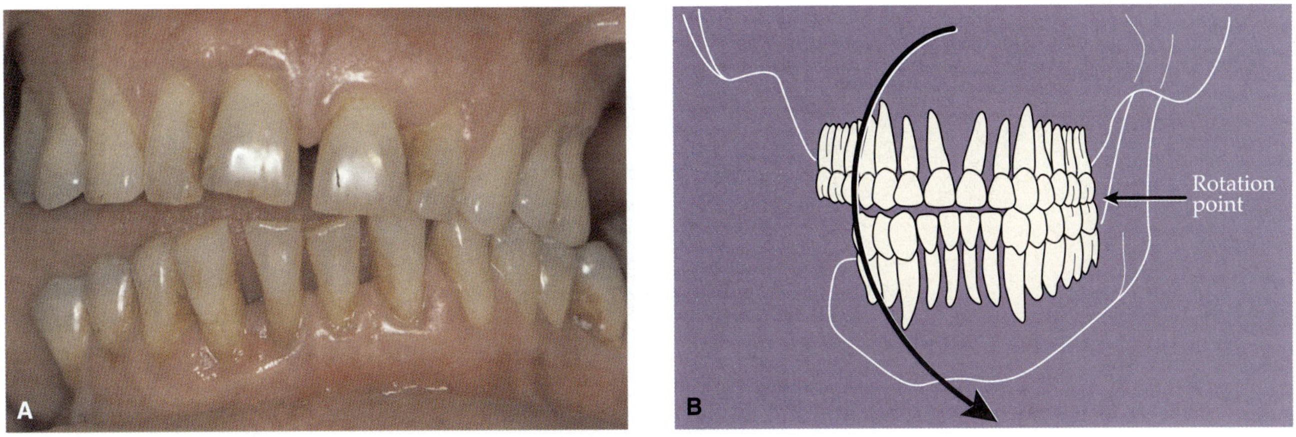

Figure 8–11. Frontal plane rotation. *A*, As the force of mandibular closure increases, the mandible rotates around occlusal contacts on the unresected side, and (*B*) the remaining teeth on the resected side drop further out of occlusion.

advantage of free tissue transfers (free flaps) over musculocutaneous flaps is the improved blood supply, enhancing wound healing and flap survival. If large mandibular segments need to be restored, the fibula is the preferred donor site unless the soft tissue deficit is unusually large. The osteotomized fibula provides sufficient length and bulk of bone, and osseointegrated implants can be placed to retain and support a prosthesis (Figure 8–14).

Secondary Surgical Procedures

Vestibuloplasty, Tongue Release, and Skin Grafts

Vestibuloplasty and tongue release are of particular value when mandibular continuity has been maintained or restored. The creation of vestibules enables the patient to pool saliva more efficiently and allows for extension of denture flanges, resulting in improved stability and retention (Figure 8–15). Creation of attached keratinized mucosa on the ridge surface with either a skin graft or a palatal graft provides additional stability for a partial or complete denture. The patient's appearance may also be improved because a prosthodontic restoration can now be molded to provide contour and support for the lower lip and cheek portions of the resected area. Improvement of speech is less noticeable in patients who lack tongue mobility.

Restoration of Mandibular Continuity

Surgically repairing mandibular discontinuity defects results in more normal mandibular move-

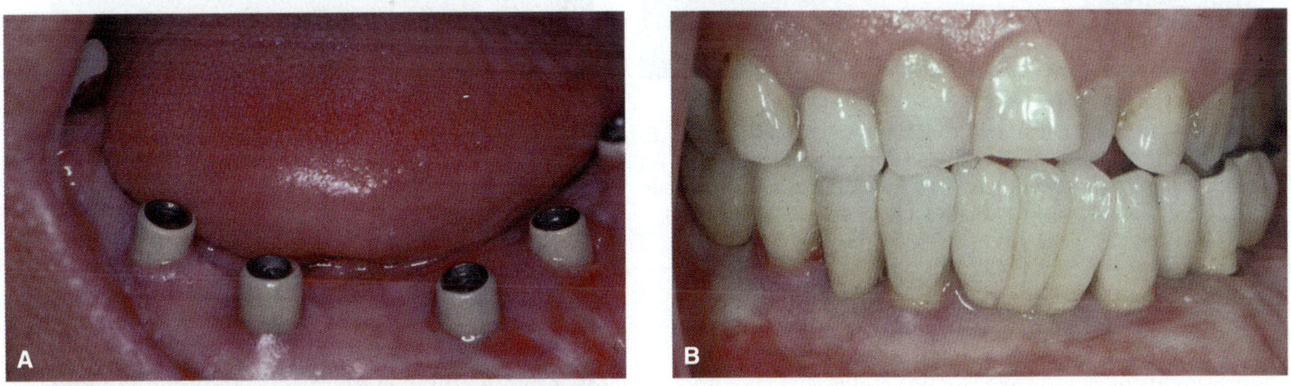

Figure 8–12. Anterior mandible defect restored with fibula free flap and an implant-supported porcelain-fused-to-metal fixed partial denture. Because the tongue is unaffected by the resection, speech and mastication are near normal. *A*, Clinical view of the implants in place. *B*, Implant-supported and -retained prosthesis in position.

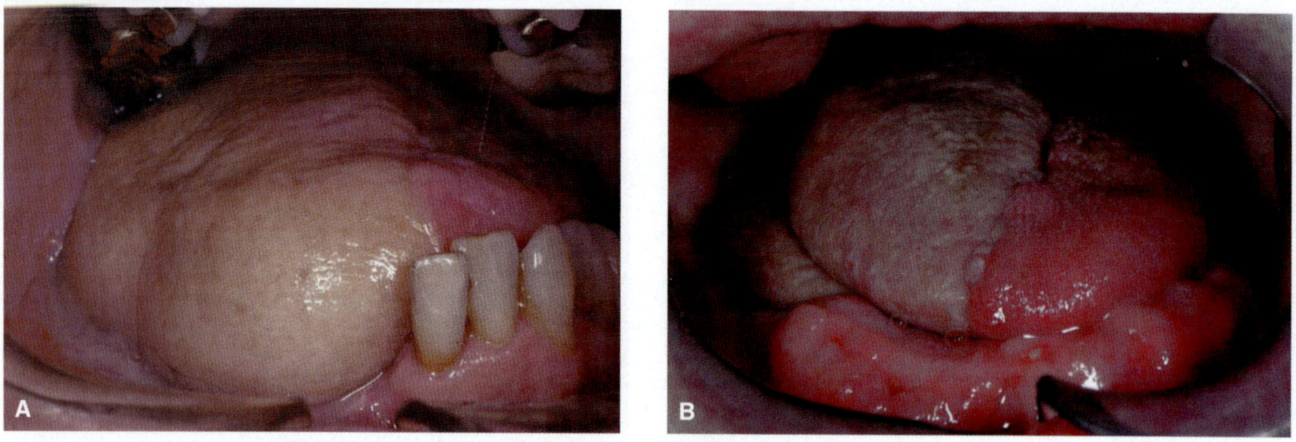

Figure 8–13. *A* and *B*, Free flaps were used to reconstruct these tongue defects.

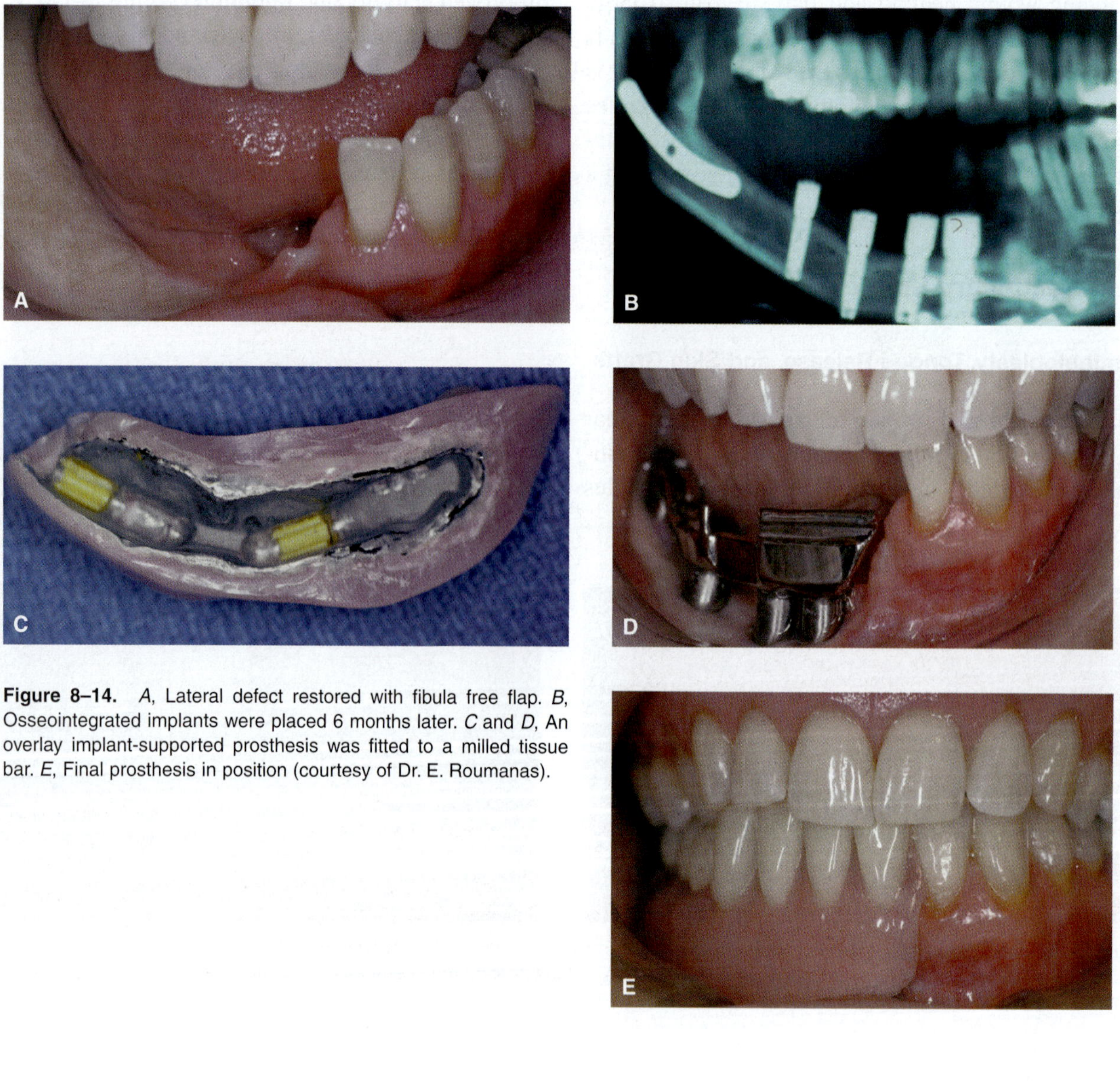

Figure 8–14. *A*, Lateral defect restored with fibula free flap. *B*, Osseointegrated implants were placed 6 months later. *C* and *D*, An overlay implant-supported prosthesis was fitted to a milled tissue bar. *E*, Final prosthesis in position (courtesy of Dr. E. Roumanas).

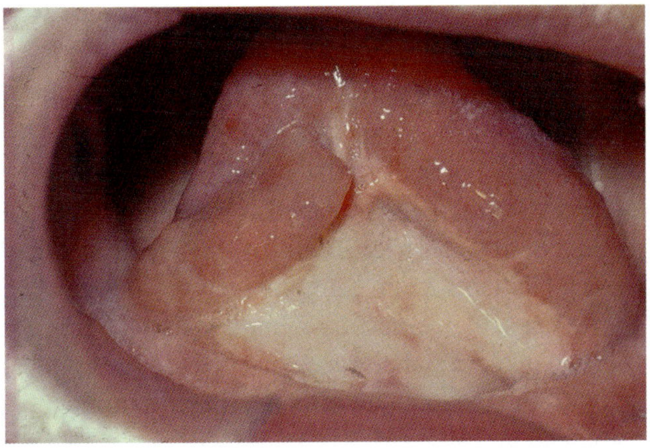

Figure 8–15. To overcome functional restrictions following surgery, tongue release and skin graft vestibuloplasty may improve tongue mobility, permit construction of dentures, and enable more effective control of saliva.

ment patterns that enable an edentulous patient to exert force on both sides of the dental arch. This increases the stability of complete dentures. In dentulous patients, a properly reconstructed mandible restores dental occlusion to normal and will partially alleviate deviation of the mandible.

Free bone grafts. Free grafts are rapidly being replaced by free flaps as a means of restoring mandibular discontinuity defects but are still being used by some clinicans. Reconstruction after extensive resection of oral malignancies with free grafts is difficult because of the lack of sufficient soft tissue to receive the graft, the decreased vascularity of the tissue bed secondary to radiation therapy and/or radical neck dissection, and the difficulty in achieving proper fixation of the graft during the healing period. The primary goals are to restore facial form and mandibular continuity, and, in selected patients, an appropriate volume and quality of bone should be provided for the placement of osseointegrated implants.

Autogenous graft sources for resected bone include the iliac crest, rib, and clavicle. Most commonly, the defects are restored either with particulate autogenous marrow housed in a metal tray or with a block of bone, both usually obtained from the iliac crest (Figure 8–16). The use of myocutaneous flaps for closure of the initial wound facilitates free bone grafting of continuity defects by

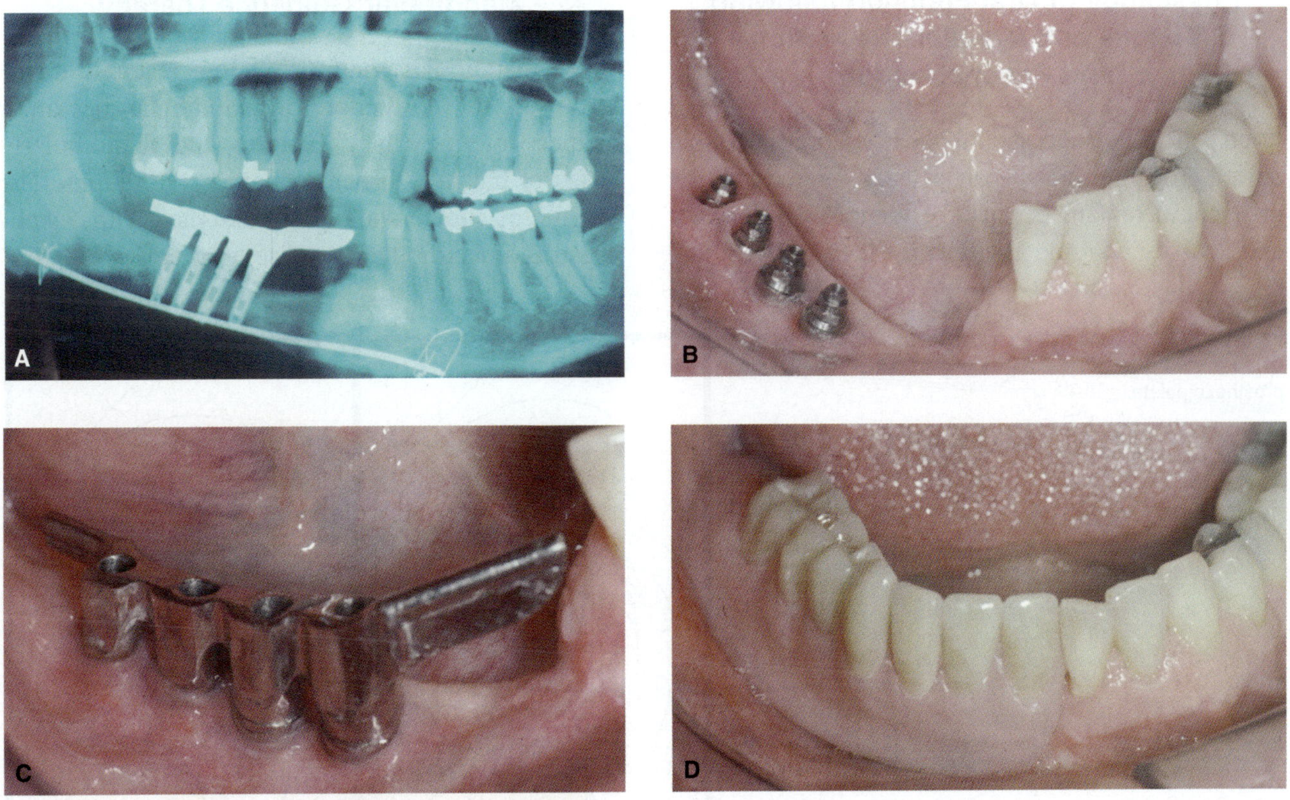

Figure 8–16. Mandibular discontinuity defect restored with free graft from iliac arrest. *A* and *B*, Osseointegrated implants were placed several years later. *C* and *D*, Milled bar and overlay prosthesis in position.

enhancing the volume and vascularity of the recipient soft tissues.

Free vascularized flaps. A major advance in mandibular reconstruction has been the development of improved techniques in microvascular surgery, which allow for composite grafting of larger volumes of tissue. In microvascular free tissue transfer (free flaps), bone, muscle, connective tissue, and skin can be autogenously grafted and remain viable. The grafting can be accomplished simultaneously with resection of the tumor with excellent results.

Numerous donor sites have been used. The radial forearm is favored for reconstruction of most extensive soft tissue defects such as tonsillar, partial glossectomy, and floor of the mouth defects. The composite fibula flap is the preferred donor site for most complex mandibular discontinuity defects (see Figure 8–14, A). Multiple osteotomies may be performed without devascularizing the bone segments to replicate the contour of the replaced mandible. Fibular thickness makes it an excellent recipient of osseointegrated implants.

Physiology of Oral Function following Tongue and Mandible Resection and Reconstruction

Even following successful reconstruction, functional deficits (deglutition, speech articulation, mastication efficiency) remain because of compromised motor and sensory control, inadequate tissue contour, and inadequate bulk of key tissues. Mastication efficiency primarily depends on the quality of tongue function and the presence of a reasonable occlusal table adjacent to the sensate, functioning portion of the residual portion of the reconstructed tongue.[5,6] Articulation of speech depends on mobility and the presence of adequate bulk of the reconstructed tongue. Patients with hemiglossectomy defects can learn to articulate, masticate, and swallow effectively if they can elevate their reconstructed tongue to interact with the palatal vault and maxillary dentition.

Palatal Speech and Swallowing Aids

If the reconstructed tongue does not possess the ability to elevate sufficiently to interact with the palatal structures, an acrylic resin template is made to engage the palatal contours and/or maxillary dentition (Figure 8–17). Their surfaces can be modified with modeling plastic or tissue-conditioning material (Figure 8–18) and eventually can be processed into acrylic resin.

Mandibular Guidance Therapy

When mandibular continuity is not restored, methods used for correction of mandibular deviation include intermaxillary fixation and mandibularly based or palatally based guidance restorations. The method of choice should be combined with a well-organized mandibular exercise program.

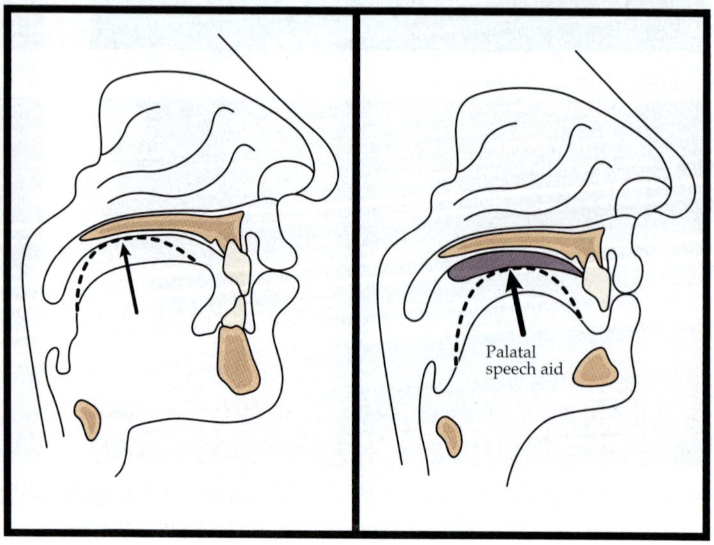

Figure 8–17. Insertion of a palatal speech aid enables the dorsum of the reconstructed tongue to valve against the prosthetic palate.

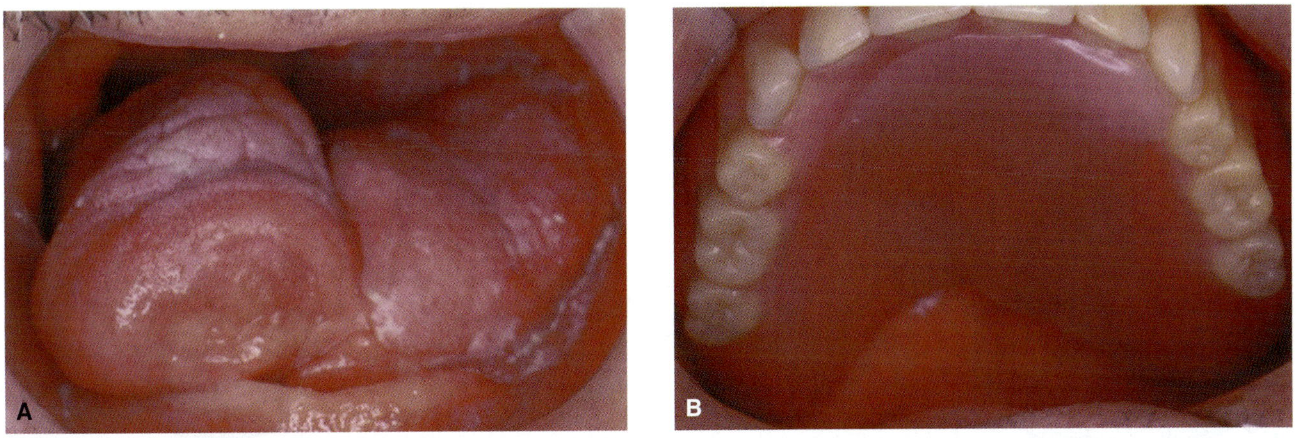

Figure 8–18. *A*, Hemiglossectomy defect repaired with a myocutaneous flap. *B*, A thick layer of tissue-conditioning material was used to fashion a palatal speech aid.

The success of mandibular guidance therapy depends on the nature of the surgical defect, early initiation, and cooperation of the patient. Patients with extensive posterior base of the tongue lesions, radical neck dissection, and radiation therapy are often unable to achieve functional intercuspal relationships. Mandibular guidance therapy is most successful when the resection involves minimal soft tissue removal or when defects are replaced with myocutaneous or free flaps. Following mandibular guidance therapy, occlusal equilibration or selective crown placement may be required to achieve optimal interocclusal relationships.

Definitive Prosthetic Restoration

The outcome of removable prostheses for patients with resections of the tongue and mandible depends on the function of the residual tongue. In some patients with poor tongue function, only appearance and oral competence can be improved, whereas in others with good tongue function, mastication is a reasonable objective.

Removable Partial Dentures

The usual principles of partial denture design and fabrication should be followed. Major connectors should be rigid, occlusal rests must direct occlusal forces along the long axis of teeth, guiding planes should be employed to provide stability and bracing, retention must be within the limits of physiologic tolerance of the periodontal ligament of the abutment teeth, and maximum support should be gained from the adjacent soft tissues. Retainers, minor connectors, and proximal plates should be designed so that they do not subject the remaining teeth to excessive lateral forces during function.

In patients with lateral discontinuity defects, it may not be possible to design a framework with retainers that disengage during function because of the altered patterns of force on the prosthesis. Viewed from the frontal plane, the arc of closure of the mandible is angular rather than vertical, with forces of occlusion confined to the nonresected side. Rotation of the mandible in the frontal plane causes the resected side to drop down out of occlusion as the force of contracture on the unresected side is increased. The location of the fulcrum line of a partial denture is not easily determined because of the difficulty in predicting movement patterns of the prosthesis during function. A typical lateral mandibulectomy defect with a suggested prosthetic design is shown in Figure 8–19. The forces of occlusion are unilateral, so the axis of rotation (fulcrum line) of the partial denture deviates from the norm. By placing the occlusal rest on the mesial of the bicuspid, it is possible to place a retainer on the bicuspid that disengages during expression of an occlusal load in the distal extension area. However, a retainer cannot be positioned in a retentive area on the opposite cuspid that disengages during occlusal function. Consequently, either this retainer must be placed on the height of contour or it must be flexible so that an occlusal load will not sub-

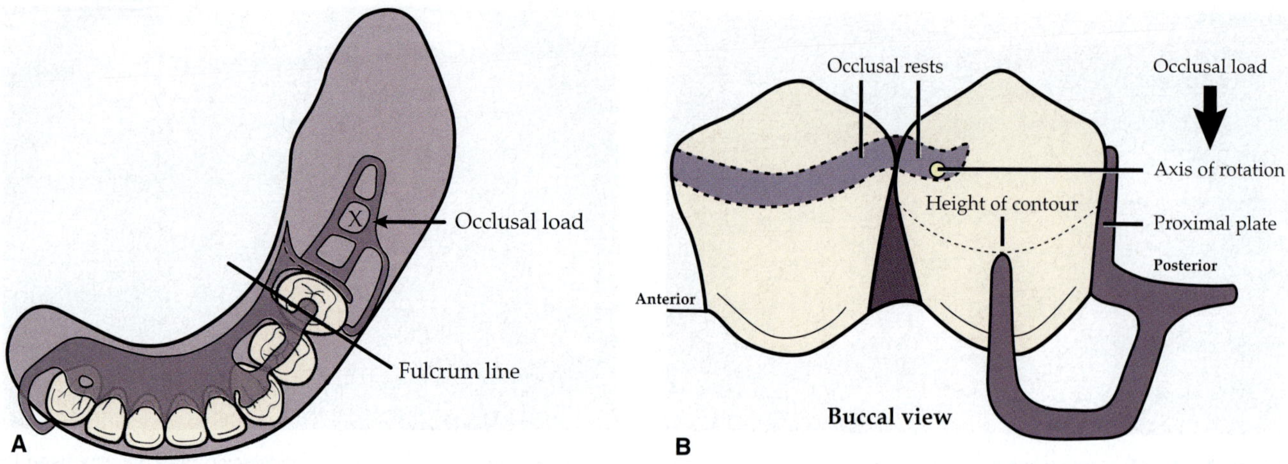

Figure 8–19. Suggested design for a partial denture. *A*, Occlusal view. *B*, Buccal view of the nonresected side. An I-bar retainer disengages when occlusal pressure is applied to the extension area.

ject the cuspid to undue stress. All partial denture frameworks should be physiologically relieved.

After the partial denture casting has been fabricated, verified, and adjusted, an altered cast impression is obtained of the edentulous areas. Particular attention should be paid to the lingual extension on the unresected side, especially the polished surfaces, which provides additional retention and stability. Maximum extension of the denture base is always attempted. Coverage of the buccal shelf on the unresected side is essential to maximize support. Centric relation records are made and occlusal schemes are developed that are consistent with the unilateral mandibular movement patterns of mandibulectomy patients (Figure 8–20).

Resection Dentures

Dentures for edentulous patients with discontinuity defects of the mandible may provide esthetic improvement by replacing teeth and improving lip and cheek contours, but unless the patient has reasonably good tongue control, mastication is generally not possible. A number of factors affect the patient's ability to function with resection dentures: (1) stability, support, and retention of the mandibular denture are compromised; (2) quality and quantity of saliva; (3) the angular pathway of mandibular closure, which induces lateral forces on the dentures, tending to dislodge them; (4) abnormal maxillomandibular relationships that may prevent ideal placement of the denture teeth over their supporting structures; and (5) impairment of motor and/or sensory control of the tongue, lip, and cheek, limiting the ability to control dentures during function. Implant-assisted resection dentures can overcome many of these difficulties, particularly those associated with compromised retention, stability, or support.

The status of the remaining tongue is probably the most important prognostic factor. If motor and/or sensory control are not significantly impaired and the tongue can be moved in several directions, resection denture stabilization and control of the food bolus during function become possible. Paradoxically, immobility of the tongue often permits a more aggressive extension of the lingual flange on the nonsurgical side, aiding stability and retention. The position of the tongue is also an important prosthodontic prognosticator relative to obtaining a peripheral seal.

Mandibular resections extending to the midline have a poor prosthetic prognosis. If the resection is limited to the ramus-molar or cuspid regions anteriorly, the prosthetic prognosis is more favorable. In some of these patients, remnants of the masseter or medial pterygoid muscle may remain attached to the mandible, enabling the development of bilaterally balanced occlusion. These patients demonstrate more normal envelopes of motion and near-normal ridge relationships, allowing for more favorable distribution of forces during mastication and swallowing.

Following impressions, centric and lateral registrations and occlusal schemes should take into con-

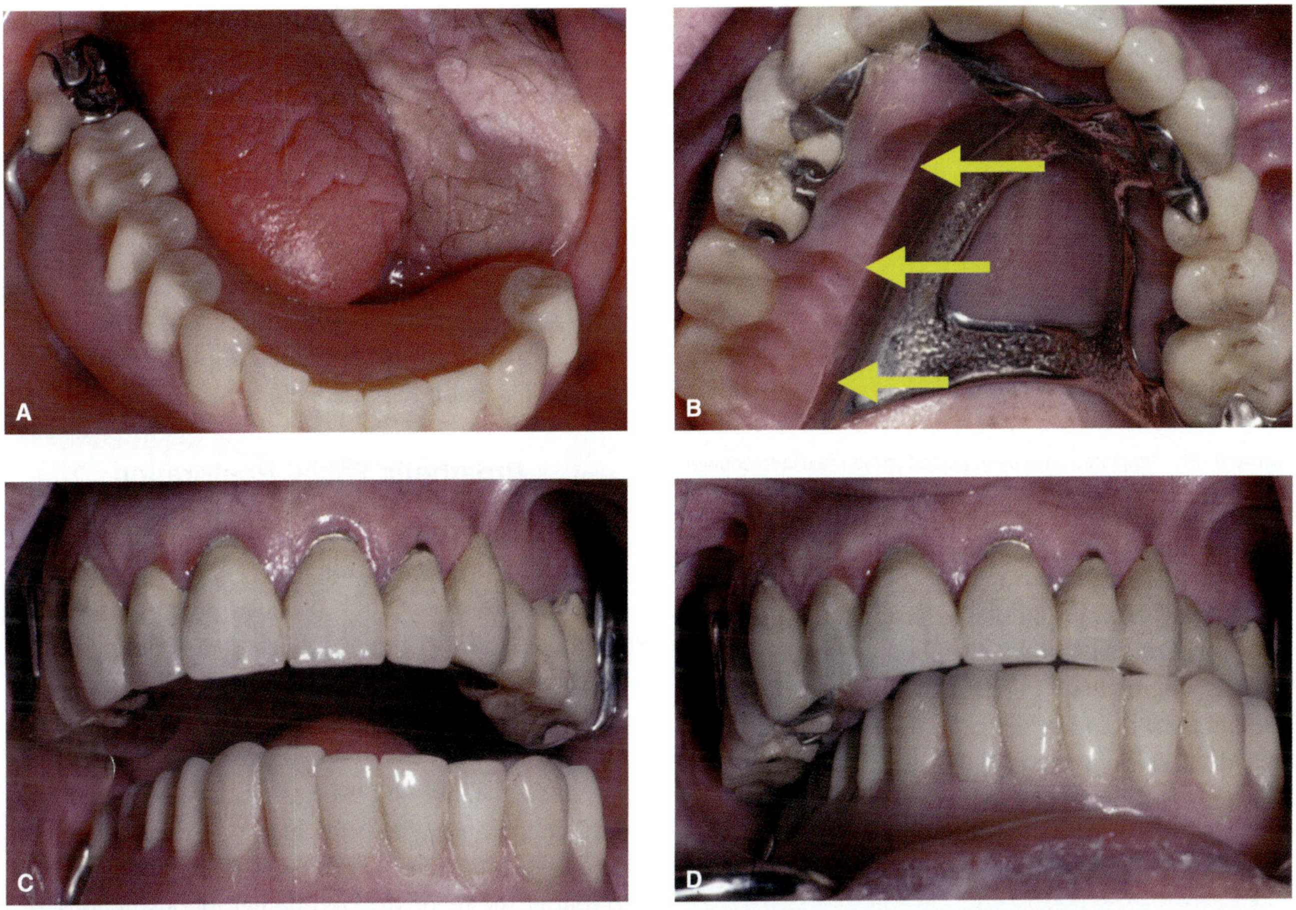

Figure 8–20. Patient with a lateral tongue mandibular discontinuity defect. The left lateral tongue was reconstructed with a myocutaneous flap. *A*, Mandibular prosthesis in position. *B*, Maxillary prosthesis in position. Note the functionally generated occlusal platform (*arrows*). *C* and *D*, Note the angular path of closure.

sideration the altered pattern of mandibular movements. Denture extensions can be verified with a disclosing wax and excessive tissue displacement eliminated with the aid of pressure-indicating paste.

Implant-Assisted Overlay Dentures

Patients with reasonable tongue bulk and mobility and with motor and sensory innervation intact on at least one side gain the most from implant-retained overlay prostheses. The tongue, then, is no longer required to control the denture, so it functions mainly to manipulate the food bolus during mastication and swallowing. If the patient's speech is intelligible, the prognosis for effective bolus manipulation with an implant-retained prosthesis is good.

In mandibular resection patients, if implants are to be placed into the mandible to retain and support an overlay prosthesis, consideration should be given to placing implants in the opposing maxilla. The unilateral occlusal forces and increased lateral forces generated during the chewing cycle tend to dislodge the upper denture. In addition, xerostomia may compromise the peripheral seal. Therefore, implants should be considered if the retention and stability of a conventional maxillary denture are marginal (Figure 8–21).

In most patients, the only implant sites available in the edentulous resected mandible are located in the symphyseal region. A minimum of two implants should be placed. However, more are desirable, if space allows, mainly for stability. Tissue bar designs must take into account the axis of rotation of the overlay denture when occlusal forces are applied in the distal extension area. A suitable design is shown in Figure 8–22.

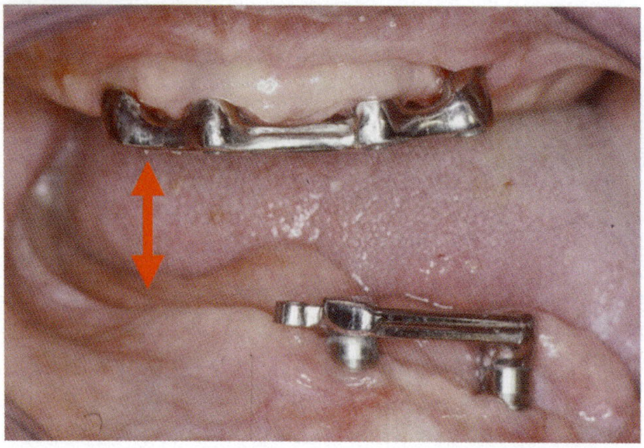

Figure 8–21. Implants have been placed in the maxilla to counteract unilateral forces of occlusion. Note frontal plane rotation.

Implant success rates in bone grafts used to restore mandibular continuity defects have been very good. Free bone grafts demonstrate a homogeneous calcification pattern that results in an excellent bone–implant interface (see Figure 8–16, A). Free flaps also provide sufficient quality and quantity of bone for excellent anchorage of implants, particularly with the fibula free flaps (see Figure 8–14, A and B).[7]

FACIAL DEFECTS

Surgical reconstruction and prosthodontic restoration have limitations. The surgeon is limited by the availability of tissue, damage to the local vascular bed, and the need for periodic visual inspection of an oncologic defect. The prosthodontist is limited by the materials available for facial restoration, movable tissue beds, difficulties in retaining large prostheses, and a patient's willingness to accept the result. The method of facial restoration should be considered before surgery, and patients should participate in the decision-making process with realistic expectations.

Surgical Reconstruction versus Prosthetic Restoration

Surgical reconstruction of small facial defects is preferable. However, it is difficult for the surgeon to contour a facial component that is as effective in appearance as a well-made prosthesis. Osseointegrated implants in facial defects have changed patient perceptions about facial prostheses because of the retention achieved. Additionally, when a large resection is necessary and recurrence of tumor is realistic, it is advantageous to be able to monitor the surgical site closely, which a prosthesis permits. Even when surgical reconstruction is deemed possible, most surgeons prefer to wait at least 1 year before surgical reconstruction. Also, surgical restoration of large defects is technically difficult and requires multiple procedures and hospitalizations, which may be further complicated if radiotherapy has been included.

Prosthetic Facial Restoration

The challenge to the prosthodontist is to fabricate an esthetically pleasing restoration (Figure 8–23). A conspicuous prosthesis may produce more anxiety and permit less social readjustment than a simple facial bandage or eye patch. The most critical period is the first 2 to 3 days after delivery. The patient must understand that a prosthesis has two different roles: for family, close friends, or business associates, it can only cosmetically replace the tissues excised; for the public at large, it generally provides enough concealment to render the reconstructed defect inconspicuous.

Materials Used for Facial Prostheses

Current materials all possess some undesirable characteristics.[8] The materials most often used are the silicone elastomers, which have achieved wide clin-

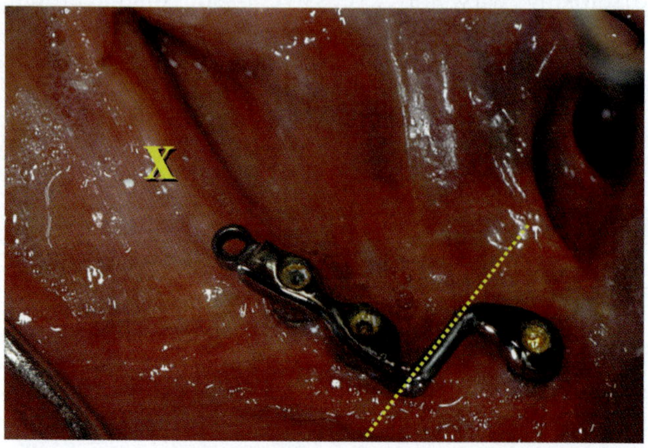

Figure 8–22. Typical tissue bar design for an edentulous lateral mandibular discontinuity defect. When occlusal load is applied in the extension area (X), the restoration rotates around the Hader bar segment (*dotted line*).

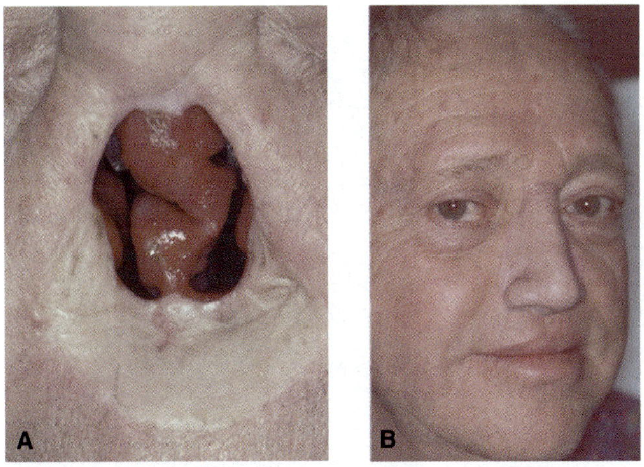

Figure 8–23. *A* and *B*, Prosthetic restoration of a nasal defect.

ical acceptance. Adhesives are used to retain most facial restorations. A major development has been the use of osseointegrated implants, resulting in extremely well-retained prostheses that permit vigorous physical activities.

Design Considerations

A presurgical moulage can be very helpful, especially if a total rhinectomy or total auriculectomy is anticipated. Impressions of the defect are usually obtained with elastic impression materials, taking care not to displace the tissues being recorded. The contours of the prostheses are sculpted in wax, both on the cast and on the patient. Surface characteristics, appropriate contour, coloration, and margin placement are equally important factors. Processing the materials is complicated and requires special instrumentation. Special flasks are necessary for processing large prostheses.

Coloration

Basic skin tones should be developed into a shade guide for each material. The base shade selected should be slightly lighter than the lightest skin tones of the patient because as additional color is added, extrinsically, the prosthesis will darken.

Combined Oral and Facial Defects

When the integrity of the oral cavity has been destroyed, food and air escape during swallowing, speech is often unintelligible, and saliva control is difficult. Additionally, it is extremely hard to adapt the margins of the prosthesis to maintain tissue contact during facial and mandibular movements. Retention of maxillary teeth or a portion of the hard palate improves the prosthetic prognosis. Placement of implants, as well as skin grafts to decrease tissue contraction and to create undercut areas for retention and stability, also improves the prosthetic prognosis.

Patients will experience less depression if as many functions as possible are restored immediately after surgery with a temporary prosthesis. These functions include swallowing food (thereby eliminating the need for a nasogastric tube or gastrostomy), controlling saliva, and speaking. The oral portion of the temporary prosthesis is constructed of acrylic resin and formed so that contact is established with healthy tissues adjacent to the defect. Functional contact with the remaining portions of the lips allows the patient to effectively seal the oral cavity. Tissue-bearing surfaces of the prosthesis are relined with temporary denture reliner at frequent intervals to accommodate tissue changes.

In constructing a definitive midface prosthesis, a custom tray is used for the master impression. Movable portions of the defect are recorded with a thermoplastic material. Record bases are fabricated, and centric relation records enable casts to be mounted on an articulator. Osseointegrated implants, eyeglass frames, adhesives, straps, teeth, and engagement of defect undercuts supply retention. The finished restoration usually provides the patient with acceptable appearance and function (Figure 8–24).

Craniofacial Implants

The use of osseointegrated implants has significantly improved patient acceptance of facial prostheses. The retention provided by implants makes it possible to fabricate large prostheses that rest on movable tissues. This enables the prosthodontist to fabricate thinner margins, which enhance esthetics by blending and moving more effectively with adjacent mobile tissues. Other benefits include elimination of the occasional skin reactions to skin adhesives, ease and enhanced accuracy of prosthesis placement, improved patient comfort, and decreased daily maintenance, which also increases the life span of the facial prosthesis.

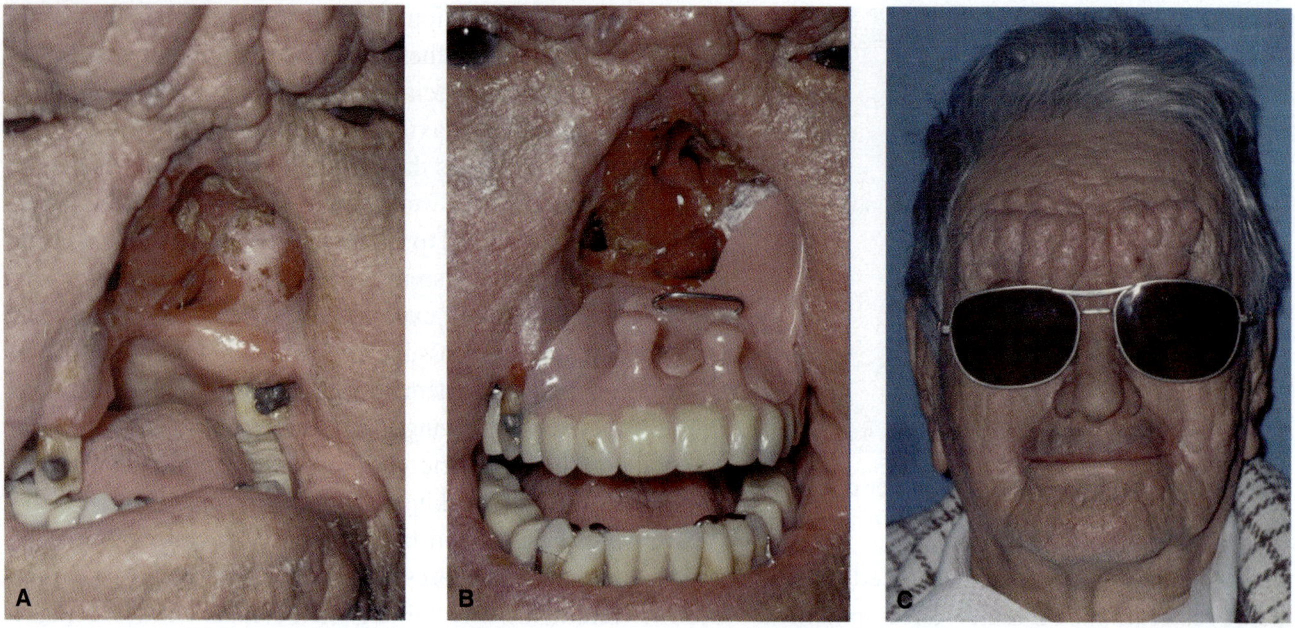

Figure 8–24. *A*, Large midfacial defect. *B*, Oral prosthesis in position. *C*, Facial prosthesis in position.

Treatment Planning

The implants must be positioned within the confines of the proposed facial prosthesis. In most patients, it is desirable to sculpt a wax replica of the future prosthesis and to use this replica to fabricate a surgical template. This template is sterilized and used as a guide during surgery to ensure proper implant position and angulation.

The number and arrangement of implants and possible bone sites are determined. In most acquired defects, radiographic studies are not necessary. In large extensive defects, computed tomographic scans and three-dimensional models may be useful in evaluating potential bone sites and important adjacent structures. The health of soft tissues circumscribing osseointegrated implants is easier to maintain if these tissues are thin (less than 5 mm in thickness) and attached to underlying periosteum. If the skin contains hair follicles or scar tissue from past reconstructive procedures, these tissues should be removed and replaced with skin grafts.

Surgical Placement

Craniofacial implant fixtures are fabricated from pure titanium. They are available in either 3 or 4 mm lengths, with a 5 mm diameter flange (Figure 8–25). The short lengths are designed to permit placement in areas with limited available bone. The flange facilitates initial stabilization of the implant and prevents penetration into interior components.

For ear defects, two or three implants are positioned posteriorly and superiorly to the ear canal (Figure 8–26). For nasal defects, the preferred fixture location is the anterior portion of the floor of the nose. Care should be taken to avoid the roots of the teeth in this area. For orbital defects, the preferred location is the lateral portion of the superior orbital rim.

Several attachment systems have been used to connect the facial prosthesis to the implants, such as bar-clips, magnets, and O-ring types. For auricular and nasal or large midfacial prostheses, we prefer the bar clip systems because they provide superior

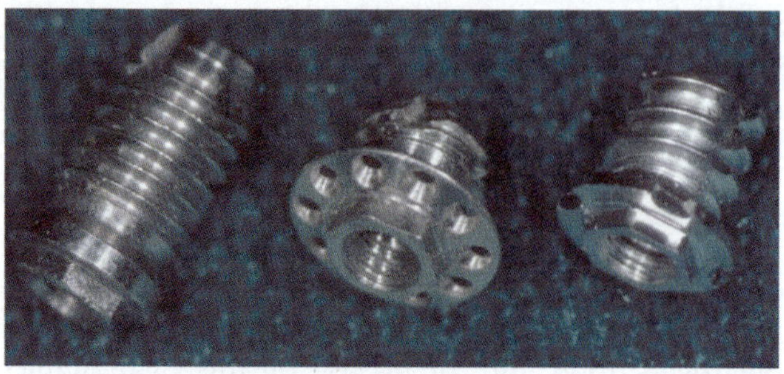

Figure 8–25. Titanium implants used in craniofacial defects.

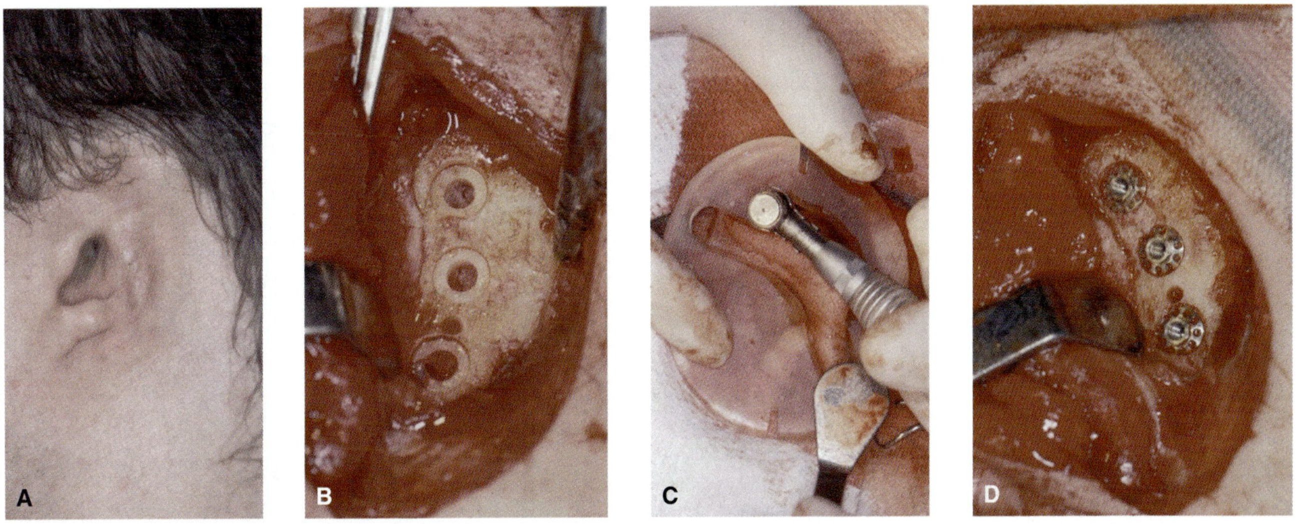

Figure 8–26. Implant placement in mastoid bone. A surgical template is used to guide implant placement.

retention (Figures 8–27 and 8–28). We prefer magnetic retention for orbital prostheses because the ease of insertion of magnetically retained prostheses outweighs the possibilities of magnet corrosion and decreased retention over time.

An acrylic resin substructure retaining the attachments is designed to fit within the contours of the silicone facial prosthesis. It should possess sufficient surface area so that the bond between the acrylic resin substructure and the silicone prosthesis will not fail during insertion or removal of the prosthesis.

Success rates for auricular sites have exceeded 90% in most studies, and few complications have been encountered. Success rates of the floor of the nose sites are around 80% and are about the same as oral implants placed in the premaxillary segment. Success rates in the orbit have been about 70%. Success rates are diminished if implant sites have been irradiated previously, particularly in the orbit (Tables 8–1 and 8–2).[9]

IMPLANTS IN IRRADIATED TISSUES

Irradiation of head and neck tumors predisposes the patient to changes in bone, skin, and mucosa, which affect the predictability of osseointegrated implants. Long-term function of osseointegrated implants depends on the presence of viable bone that is capa-

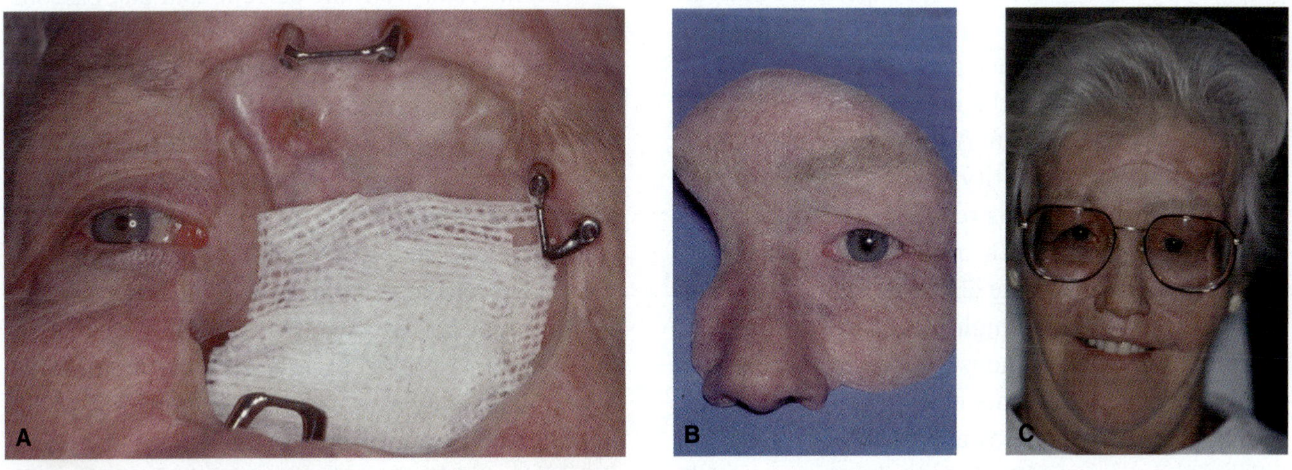

Figure 8–27. Large midfacial defect restored with an implant-retained prosthesis. *A*, Tissue bars in position. A Hader bar retention system was used. *B*, Finished prosthesis. *C*, The prosthesis snaps into position.

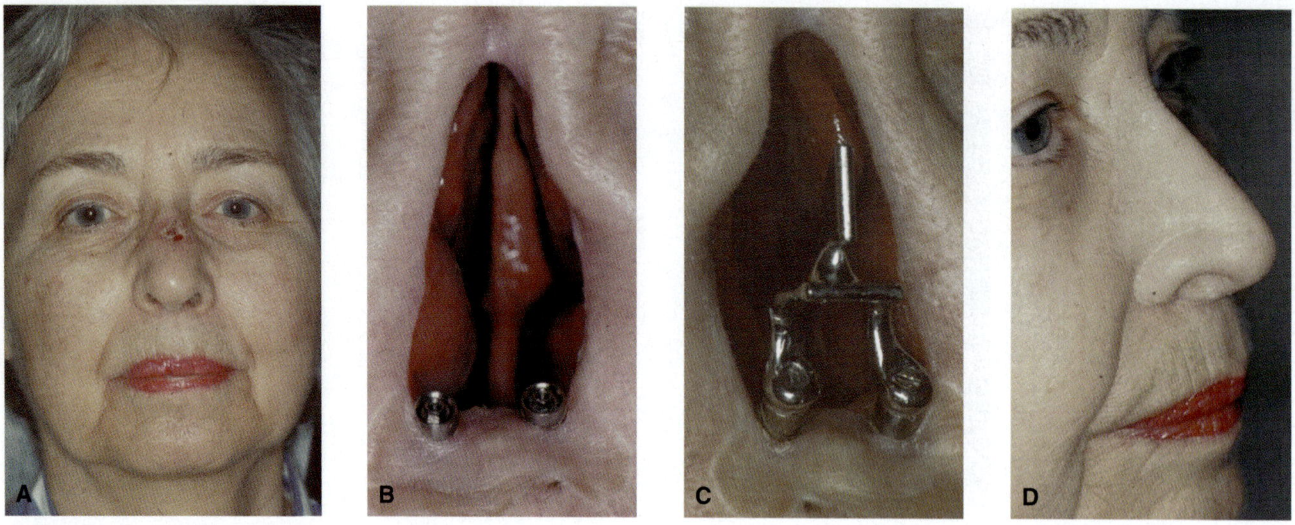

Figure 8–28. *A*, Patient presented with squamous carcinoma. *B*, Tissue bar for rhinectomy defect with Hader bar attachments arranged vertically and horizontally. *C*, Implants were placed at the time of surgical resection. *D*, Prosthesis in position.

ble of remodeling and turnover as the implant is subjected to stresses associated with supporting, retaining, and stabilizing prosthetic restorations. The viability of irradiated bone may not be sufficient to ensure a long-term predictable result, particularly in anatomic sites such as the supraorbital rim and the mandible. Even in the maxilla, remodeling and turnover of bone subjected to high-dose radiotherapy (above 5,000 cGy) may be adversely affected to the point where an implant subject to functional stresses cannot be sustained.

Predictability of Implants in Irradiated Bone

Preliminary reports and our own experience indicate that the success/failure rate of osseointegrated implants in irradiated bone appears to depend on the anatomic site selected, the dose to the site, and the use of hyperbaric oxygen. Animal experiments have shown that the quantity of the bone at the bone–implant interface is reduced.

The early trends seen in recent clinical reports appear to substantiate the concerns raised in the animal studies; namely, a high percentage of implants in irradiated tissues demonstrate advanced bone loss at an early stage. Implants in irradiated tissues used to retain facial prostheses appear to have a significantly lower success rate than implants in nonirradiated tissues (see Tables 8–1 and 8–2).

In the maxilla as well, the implant failure rate in irradiated patients has been slightly higher than in normal patients. Roumanas and colleagues reported on the results of 33 implants placed in the irradiated maxillae of 13 patients.[2] All patients received at least 5,000 cGy to the implant sites. Eleven of the 33 failed and were removed and two others were buried beneath the mucosa, for a success rate of 60.6%. Many of the remaining implants demonstrated moderate to severe bone loss around the remaining implants (bone loss extending to at least the level of the fourth thread). Because of these results, some clinicians have attempted to improve the viability of bone with hyperbaric oxygen treatments prior to implant placement.

It seems clear from the current data that osseointegration is impaired in bone that has received doses in excess of 5,000 cGy. Success rates, based on short-term clinical reports, are reduced compared with nonirradiated sites, particularly in the orbit (Figure 8–29). The success rates are lower than in normal individuals, even in the maxilla, with its excellent blood supply. In addition, preliminary animal studies appear to indicate that the bone–implant interface may be significantly compromised, making the implant less able to tolerate functional loads. Hyperbaric oxygen appears to help revitalize the bone, leading to improved success rates, but long-term clinical follow-up data are still lacking. In addition, its high cost precludes its use in most patients.

Table 8–1. NONIRRADIATED CRANIOFACIAL IMPLANTS—UCLA STUDY*

Implant Sites	Patients Treated	Placed	Number of Implants: Uncovered	Buried	Failed	Survival Rate (%)
Auricular	35	111	97	8	5	94
Nasal	16					
Piriform		27	25	0	5	80
Glabella		6	6	0	4	33
Orbital	9	28	25	2	7	70
Overall	60	172	153	10	21	85

*Implant-retained prostheses for facial defects: an up to 14-year follow-up report on the survival rates of implants at the University of California-Los Angeles. Adapted from Roumanas E et al.[9]

Risk of Osteoradionecrosis

The risk of osteoradionecrosis in the mandible is probably best determined by an analysis of the bone necrosis rate seen in postradiation extractions. Based on these data, it should be relatively safe to place implants in irradiated mandibular sites if the dose is less than 5,500 cGy. The risk would be quite high for doses above 6,500 cGy. In such patients, if implants are desirable, we recommend a course of hyperbaric oxygen. It should be noted that most patients with oral or pharyngeal tumors do not receive radiation to the symphyseal region. Therefore, implants can be placed with a high degree of predictability in this region in most irradiated patients.

In the maxilla, the risk of bone necrosis is probably negligible. The use of hyperbaric oxygen can be justified only on the basis of improving success rates.

Irradiation of Existing Implants

Irradiation of titanium implants already in place results in backscatter; therefore, the tissues on the radiation source side of the implants receive a higher dose than the other tissues in the field. The dose is increased about 15% 1 mm from the implant. Because of backscatter and the increased numbers of elderly patients receiving implants, clinicians ask if osseointegrated implants should be removed in patients about to be irradiated for head and neck tumors. Available evidence suggests that all abutments and superstructures be removed prior to radiation and skin and/or mucosa should be closed over the implant fixtures. When healing is complete, radiation therapy can begin. Following completion of radiation, abutments and the superstructure are reattached and the prosthesis is remade or readapted.

PROSTHODONTIC TREATMENT OF THE IRRADIATED PATIENT

The risk of developing an osteoradionecrosis is minimal in patients who have been edentulous for some time before undergoing head and neck radiation therapy. The risk of bone necrosis increases in those patients who have teeth removed just before or after

Table 8–2. IRRADIATED CRANIOFACIAL IMPLANTS—UCLA STUDY*

Implant Sites	Patients Treated	Placed	Number of Implants: Uncovered	Buried	Failed	Survival Rate (%)
Auricular	2	6	6	0	0	100
Nasal	4					
Piriform		8	6	0	1	83
Glabella		2	2	0	2	0
Orbital	6	19	15	0	11	27
Overall	12	35	29	0	14	52

*Implant-retained prostheses for facial defects: an up to 14-year follow-up report on the survival rates of implants at the University of California-Los Angeles. Adapted from Roumanas E et al.[9]

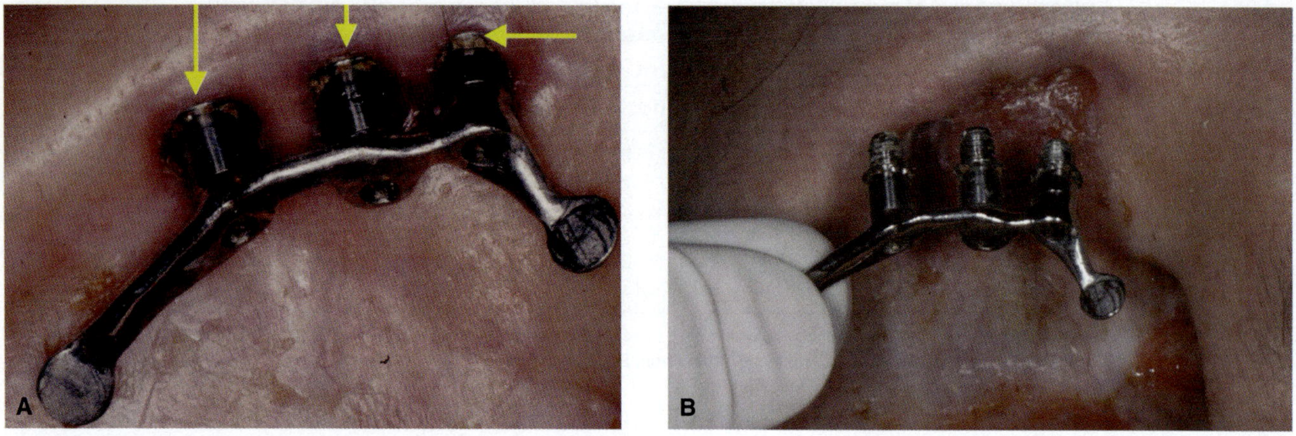

Figure 8–29. Implants in the irradiated orbit. *A*, Tissue bar retained by osseointegrated implants 2 years postdelivery. Note exposure of implant flanges. *B*, One year later, the implants failed.

radiotherapy (see Chapter 7, "Complications of Treatment").

Timing of Denture Placement

Empirical recommended insertion times have ranged up to 3 years. In our study of 92 patients who were edentulous before the onset of cancer, prostheses were inserted, on average, 15 months after radiation was completed; 45 patients received dentures within 6 months. None of the 92 developed a denture-related osteoradionecrosis. These data and our clinical experience indicate that dentures can be fabricated soon after completion of radiation therapy in most patients. If the radiation fields cover little of the mandibular denture-bearing surface, dentures can be inserted as soon as the mucositis resolves. An irregular mandibular ridge, especially in a patient whose mandible was wholly within the radiation field, may prompt the clinician to defer dentures indefinitely.

In summary, for edentulous patients who were experienced denture wearers before radiotherapy, there is little risk of developing significant complications from wearing dentures. For those who had teeth extracted within the radiation field before radiotherapy and were not experienced denture wearers, the risk of bone necrosis is higher. Therefore, placement of dentures depends on patient needs, the status of the mucosal and bony bearing surfaces, and the amount and fields of radiation. Some patients in this group may never be candidates for complete dentures.

Prosthodontic Procedures: Complete Dentures

Boggy mucosa with prominent telangiectasia and fibrosis implies that prosthodontic restorations will be poorly tolerated and mucosal integrity is at risk. In the case of floor of the mouth lesions, it may be prudent to somewhat limit extension of the mandibular-lingual flange (Figure 8–30). Scar tissue is most unyielding, and the slightest overextension can result in a mucosal perforation and perhaps lead to bone or soft tissue necrosis (see Chapter 7).

Excessive trismus is occasionally observed in patients whose radiation field includes the temporomandibular joint and muscles of mastication. If there is trismus, it may be necessary to reduce the vertical dimension of occlusion, and this will make intake of food easier. Xerostomia and viscous saliva compromise retention as well as increase friction at the denture–mucosa interface, causing mucosal irritation. Here the use of a denture adhesive powder is recommended to facilitate retention. Patients with mandibular ridges having severe bilateral undercuts, mandibular tori, or excessive ridge resorption with little attached mucosa are poor candidates for complete dentures after radiation therapy.

Impressions

Conventional border molding using a custom tray and modeling plastic is advocated. If xerostomia is particularly profound, a thin coating of petroleum

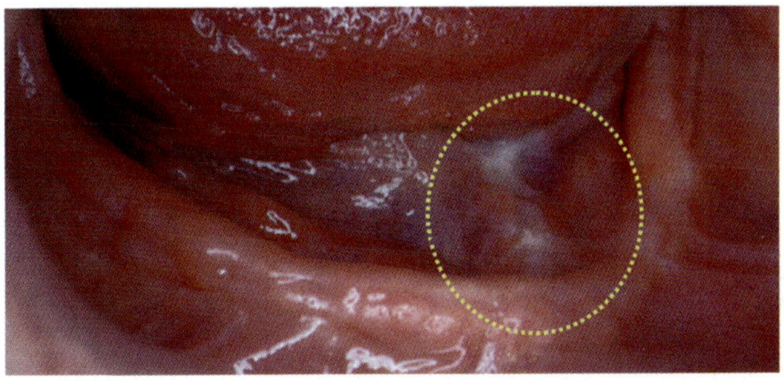

Figure 8–30. Patient received 6,800 cGy for a squamous carcinoma of the anterior floor of the mouth. Note scar associated with tumor site (*oval*). Overextension of a denture flange can result in a mucosal perforation and perhaps lead to soft tissue or bone necrosis.

may be applied over the soft modeling plastic to prevent its sticking to dry mucosa. Displacement of the tissues of the floor of the mouth in an attempt to obtain a peripheral seal is not advocated. Efforts in developing the lingual flange should be directed toward gaining stability and support rather than retention. The elastic impression materials are most suitable in refining the impression.

Vertical Dimension

The completed impressions are boxed and poured in dental stone. Conventional record bases are prepared and used to determine the vertical dimension of occlusion. The usual methods of determining vertical dimension (phonetics, closest speaking distance, swallowing, neuromuscular perception, and recording vertical dimension at rest) and centric relation apply. A variety of materials are suitable media for obtaining the final registrations. Graphic recording devices can likewise be employed successfully.

Occlusal Forms

On a theoretical basis, we favor monoplane or lingualized occlusal schemes, with bilateral balance obtained with posteriorly situated balancing ramps if needed. In arranging posterior teeth, there should be proper buccal horizontal overlap to avoid tongue and cheek biting.

Delivery and Postinsertion Care

Occlusal discrepancies should be eliminated before removing processed dentures from their casts. Pressure-indicating paste is used to identify areas of excessive pressure, and disclosing wax is useful in verifying extension of denture flanges. The dentures should be remounted on a suitable articulator, with new maxillomandibular records taken at the time of delivery. Instructions are provided about removing dentures if soreness develops, limiting denture use initially during mastication, and not wearing them during sleeping hours. During the first week, 24- and 48-hour recall appointments are recommended. Commercial denture cleansers are effective tools for removing plaque deposits and food particles from denture surfaces. Careful follow-up is essential.

SELECTED REFERENCES

1. Beumer J, Curtis T, Marunick M, editors. Maxillofacial rehabilitation: prosthodontic and surgical considerations. St. Louis: Ishiyaku EuroAmerica; 1996.
2. Roumanas E, Nishimura R, Davis B, Beumer J. Clinical evaluation of implants retaining edentulous maxillary obturator prostheses. J Prosthet Dent 1997;77:184–90.
3. Schwartzman B, Caputo A, Beumer J. Occlusal force transfer by removable partial denture designs for a radical maxillectomy. J Prosthet Dent 1985;54:397–403.
4. Urken ML, Weinberg H, Vickery C, et al. The combined sensate radial forearm and iliac crest free flaps for reconstruction of significant glossectomy–mandibulectomy defects. Laryngoscope 1992;102:543–58.
5. Curtis D, Sharma A, Finzen F, et al. Tongue and cheek function in the hemimandibulectomy patients. J Dent Res 1994;73:187.
6. Marunick M, Mathog R. Mastication in patients treated for head and neck cancer: a pilot study. J Prosthet Dent 1990;63:566–73.
7. Roumanas E, Markowitz B, Lorant J, et al. Reconstructed mandibular defects: fibula free flaps and osseointegrated implants. Plast Reconstr Surg 1997;99:356–65.
8. Ma T. Clinical overview of materials for extraoral maxillofacial prosthetics. Trans Acad Dent Mater 1992;5:9–23.
9. Roumanas E, Freymiller E, Chang TL, et al. Implant-retained prostheses for facial defects: an up to 14-year follow-up report on the survival rates of implants at UCLA. Int J Prosthodont 2002;15:325–32.

9

Leukemia and Lymphoma

MARK M. SCHUBERT, DDS, MSD
DOUGLAS E. PETERSON, DMD, PhD
SOL SILVERMAN JR., MA, DDS

Diseases of myeloproliferation (leukemias) and lymphoproliferation (lymphomas and multiple myeloma) account for almost 106,300 new cases of cancer each year in the United States and represent approximately 8% of all malignancies. These myelo- and lymphoproliferative malignancies make up a diverse group of diseases that can significantly affect oral health in a number of different ways. Additionally, dental diseases and conditions can adversely affect the course of disease and its treatment.

In approximately 25% of cases, initial signs and symptoms may appear in the oral cavity or neck. These oral manifestations may cause the patient to seek dental consultation, or the manifestations may be detected on routine examination. Special precautions may be required during selected oral and dental procedures to minimize or avoid serious adverse reactions owing to the patient's compromised immune and hematopoietic status. Therefore, knowledge of these disorders, including general signs and symptoms, pathogenesis, treatment, complications, and prognosis, is extremely important. Therapies used to treat these diseases have a profound effect on oral health, including significant morbidity.[1]

LEUKEMIAS

Leukemias represent a cohort of neoplastic disorders of the hematopoietic tissue that are characterized by proliferation of abnormal white cells.[2] They occur in all races, almost equally in males and females, and may develop at any age but are more common in adults. More than 30,000 new cases of leukemia are diagnosed each year in the United States, accounting for almost 22,000 deaths. The etiology of leukemia remains unknown, but genetic and environmental factors increase risk. Although viral etiology is well established in many animal models, a link between a virus and this disease in humans is less clear.[3] A rare form of adult T-cell leukemia/lymphoma has been correlated to exposure to a retrovirus known as human T-cell lymphotrophic virus type 1. Infection and hemorrhage are the chief causes of death.

The leukemias are typically grouped into acute and chronic diseases, primarily based on the degree of maturation of the white cells. These cohorts are then subclassified according to the cell types involved. Acute leukemias have a more rapid onset and course leading to death within 3 to 6 months if not treated. By comparison, chronic leukemias tend to have a more gradual onset and protracted course, although acceleration of disease can eventually occur and result in fatality.

Malignant transformation of precursor blood cells in the leukemias is clonal in nature.

The proliferation of the leukemic clone from a precursor cell within bone marrow does not occur at a significantly more rapid rate than proliferation of normal myeloid precursor cells. However, leukemic cells have limited ability to differentiate and mature; they increase their numbers by undergoing many more mitotic cycles than is normal. The stage of maturation and subsequent degree of overproliferation of the leukemic cell will affect the characteristic disease course and response to therapy. Less mature forms tend to have more rapid progression and be less responsive to therapy.

Proliferation of leukemic cells in the marrow, in addition to compressing the anatomic space within which nonleukemic cells are developing, can actually suppress cell division and maturation of the normal hematopoietic cells. As the leukemia progresses, increasing numbers of immature white cells or blasts begin to appear in the peripheral blood, thus reflecting the ongoing leukocytosis. Leukemic suppression of the production of other blood cells leads to progressive anemia owing to decreased erythrocyte production, reduction in platelets (thrombocytopenia), and reduction in normal white blood cells (WBCs), including polymorphonuclear leukocytes (neutropenia) (Figure 9–1).

ACUTE LEUKEMIAS

Acute leukemias result in a rapid and fulminant disease course that, if left untreated, leads to death in a few weeks to months. Potentially any of the myeloid cell lines can be involved. Acute leukemias are divided into two major types: acute lymphocytic leukemia (ALL) and acute myelogenous leukemia (AML, or occasionally designated acute nonlymphocytic leukemia [ANL]). In children between 1 and 14 years of age, ALL is the most frequent form of cancer and is the leading disease-cause of death. The primary treatment of ALL includes high-dose chemotherapy plus either central nervous system radiation or intrathecal methotrexate. Maintenance chemotherapy is administered over several years (eg, 3 years). This protocol has been shown to achieve 3-year disease-free survival for 50 to 80% of patients, with 75% of these patients remaining in remission indefinitely with no further treatment. For those patients who relapse, hematopoietic cell transplantation (HCT) has become a reasonable and effective treatment choice.

AML has shown the strongest causative link to exposure to toxins and to a variety of congenital and hematologic disorders. AML occurs in all decades of life but is primarily found in patients over the age of 30 years.[4] AML cells are not as sensitive to chemotherapy as ALL cells and thus require more aggressive intial treatment. Induction therapy, using highly intensive chemotherapy, is administered to clear the marrow of leukemic blast cells, followed by continuing chemotherapy to further consolidate the remission. Untreated survival time for AML is approximately 2 months. Induction therapy can produce a short-term remission in 50 to 70% of patients, but long-term survival is typically only 1 or 2 years. Advances in long-term survival have been achieved with HCT (see below). Long-term survival figures have changed from less than 10% for chemotherapy protocols to 40 to 50% with marrow transplantation.

Signs and symptoms of acute leukemias are related to progressive marrow failure and the increasing burden of leukemic cells. Neutropenia and functional abnormalities in the leukemic cells

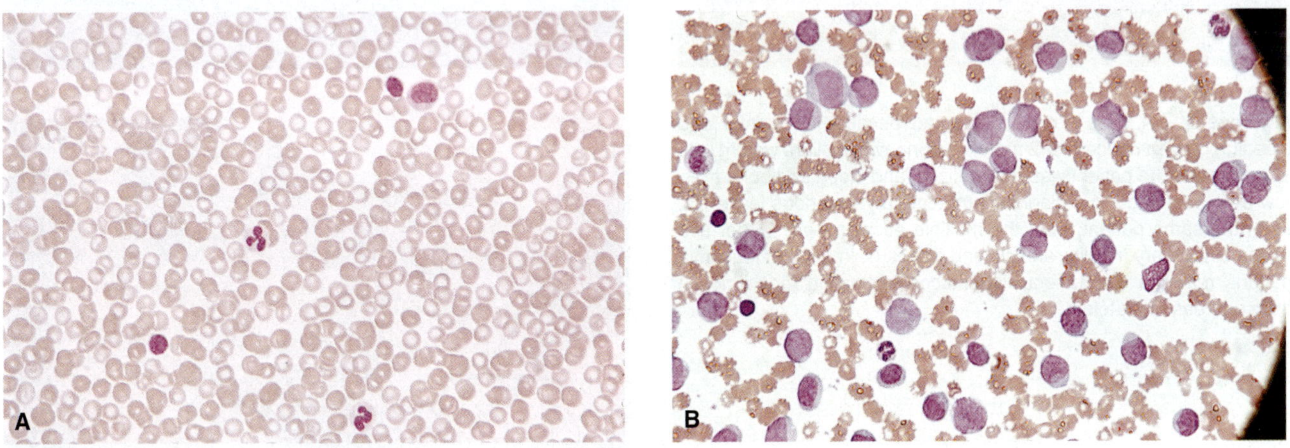

Figure 9–1. *A*, A normal differential smear. Note two normal-appearing polymorphonuclear leukocytes, two lymphocytes, one monocyte, and the approximately 700-to-1 ratio between normal-appearing red blood cells (RBCs) and white blood cells (WBCs). *B*, A differential smear from a patient with myelogenous leukemia. Note the immature myeloblasts and myelocytes and the altered RBC-to-WBC ratio.

result in progressive acute local and systemic infections, with associated fever and chills.

Symptoms of anemia owing to a profound decline in the number of erythrocytes include fatigue, dyspnea on exertion, weakness, malaise, and pallor. Bleeding complications include petechiae and purpura, epistaxis, and gingival bleeding (Figure 9–2). Other symptoms include anorexia, heachache, and joint/bone pain.

CHRONIC LEUKEMIAS

Chronic leukemias result from the proliferation of malignant lymphocytes in the case of chronic lymphocytic leukemia (CLL) and malignant myelogenous cells in chronic myelogenous leukemia (CML). Because malignant transformations occur in more mature myeloid cell types, chronic leukemias are characterized by a more indolent course than acute leukemias, and survival times are longer. The onset of CML and CLL can be insidious, and these diseases are often first detected during routine medical evaluations or examinations for other health reasons.

CML occurs primarily in individuals over the age of 20 years, with its frequency increasing with each succeeding decade.[5] CML is characterized by three stages: (a) a chronic phase with an insidious but persistent high WBC count, which can last many years; (b) an accelerated phase, in which WBC counts begin to increase despite the use of previously effective chemotherapy; and, finally, (c) blast crisis, in which the disease essentially manifests in ways comparable to acute leukemia. Once a patient progresses to the blast crisis phase, standard chemotherapy is ineffective, and survival times range from 2 to 10 months. In CML, the use of intensive chemoradiotherapy followed by HCT induces complete remission in 40 to 50% of patients.

CLL is a type of leukemia most commonly observed in the elderly population; for example, the median age at diagnosis is 70 years, and the disease is rarely found in patients under the age of 35 years.[6]

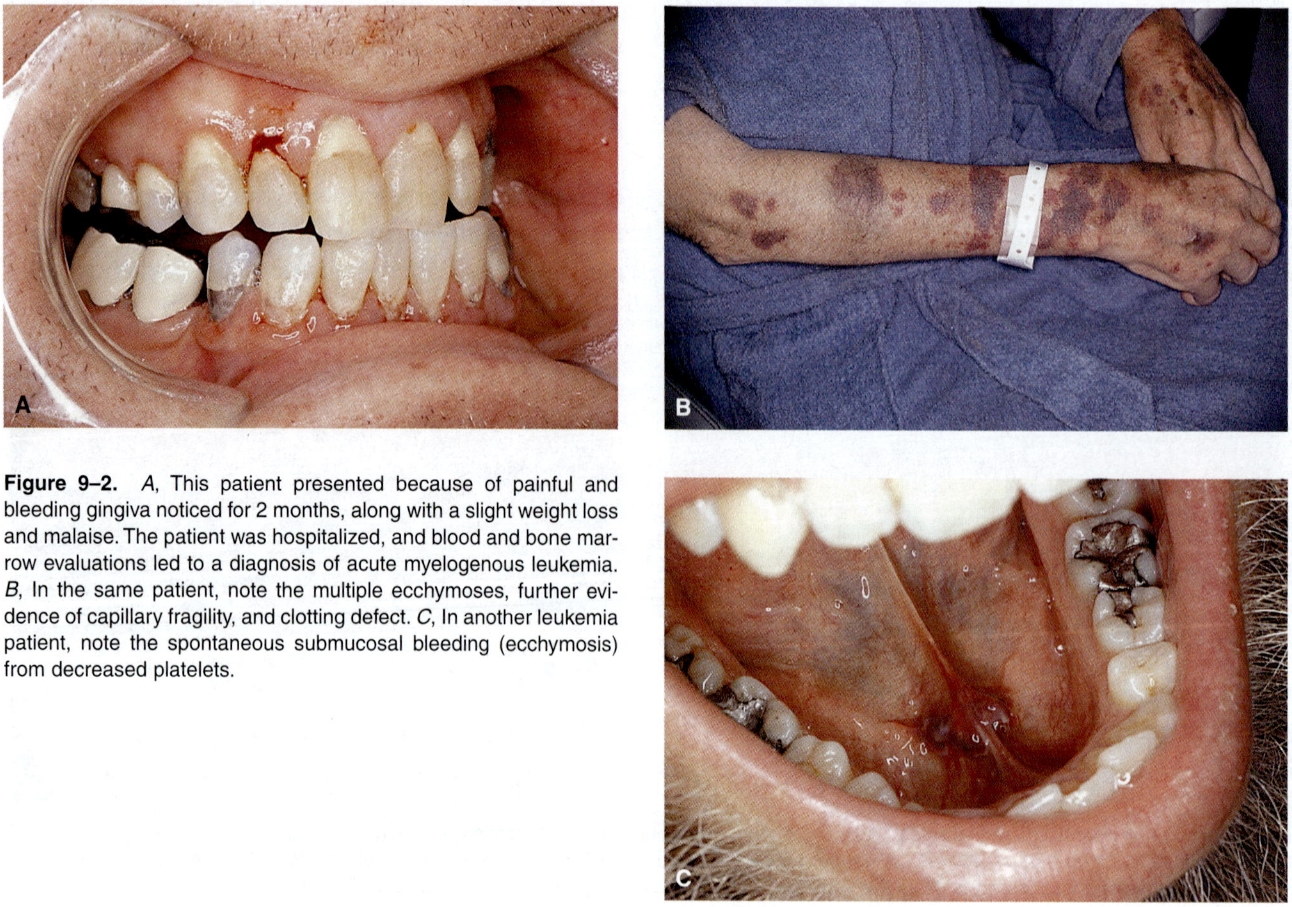

Figure 9–2. *A*, This patient presented because of painful and bleeding gingiva noticed for 2 months, along with a slight weight loss and malaise. The patient was hospitalized, and blood and bone marrow evaluations led to a diagnosis of acute myelogenous leukemia. *B*, In the same patient, note the multiple ecchymoses, further evidence of capillary fragility, and clotting defect. *C*, In another leukemia patient, note the spontaneous submucosal bleeding (ecchymosis) from decreased platelets.

Adults with CLL may live for long periods of time, often showing little clinical evidence of the disease. CLL is more aggressive in younger patients, resulting in shorter survival times. The signs and/or symptoms of CLL progress with the accumulation of B lymphocytes. Neoplastic B lymphocytes (95% of cases) or, less often, T lymphocytes aggregate chiefly in lymph nodes, spleen, blood, and marrow. There is a progressive decline in immunoglobins, but these patients can maintain adequate red blood cells (RBCs), neutrophils, and platelets until relatively late in the course of this disease. Therapy (chemotherapy alone or in combination with radiation) is generally delayed until the tumor burden affects organ health and/or produces symptoms.

The most common systemic complaints of patients with chronic leukemia are fatigue, malaise, occasionally fever or infection, lymphadenopathy, night sweats, and weight loss. Cervical lymphadenopathy and gingival bleeding may be early signs that prompt a patient to seek dental evaluation before medical consultation is sought.

LEUKOPENIA

Leukopenia, a deficiency in the number of circulating WBCs, commonly occurs in response to immunosuppressive drugs used for control of disease. Patients with leukopenia are less able to cope with infection and therefore require special precautions against infectious agents.

Classification and Findings

The leukopenias may be classified in different ways. The relative or absolute reduction of polymorphonuclear leukocytes (neutrophils) is known as neutropenia. In neutropenia, the lymphocytes and monocytes may also be slightly reduced. Marked suppression of all WBCs, along with RBCs, is termed pancytopenia.

The variable signs and symptoms of leukopenia include weakness, malaise, chills, and fever. These individuals are susceptible to infection. Painful mouth and oropharyngeal ulcerations often occur (Figure 9–3). The pathogenesis of these lesions (often referred to as neutropenic ulcerations) is thought to be a poor response to trauma, allowing local and acquired bacterial flora to cause infections.

In view of the poor resistance in these patients, there is a high risk of subsequent septicemia and a deterioration in clinical status unless the leukopenia can be reversed. Persons with leukopenia are also prone to oral fungal (*Candida*) and viral (herpes family) infections, which may further complicate their diagnosis and management. The viral infections could be in the form of herpes simplex gingivostomatitis, cold sores, varicella zoster (shingles), and/or lesions caused by cytomegalovirus (CMV).

Diagnosis and Prognosis

Diagnosis of leukopenia often initially can be documented by a complete blood count, including the total number of white cells. With associated infections, erythrocyte sedimentation rates also rise. RBCs are generally not affected. Bone marrow biopsy and hematologic testing will generally confirm the diagnosis. In drug-induced leukopenias, the platelets are usually reduced, increasing the risk of bleeding. If causative factors can be corrected or, in the case of chemotherapy-induced leukopenia, once the drug is withdrawn, subsequent recovery of the myeloid stem cells will lead to remission of clinical signs and symptoms. The most severe oral problems occur when the total WBC count falls below 2,000 cells per mm^3 from normal values, which are above 5,000 cells per mm^3.

Because neutropenia and thrombocytopenia place these patients at risk when they undergo dental procedures, consultation with the physician is recommended before any invasive intervention procedure. Often temporary withdrawal of the chemotherapeutic agent is required to increase the blood count. With or without this step, antibiotic coverage is recommended when a possible bacteremia is anticipated, and precautions should be taken against bleeding. It is important to realize that the least invasive means of managing a dental problem is usually indicated in these instances. Sometimes blood component transfusions are indicated. The patient's hematologic status often determines the extent of dental care that can be performed. Some patients who are in clinical remission (normal peripheral blood counts, clinically healthy) can receive comprehensive dental care with excellent tolerance; however, the recommended precautions should still be taken because the basic ability of these patients to cope with infection is still diminished. Patients in complete remission (including normal marrow) are often considered and treated as normal.

ORAL MANIFESTATIONS AND CARE OF PATIENTS WITH LEUKEMIA

The oral cavity may be one of the first sites of signs and/or symptoms that ultimately lead to the diagnosis of these diseases. The immunologic and hematologic deficiencies of leukemias are linked to oral manifestations that include unexplained acute periodontal abscesses and necrotizing ulcerative gingivitis, mucosal purpura, gingival edema with or without erythema and/or spontaneous gingival bleeding, excessive bleeding after a surgical procedure, and cervical lymphadenopathy. Oral candidiasis and herpetic stomatitis can also be present. Additionally, these signs may be associated with complaints of weakness, malaise, intermittent fevers, anorexia, and pallor. Unexplained bleeding or periodontal infections that do not respond to routine therapy, especially in the presence of systemic symptoms, warrant consideration of a blood dyscrasia (Figure 9–4).

Leukemic infiltrates can occur in the region of the head and neck and oral cavity. Those occurring in lymph nodes and skin/subcutaneous tissues are referred to as chloromas and can mimic local infections or reactive adenopathy. Gingival swelling owing to leukemic infiltrates is seen primarily with AML, is less common with CML, and rarely is present in ALL. Preexisting gingivitis and periodontitis predispose to gingival infiltrates. The appearance of gingival infiltrates is variable, resembling generalized gingival swelling, necrotic ulcers, purpuric lesions, hemangiomas, or granulomas and spontaneous gingival bleeding (Figures 9–5 and 9–6). Treatment requires

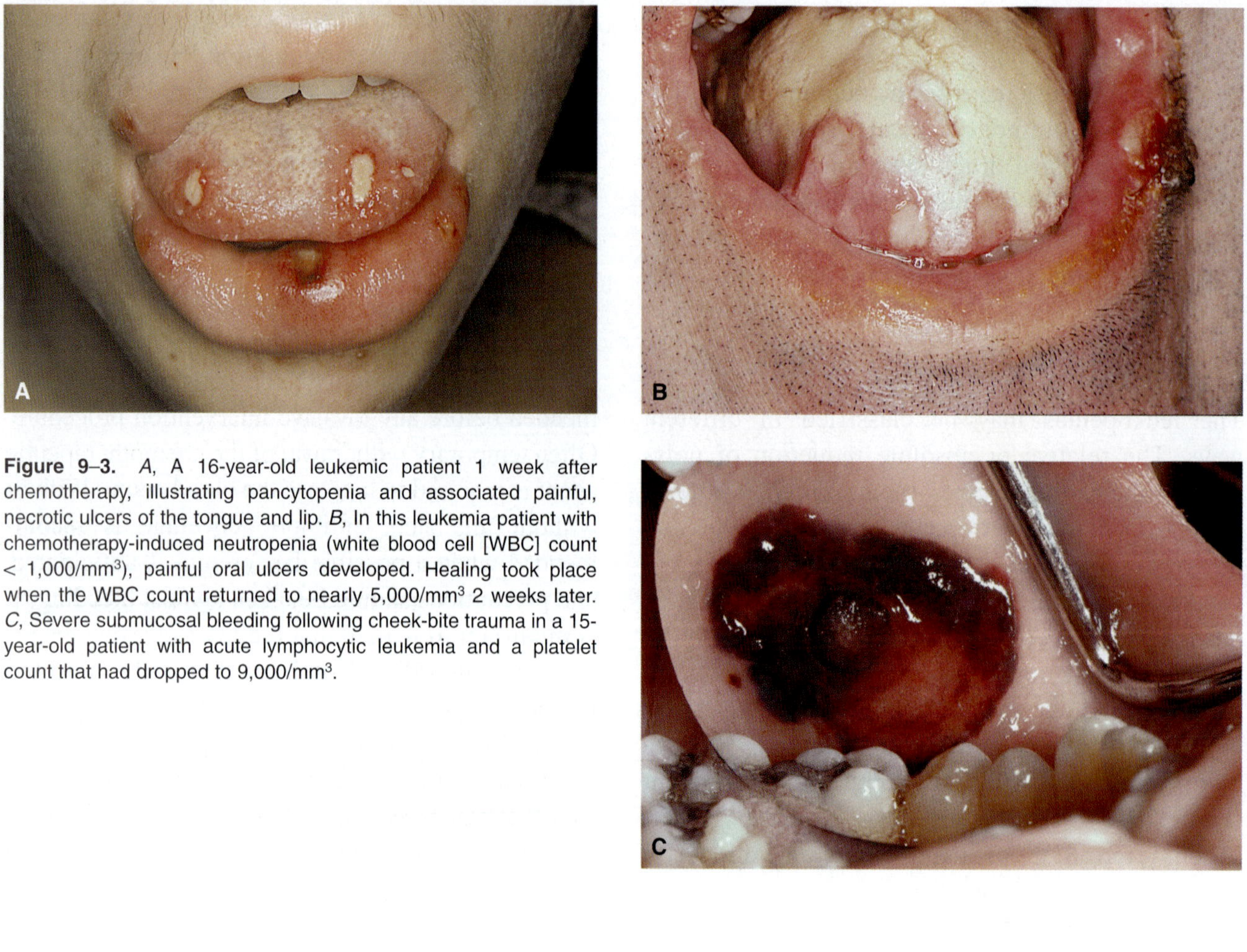

Figure 9–3. *A*, A 16-year-old leukemic patient 1 week after chemotherapy, illustrating pancytopenia and associated painful, necrotic ulcers of the tongue and lip. *B*, In this leukemia patient with chemotherapy-induced neutropenia (white blood cell [WBC] count < 1,000/mm^3), painful oral ulcers developed. Healing took place when the WBC count returned to nearly 5,000/mm^3 2 weeks later. *C*, Severe submucosal bleeding following cheek-bite trauma in a 15-year-old patient with acute lymphocytic leukemia and a platelet count that had dropped to 9,000/mm^3.

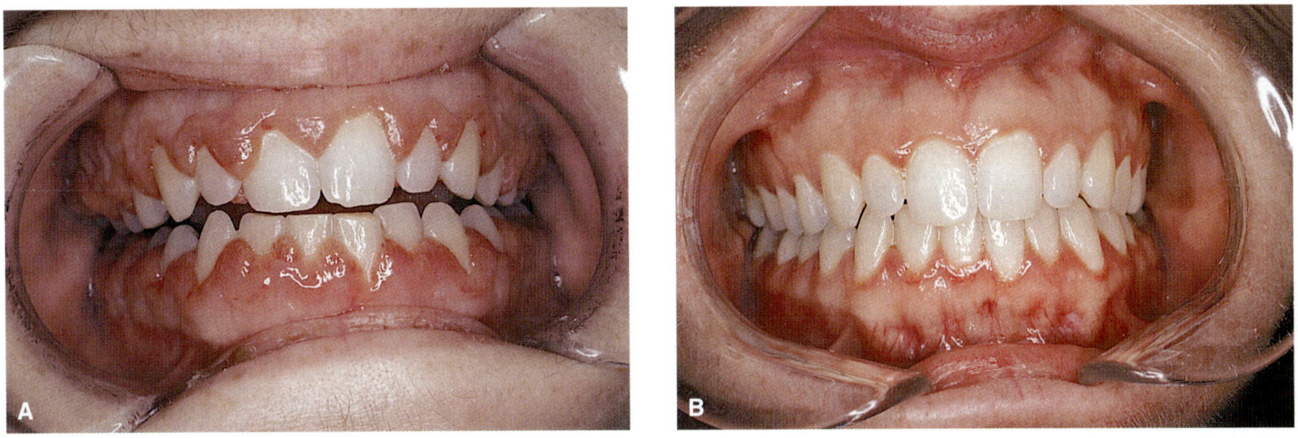

Figure 9–4. Acute myelogenous leukemia first indicated by oral signs and symptoms of gingival swelling and pain in a 26-year-old woman. *A*, Gingival swelling and erythema accompanied by pain and slight bleeding had been noticed for 3 months. The patient also complained of malaise, fever, and slight weight loss. Laboratory findings included the following: white blood cell count 80,000/mm^3, hemoglobin 9.2 g/100 mL, scarcity of platelets, and many immature cells in the monocyte series. *B*, Induction chemotherapy achieved a temporary remission leading to a general feeling of well-being, and her gingiva showed a great improvement. Six months after chemotherapy and a bone marrow transplant (sister donor), the patient had no evidence of active leukemia, and her gingiva appeared almost normal.

maintanence of excellent oral hygiene (brushing, flossing, antimicrobial oral rinses) but generally depends on systemic antileukemic chemotherapy or even low-dose radiation therapy to eliminate any infiltrating leukemic cells.

Oral Infections

Oral infections represent one of the most serious oral complications for the leukemic patient. Bacterial, viral, and fungal infections can cause local tissue damage and pain. In addition, and when a patient is immunocompromised, there is significant risk of a life-threatening septicemia.

Fungal Infections

Oral *Candida* infections are relatively common in leukemia patients, with pseudomembranous (white) candidiasis being the most frequent form (Figure 9–7, A). As immunosuppression becomes more profound, atrophic (red) and invasive candidiasis can occur. During periods of profound immunosuppression, other invasive fungal infec-

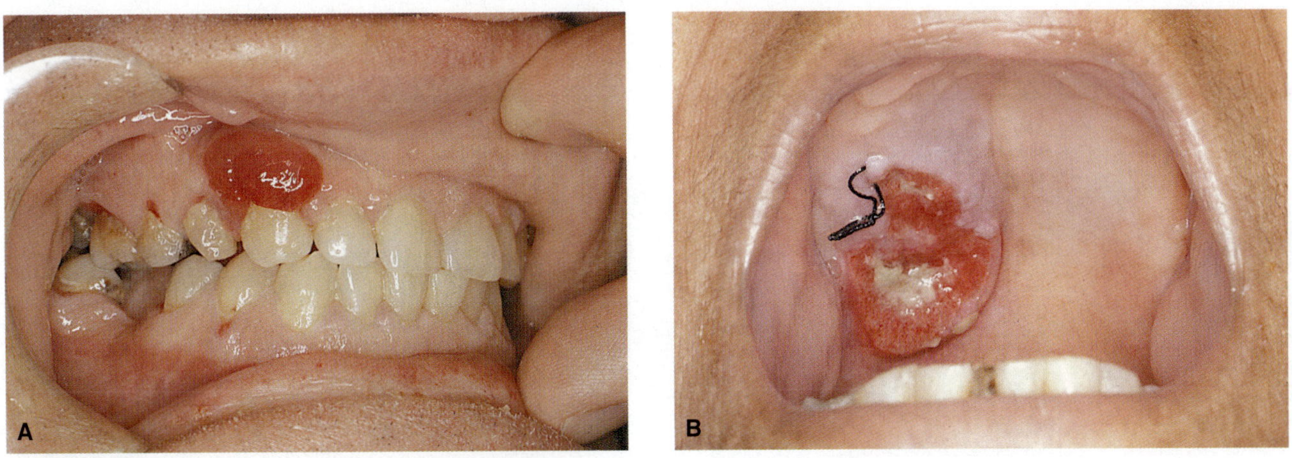

Figure 9–5. Leukemic infiltrates in the mouth. These infiltrates are an accumulation of immature cells similar to those found in the marrow. *A*, Mildly symptomatic infiltrate of maxillary gingiva, which bled in response to mild irritation. *B*, Large leukemic infiltrate in the palate of a patient with chronic lymphocytic leukemia. The lesion was controlled by a combination of chemotherapy and localized irradiation (600 cGy in two treatments).

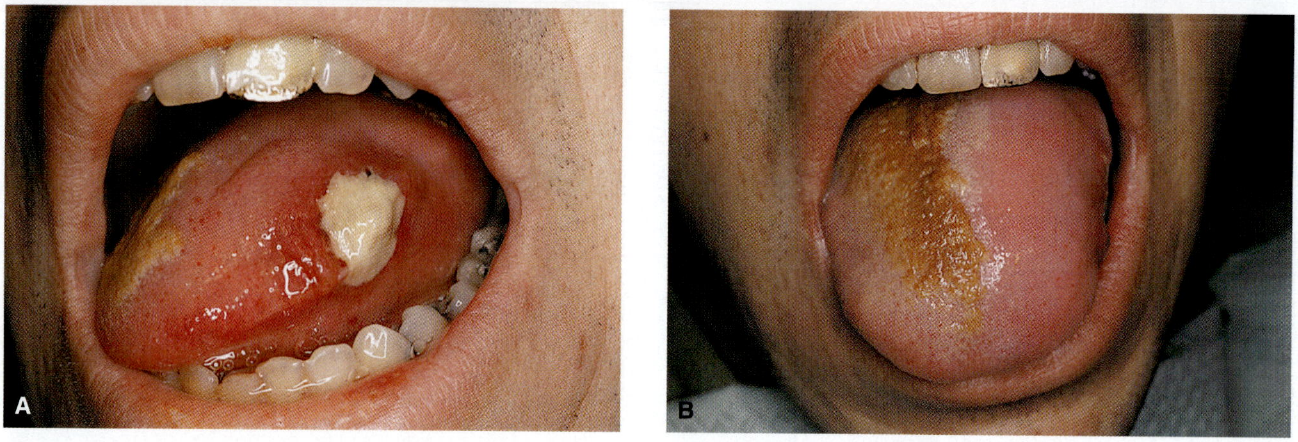

Figure 9–6. *A*, A very painful leukemic infiltrate of the tongue in an adolescent with acute myelogenous leukemia. *B*, Low-dose irradiation in three fractions led to a complete response.

tions (aspergillosis, histoplasmosis, and mucormycosis) become a concern (Figure 9–7, B). Infections often cannot be controlled until the patient's leukopenia improves.

A variety of topical agents are available for the management of oral candidiasis, including nystatin products (rinses, pastilles, and powders), clotrimazole troches, and amphotericin rinses.[7] The use of prophylactic topical oral antifungal agents has not been shown to be effective in preventing oral fungal colonization in these patients. However, clinical signs and symptoms can be controlled with these agents (see Chapter 7, "Complications of Treatment"). Systemic therapy with fluconazole, itraconazole, ketoconazole, or amphotericin B can be effective in managing superficial and invasive oral fungal infections.[8]

Viral Infections

Viral infections are responsible for significant morbidity in patients who are immunosuppressed (Figure 9–8). Reactivation of the herpes simplex virus (HSV), when there is a deficiency in cellular immunity, can result in severe oral lesions. The ulcerations can appear atypical and become very large and painful. They may persist as long as the patient is immunocompromised or until therapy is instituted. Lesions caused by the varicella-zoster virus (VZV), CMV, adenovirus, and coxsackievirus are occasionally seen.

In patients with mild HSV lesions, treatment can often be supportive and palliative. Mild-to-moderate disease is usually treated with oral acyclovir, valacyclovir, or famciclovir. However, as the severity of

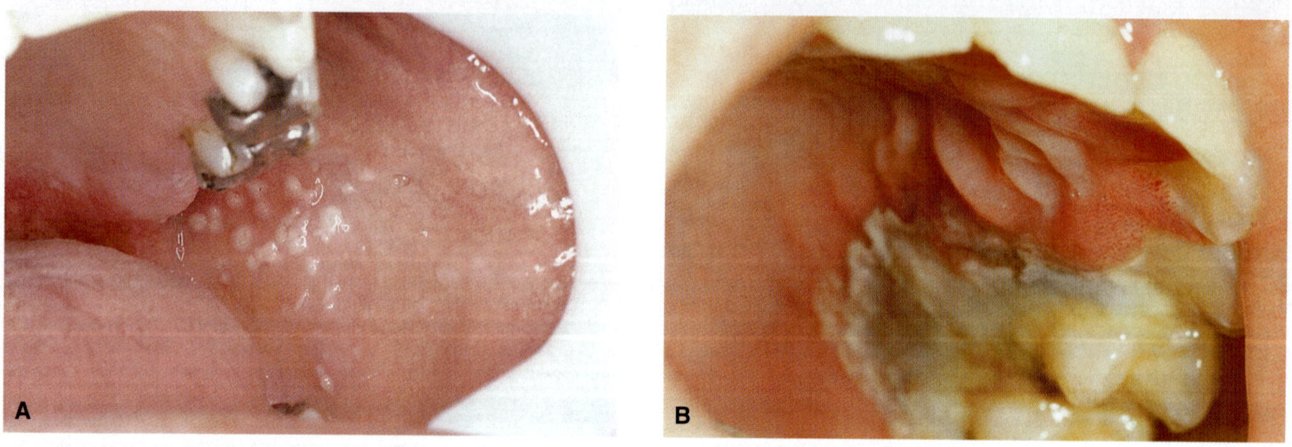

Figure 9–7. *A*, Pseudomembranous candidiasis occurring in response to chemotherapy-induced neutropenia and xerostomia. *B*, Mucormycosis (zygomycosis, phycomycosis) involving the palate of a leukemia patient 35 days post–allogeneic transplantation. Treatment entailed surgical resection of bone and mucosa along with intensive systemic antifungal therapy with amphotericin.

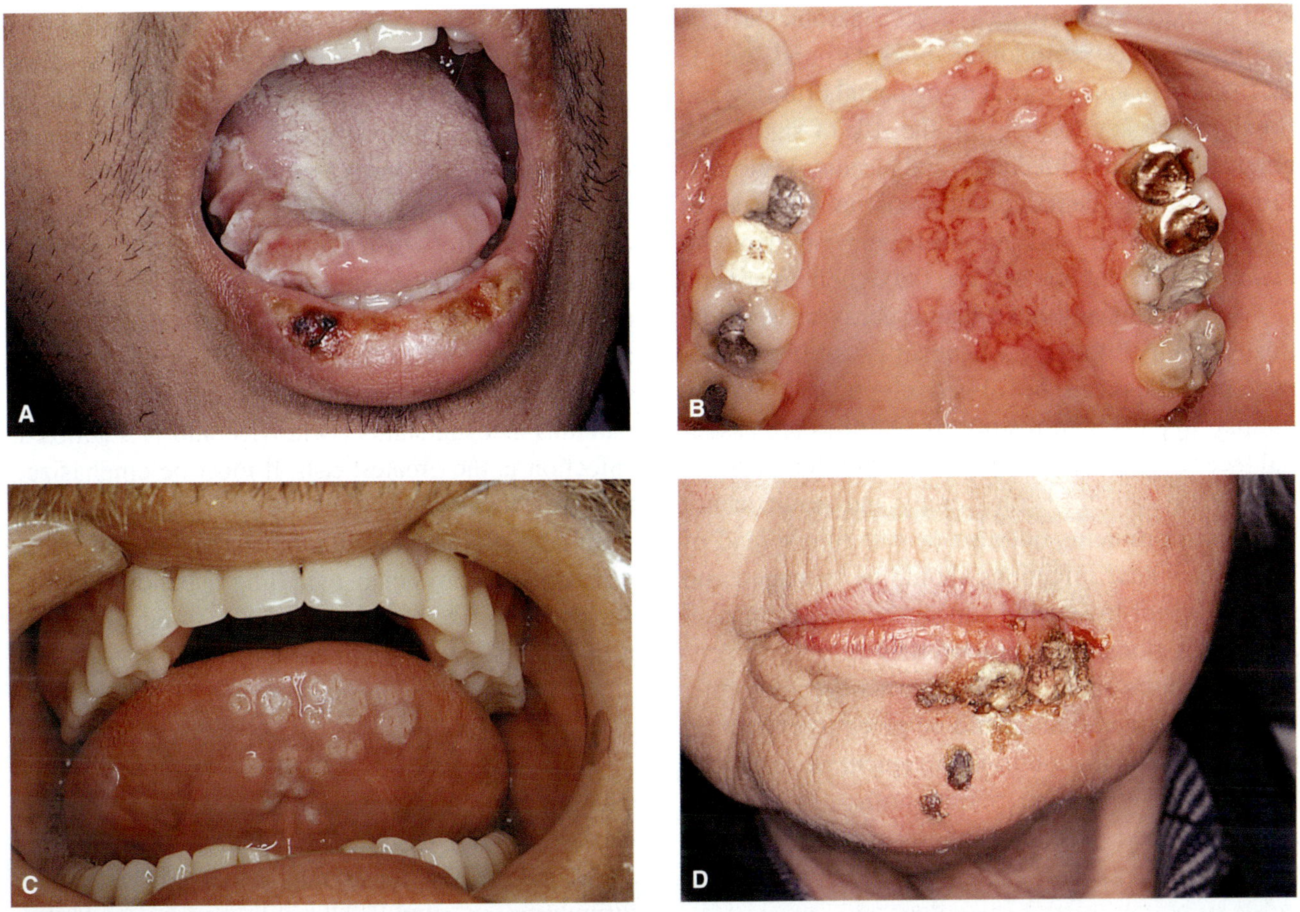

Figure 9–8. Herpes-family virus infections in immunosuppressed leukopenic patients. *A*, Recurrent herpes simplex infections of lip and tongue from reactivated virus. *B*, Recurrent herpes simplex infection of the palate, day 5. *C*, Primary herpetic gingivostomatitis in a leukemic patient being controlled with periodic chemotherapy, day 7. *D*, Varicella-zoster (shingles) in an immunosuppressed lymphoma patient. Note the unilateral distribution of the painful ulcerations.

immunocompromised status increases or if patients develop more extensive disease, consideration for parenteral antiviral therapy with acyclovir or a very high oral dosage is preferred. HSV and VZV can be treated with either acyclovir/valacyclovir or famciclovir.

CMV infection is treated with ganciclovir. Patients who have positive antibody titers to HSV and CMV are typically given a prophylactic antiviral drug to suppress viral reactivation prior to chemotherapy.

Human papillomavirus skin infections are commonly noted following HCT (see below) and can occasionally be seen in the oral cavity as verrucous-appearing lesions.

Bacterial Infections

Bacterial infections can be caused by organisms normally found in the oral cavity, as well as by opportunistic and acquired pathogens such as *Pseudomonas, Klebsiella, Serratia,* and *Escherichia* spp. Staphylococcal and streptococcal species can cause significant oral infections. Identification of the source of infection and appropriate selection of antimicrobial agent(s) are critical to effective management.

Gingival and periodontal infections are a major concern for patients being treated for leukemia. They can account for fevers of undetermined origin and bacteremias. One study showed that 25% of all acute infections experienced by AML patients while undergoing induction therapy arose in a site of preexisting periodontal disease. Improved infectious disease protocols (antibiotics, oral care) for immunosuppressed patients have reduced the frequency and severity of this problem. When periodontal infection occurs, treatment considerations should include broad-pectrum antibiotics, chlorhexidine rinsing, irrigation with peroxide agents (which affect anaerobic bacteria colonizing the periodontal pocket), and gentle mechanical plaque removal using dental brushing and flossing. The key to reducing the risk of significant gingiva-associated infections (and bleeding) is to perform thorough dental prophylaxis in advance of myelosuppression and to implement protocols to maintain excellent oral hygiene throughout treatment.

Moderate or advanced dental decay needs to be treated prior to therapy whenever possible. Temporary materials can be effectively placed. Again, optimal hygiene and the use of fluorides are essential (see Chapter 7). Pulpal/periapical infections can complicate cancer chemotherapy and result in not only local problems but also in systemic spread of infection. These infections should be managed and resolved prior to starting cancer therapy. Empirical antibiotics along with appropriately aggressive dental procedures should be used whenever possible. Careful consideration should be given to extraction of teeth with endodontic involvement or instances of moderate to severe periodontitis.[9] Prophylatic antibiotics and platelet support may be required prior to surgery.

Summary Overview of Oral and Dental Care

When it is suspected that a patient may have leukemia, conservative empirical care should be prescribed while diagnostic blood work or appropriate referral is made to evaluate the possibility of a blood dyscrasia. As the leukemic cell burden increases, the normal marrow function becomes impaired, and mature WBC, RBC, and platelet counts decrease, patients become increasingly prone to infection, bleeding, and anemia. Whenever possible, patients should receive dental treatment to eliminate any active infections as well as conditions that increase the risk for oral bleeding. During chemotherapy for leukemia, all blood counts drop dramatically, and it is generally not feasible to perform any dental treatments without aggressive supportive care, and, even then, treatment is generally not advised. In the immediate recovery period following chemotherapy, all counts can remain depressed for weeks to months, making the patient especially susceptible to infections, bleeding complications, and mucositis.

It is important to keep patients free from oral foci of infection. Initially, temporary conservative management strategies for dental disease should focus on managing dental problems as noninvasively as possible. Bland mouthrinses, antibiotics, and analgesic agents can be used. Aspirin and other nonsteroidal anti-inflammatory drugs should not be used owing to their negative effects on platelet aggregation. Temporary restorations and noninvasive periodontal therapy are indicated. Curettage, extractions, or other "aggressive" therapies should be avoided until the patient's medical status is clarified and/or stabilized. Infection is the greatest risk. It must be emphasized that any "invasive" or questionable dental procedure should be coordinated with the medical oncologist or primary care physician regarding a patient's status, ability to tolerate dental procedures, timing, and suggested prophylactic regimens.

Oral Mucositis

Chemotherapeutic agents used to eradicate malignant white cell production can also affect normal cells, particulary those that have relatively high turnover rates, such as bone marrow, hair follicles, and gastrointestinal and oral mucosae.[10]

Damage to the oral mucosal epithelium from chemotherapy and radiation results in mucosal thinning, ulceration, and submucosal inflammation—a condition referred to as oral mucositis (Figure 9–9).[11] Additionally, gastrointestinal damage can cause emesis, which can result in chemical (ie, acidic) damage to oral tissues. Oral mucositis causes significant pain, interferes with oral hydration and eating, and increases the risk of local and systemic infection (bacteremia). Different chemotherapeutic agents cause different degrees of toxicity to oral mucosa (see Chapter 6, "Treatment"). This toxicity is exacerbated by neutropenia as well as by physical or chemical trauma.

A stepped approach to the management of mucositis can be used, with progression to various levels (see Chapter 7). Bland oral rinses (0.9% saline, sodium bicarbonate) can be soothing and help with dryness for patients with mild-to-moderate mucositis. Other topical agents to provide temporary relief of mucositis pain include antacid solutions and saliva substitutes.

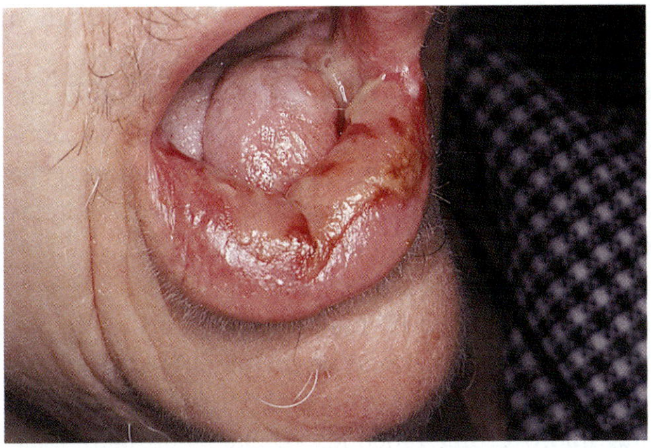

Figure 9–9. This leukemia patient developed a painful mucositis 1 week after chemotherapy. His white blood cell count had dropped to below 1,000 cells/mm^3.

Topical anesthetics can be introduced as mucositis pain increases. Agents including viscous lidocaine, diphenhydramine, and doxepin solutions can be sprayed and swished, held for 1 to 2 minutes, and expectorated as often as needed. Many centers commonly use a combination solution containing topical anesthetics, coating agents, antifungals, and antihistamines. However, consideration should be given to the cost-benefit ratio of these combination rinses versus the use of the various agents individually. The specially formulated combination mouthrinses (concoctions usually unique to a hospital) are usually expensive and contain ineffective dosages of each component. However, they do offer relief to some patients. Whenever topical anesthesia is used, patients need to be instructed (a) not to eat for 30 minutes following use, (b) to avoid posterior oropharyngeal anesthesia that could increase the risk of aspiration owing to elimination of the gag reflex, and (c) that swallowing of anesthetics could result in systemic toxicity. The use of topical corticosteriods is unlikely to cause immunosuppression but may increase the risk for infection.

It is important to introduce systemic analgesics as soon as pain management with the above agents is deemed inadequate. Long-acting opiates formulated for timed release or in patches, or those administered by computerized patient-controlled analgesia methods, are optimal in most cases.

Research efforts are under way to identify agents or techniques that are capable of reducing or preventing oral mucositis. Examples include prostaglandin analogues, L-glutamine, and benzydamine hydrochloride mouthrinses. The efficacy of oral sucralfate suspension (a coating agent) is not clear. Use of cytokines and growth factors (eg, epidermal growth factor, transforming growth factor β3, interferon-α, and keratinocyte growth factors) either to directly reduce mucosal damage or improve mucosal healing appears promising. Other approaches involve antimicrobial proteins such as defensins (Iseganin) and topical antibiotics to reduce the influence of oral microflora on damaged mucosa. Low-energy lasers to stimulate mucosal repair appear to be of some limited promise.

Invasive Procedures

Prior to invasive dental and surgical procedures in patients with leukemia or undergoing chemotherapy, the patient's immune and coagulation status has to be carefully assessed and antibiotic and platelet support used accordingly. However, each case needs to be analyzed and the patient's physician and other appropriate specialists consulted. It is important to consider the risk of undertaking dental treatments versus not carrying out the proposed therapy.

Extractions should be carried out atraumatically and sockets closed primarily, following conservative alveolectomy. If there is documented infection associated with the tooth, antibiotics should be administered for 7 to 10 days following surgery. Whenever possible, 10 to 14 days should be allowed following extraction prior to beginning myelosuppressive chemotherapy. If extraction is not possible, initial endodontic therapy can be started, along with systemic antibiotic coverage. If still necessary, extractions can be performed once the hematologic status has returned to normal. Appropriate treatment to eliminate the risk of infection is important because pathogens can readily disseminate directly from the dental pulp and periapical tissues into the systemic circulation.

The value of topical chlorhexidine to reduce bacterial colonization and infection in immunosuppressed cancer patients remains unclear. Use of chlorhexidine rinses to augment oral hygiene appears to have value when routine brushing and flossing are not possible. Chlorhexidine has been reported in some studies to reduce the severity and/or duration of mucositis but has shown no benefit in several others. Furthermore, chronic use has been shown to predispose to overgrowth by gram-negative pathogens and thus should be avoided.

Removable prosthetic appliances should be adjusted to prevent oral mucosal trauma. Denture-soaking cups can readily become colonized with a variety of pathogens, including *Pseudomonas aeruginosa, Escherichia coli, Enterobacter* spp, *Klebsiella* spp, *Staphylococcus aureus,* and *Candida* species (*C. albicans, C. tropicalis, C. glabrata,* etc). Soaking solutions should be changed daily to minimize bacterial colonization. It is reasonable to have patients restrict denture use during chemotherapy.

Oral Hemorrhage

Bleeding in patients receiving cancer therapy can result from thrombocytopenia, disseminated intravascular coagulation, and liver disease, especially in the presence of gingivitis/periodontitis, viral infections, or other ulcerative lesions. Spontaneous mucosal petechiae and gingival bleeding can occur when the platelet level drops below 20,000 cells per mm^3 (Figure 9–10). Trauma associated with oral function can also induce hemorrhage. Bleeding can be alarming to patients and caregivers but is rarely a serious or debilitating complication. Local therapy for bleeding is directed toward establishing an adequate clot. Direct pressure applied by gauze soaked in topical thrombin can be used. Ice can provide temporary vasoconstriction, or vasoconstricting drugs such as cocaine solutions or epinephrine can be applied. Rebound vasodilation can occur as the drug's effect wears off. Collagen products to promote clot formation (eg, microfibrillar collagen) are helpful to organize and stabilize clots. Platelet transfusions are usually required when platelet counts are profoundly suppressed in the face of active bleeding that does not respond to local therapy.

Salivary Gland Dysfunction

Hyposalivation in chemotherapy patients varies with different agents and protocols. Salivary gland damage occurs during the first 3 weeks after chemotherapy begins, with gradual healing after the cessation of therapy. Salivary dysfunction associated with cancer chemotherapy is generally reversible. Drugs that can cause xerostomia may contribute to xerostomia (eg, anticholinergics, antiemetics, or tricyclic antidepressants). Mouth breathing or oxygen administration contributes to oral dryness.

Management of salivary gland dysfunction is similar to that induced by radiotherapy (see Chapter 7). Sialogogues (pilocarpine or cevimeline) can help to stimulate salivary secretions and relieve symptoms and improve oral functions. Dietary considerations, such as using moist foods (eg, flavored gelatins) or sauces and gravies, can improve the comfort of eating. Dry or cracked lips should be kept lubricated with lip-moisturizing agents or lanolin-based creams.

Risk of decay increases from a loss of salivary remineralizing elements, antimicrobial proteins, and a shift to the more cariogenic bacterial flora. Management includes effective plaque removal (brushing and flossing), diet modifications to reduce cariogenic foods, topical antimicrobial rinses (chlorhexidine), and daily topical fluoride use (eg, 1.1% neutral sodium fluoride or 0.4% stannous fluoride gel) that can be applied by brushing, rinsing, or vinyl trays.

Neurotoxicity

Neurotoxicity can be associated with the use of the *Vinca* alkaloids (vincristine and vinblastine). These chemotherapeutic agents can cause severe, deep-

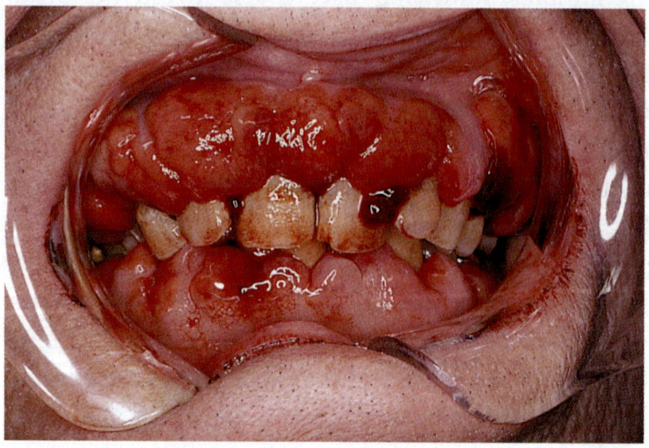

Figure 9–10. Unresponsive acute myelogenous leukemia. Note gingival infiltrates and spontaneous bleeding. The patient had profound neutropenia and thrombocytopenia.

seated, throbbing mandibular or maxillary pain that can mimic dental pathology (eg, toothaches). Usually, this type of neurotoxicity is transient and subsides soon after reducing or stopping the chemotherapy. Opioid-containing analgesics are usually effective for controlling this type of pain.

Occasionally, tooth hypersensitivity, especially to thermal stimuli, arises several weeks following chemotherapy or HCT. Symptoms are usually only mild to moderate in severity and resolve spontaneously within a few weeks to months. Desensitizing toothpastes and/or topical fluorides may help reduce symptoms and speed recovery.

Taste dysfunction represents a neurosensory toxicity of the cancer therapy. The taste bud receptor is a neuroepithelium-derived cell with a turnover rate of approximately 10 days. Affected buds usually regenerate. Cancer chemotherapy can occasionally cause a bad taste (termed venous taste phenomenon) that results from the diffusion of the drug into the oral cavity.

Temporomandibular dysfunction can manifest as facial pain, headache, and, occasionally, ear pain. Patients are clearly prone to clenching/bruxism as a result of stress, sleep dysfunction, and/or, occasionally, central nervous system toxicity caused by certain medications. Muscle relaxants or anxiety-reducing agents plus local physical therapy (moist heat applications, massage, and gentle stretching) will often resolve these symptoms. Occlusal splints to be used while sleeping may be helpful for patients with more persistent clenching/bruxism tendencies.

Alterations in Dental and Skeletal Growth and Development

High-dose chemotherapy can damage developing dental and skeletal structures, resulting in hypoplastic dentin and/or enamel, shortened and/or conical roots, taurodontic-like teeth, microdontia, incomplete enamel formation, and complete agenesis of teeth (Figure 9–11). Eruption patterns can be altered. Shortened root length leads to decreased alveolar height. Development can be reduced owing to damage to growth centers in the maxilla and mandible. However, it is useful to note that these changes in overall facial/jaw size are symmetric and do not result in signficant maxillary and/or mandibular discrepancies. The addition of radiation to treatment protocols (eg, cranial or total-body irradiation [TBI]) significantly increases the risk of damage to developing teeth and jaws.

MALIGNANT LYMPHOMAS

The term malignant lymphoma refers to a number of clinically related disorders caused by neoplastic proliferations of the lymphoreticular system. Although these diseases usually present with lymphadenopathy or splenomegaly, extranodal sites, including the oropharynx (Waldeyer's ring), the gingiva, and other oral tissues, can be involved with disease and cause signs and symptoms.[12] In fact, the recognition of such lesions may lead to the initial suspicion and diagnosis. The diseases to be considered here are Hodgkin's disease (HD), non-Hodgkin's lymphomas (NHLs) (including Burkitt's lymphoma [BL] and mycosis fungoides [MF]), and multiple myeloma.

HODGKIN'S DISEASE

HD is a lymphoproliferative disorder. The diagnosis of HD is based on the histologic presence of the multinucleated Reed-Sternberg giant cells in a biopsied lymph node. Staging on the basis of clinical findings and molecular resonance imaging is critical

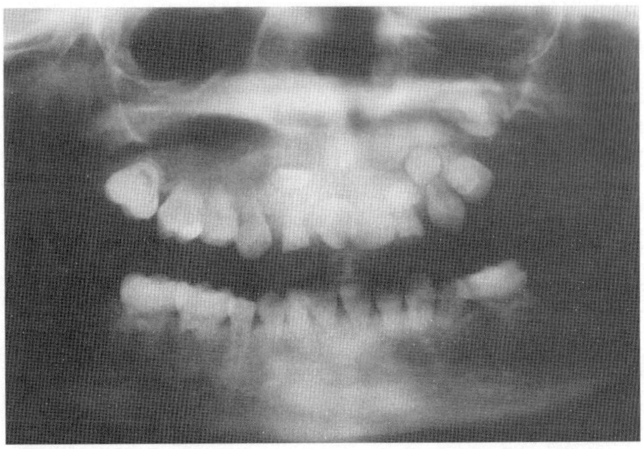

Figure 9–11. Panograph jaw radiograph in a 13-year-old patient who had undergone hematopoietic cell transplantation for acute lymphocytic leukemia at 18 months of age. Damage to the dentition from chemotherapy and total-body irradiation (shortened roots, misshaped crowns, impactions, and agenesis).

to treatment and prognosis. At the present time, the etiology of this disease is not known, although there is evidence of a genetic tendency in individuals with certain human leukocyte antigens (HLAs). There is a characteristic bimodal age and incidence curve with one peak in early adult life and a second sustained increase in the fifth decade. HD is seen in all races. Each year it afflicts about 7,000 Americans and kills approximately 1,400.

Signs and Symptoms

Complaints may include fever, unexplained weight loss, excessive sweating, pruritus, and fatigue. However, the most important sign is painless lymph node enlargement, with most patients presenting with adenopathy in the supraclavicular or cervical area. Although not common, oral and nasopharyngeal lesions have been reported. Diagnosis is made by biopsy.

Pathogenesis, Treatment, and Survival

HD appears to start in regional lymph nodes and spreads in a somewhat unpredictable but orderly way as it progresses. In 60 to 80% of cases, HD starts in the head and neck region. With disease progress, nodal involvement is noted to extend from supraclavicular nodes to mediastinal (above the diaphragm) nodes to abdominal (below the diaphragm) nodes. Survival times vary from months to many years.

Localized cervical disease has the best prognosis. Histopathologic classifications of HD-involved lymph nodes (lymphocyte predominant, nodular sclerosis, mixed cellularity, and lymphocyte depleted) correlate well with the clinical stage and aggressiveness of disease. Prognosis varies with disease stage; the 5-year relative survival rate for stage I disease approximates 90% and drops to about 60% in stage IV disease. Treatment ranges from minimal supportive care to intensive combinations of radiation and chemotherapy. Remissions and recurrences are common. A complication of combined treatment is the risk of developing acute leukemia. The use of HCT to control otherwise incurable disease has had success.

Dental Implications

The dentist becomes involved in two ways. First, the initial signs usually include cervical lymphadenopathy with associated symptoms (Figure 9–12). The head and neck may be the only area involved early in the disease. Therefore, careful evaluation of persistent lymphadenopathy is important for early recognition and accelerated proper staging and treatment. Second, these patients have varying degrees of impaired immunity and thus require optimal oral health to keep their teeth and periodontal structures from acting as foci for infection. Precautions regarding anemia, thrombocytopenia, and neutropenia apply to HD patients just as they do to patients with leukemia. Oral complications of HD treatment are similar in range (although generally less severe than in leukemia) and also are managed similarly. Radiotherapy alone is used to treat limited disease, mainly stages I and II. Chemotherapy is added to radiation therapy where advanced-stage disease exists. Head and neck radiation fields to treat cervical lymph nodes include the salivary glands as part of mantle field radiation. The total radiation dose is usually moderately low (400 to 500 cGy); therefore, most patients will generally recover some degree of salivary flow, which may or may not be satisfactory.[13] Although there is still some risk for osteonecrosis

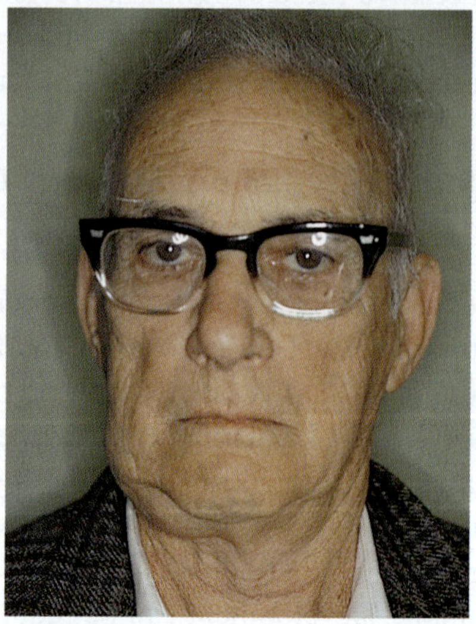

Figure 9–12. Submandibular swelling in patient with Hodgkin's disease. Evaluation showed the mass to be a tumor-filled lymph node that was the first clinical manifestation of widespread Hodgkin's lymphoma.

following these doses, it is not as significant as that seen with radiation protocols for head and neck squamous cell carcinomas (see Chapter 7).

NON-HODGKIN'S LYMPHOMA

NHL represents a heterogeneous group of malignant disorders of lymphoid derivation involving a wide range of disorders with associated important variations in patient age at the time of diagnosis, primary cell of origin, and therapeutic response. NHL can range in severity from relatively indolent to aggressive and rapidly fatal lymphoproliferative disease. Almost 54,000 new cases of NHL are diagnosed each year in the United States, and over 24,000 will succumb to their disease. Gender distribution is about equal, with a slight male bias. The etiology of these lymphomas remains unknown, although radiation, chemotherapy, viral infection, and immune deficiencies have been associated factors.

Different types of B-cell lymphomas have been linked to the Epstein-Barr virus (EBV) in many cases. Additionally, NHL is the second most common, as well as the fastest increasing, malignancy associated with human immunodeficiency virus (HIV) infections (see Chapter 12, "Human Immunodeficiency Virus–Associated Malignancies"). Overall, the 5-year survival rate for persons with NHL is 30 to 40%.

Clinical Features

NHL occurs in people of all races and in all age groups, arising in any lymphoid aggregate. Lymphadenopathy, sometimes painful, is the usual initial finding and very frequently occurs in the head and neck area. The early clinical signs and symptoms of NHL include malaise, fever, weight loss, and sweating. The diagnosis is made by biopsy.

Extranodal disease occurs in about 25% of patients with NHL. The two most common sites are the stomach and the head and neck region. In the head and neck region, intraoral NHL is uncommon, occurring most frequently in older and/or immunocompromised persons. When NHL occurs as localized extranodal involvement of the head and neck, nearly three-fourths involve Waldeyer's ring (nasopharynx) and one-fourth involves the paranasal sinuses. Although any mucosal site can be involved, the most frequent oral sites are the soft and hard palate (Figure 9–13). Malignant lymphomas are usually multifocal, even from the beginning, with a range from localized nodal disease to disseminated disease involving the bone marrow. Classification and staging depend on the immunophenotype and morphology of cells, tissue architecture, cytogenetic abnormalities, and the extent of disease. In addition, the testing has clinical relevance regarding treatment planning.

Treatment

Treatment usually depends on multidisciplinary treatment plans, with combination chemotherapy serving as the primary form of therapy because NHL is more often manifested as widely disseminated disease. NHL is dispersed through hematogenous routes and is not manifested with the orderly contiguous nodal involvment seen with Hodgkin's lymphoma. Radiation therapy is usually used adjunctively to chemotherapy even to treat localized disease. Involvement of Waldeyer's ring is often managed with radiation doses ranging between 400 and 450 cGy. Surgery is often used to explore the extent of disease, establish a diagnosis, and reduce tumor mass to aid treatment or restore function. HCT is used to treat patients with resistant or recurrent disease. Because of the poor prognosis, the treatment tends to be aggressive.

Dental Management

The dentist may be involved in the early diagnosis because of symptomatic or asymptomatic masses in the head and neck area or radiographic changes (see Figures 9–13 and 9–14). Frequently, the signs are not impressive and are thought to be benign because the tumor may be slow growing, small, and not bothersome. Diagnosis is established by biopsy. Any cervical mass greater than 1 cm that persists for longer than 1 month must be further evaluated to rule out tumor.

Because many patients with NHL may be scheduled to receive head and neck irradiation, chemotherapy, or both, precautions against oral sepsis and

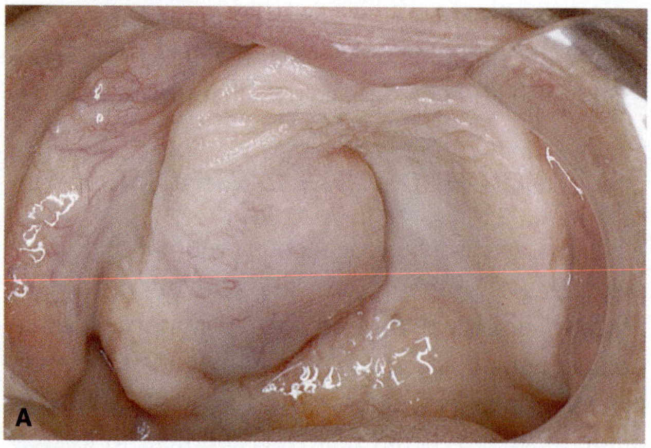

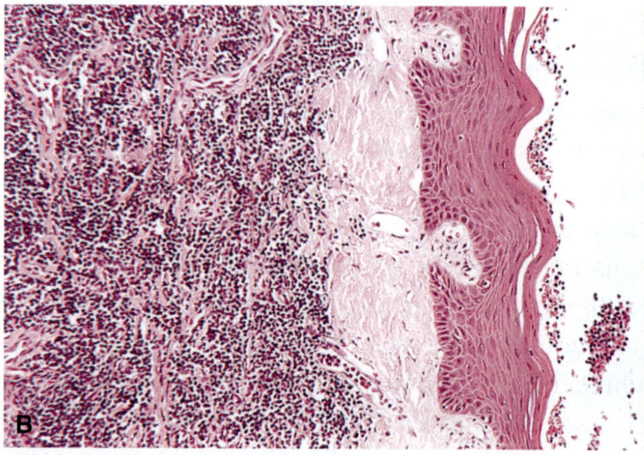

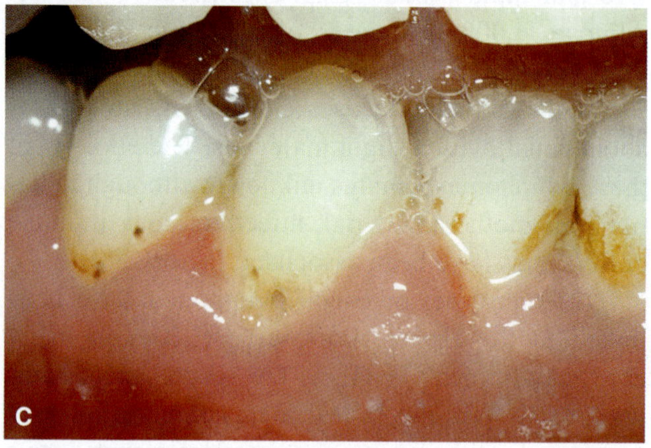

Figure 9–13. Malignant lymphoma in the palate. The patient's only complaint was that this swelling of about 3 months duration made her denture unstable. *A*, Rubbery, firm, palatal swelling. *B*, Biopsy revealed malignant lymphocytic cellular infiltrate under normal-appearing epithelium. *C*, Non-Hodgkin's lymphoma presenting as firm gingival swellings.

bleeding are critical. Because the radiation used rarely exceeds 500 cGy, osteoradionecrosis is not a common complication. However, xerostomia is common and demands special attention to oral hygiene, saliva stimulants and substitutes, fluoride mouthrinses or applications, and diet (see Chapter 7). A burning sensation in the mouth (stomatopyrosis) may be caused by drug toxicity, xerostomia, candidiasis, or anemia.

MULTIPLE MYELOMA

Multiple myeloma, a plasma cell dyscrasia, occurs with equal frequency in men and women and rarely occurs in patients under the age of 40 years. Currently, in the United States, there are almost 15,000 new cases each year and about 11,000 deaths. The average survival time from diagnosis is poor—approximately 2 years.

The plasma or myeloma cells, specialized for production of immunoglobin, proliferate to an abnormally high degree in bone. This leads to marrow replacement, anemia, decalcification, and hypercalcemia, and subsequent complications of osteopenia, multiple fractures (especially spine and long bones), and pain. Dental radiographs can often demonstrate the characteristic punched-out radiolucencies in the mandible and less often in the maxilla, associated with bony involvement by the multiple myeloma cells of marrow spaces. The inadequate production of blood cells and platelets causes leukopenia and thrombocytopenia. Normal immunoglobulin production is decreased, compromising immunocompetence. Early signs and symptoms include weakness, weight loss, recurrent infections, bone pain, and anemia. Jawbone lesions can occur (see Figure 9–14, C). Although extramedullary solitary plasmacytomas can occur in the oropharynx, these lesions are not related to generalized myeloma. Amyloid protein may form in the tongue or gingiva, causing swelling and pain (see Figure 9–14, D).

The diagnosis of multiple myeloma is made through bone marrow morphologic findings and

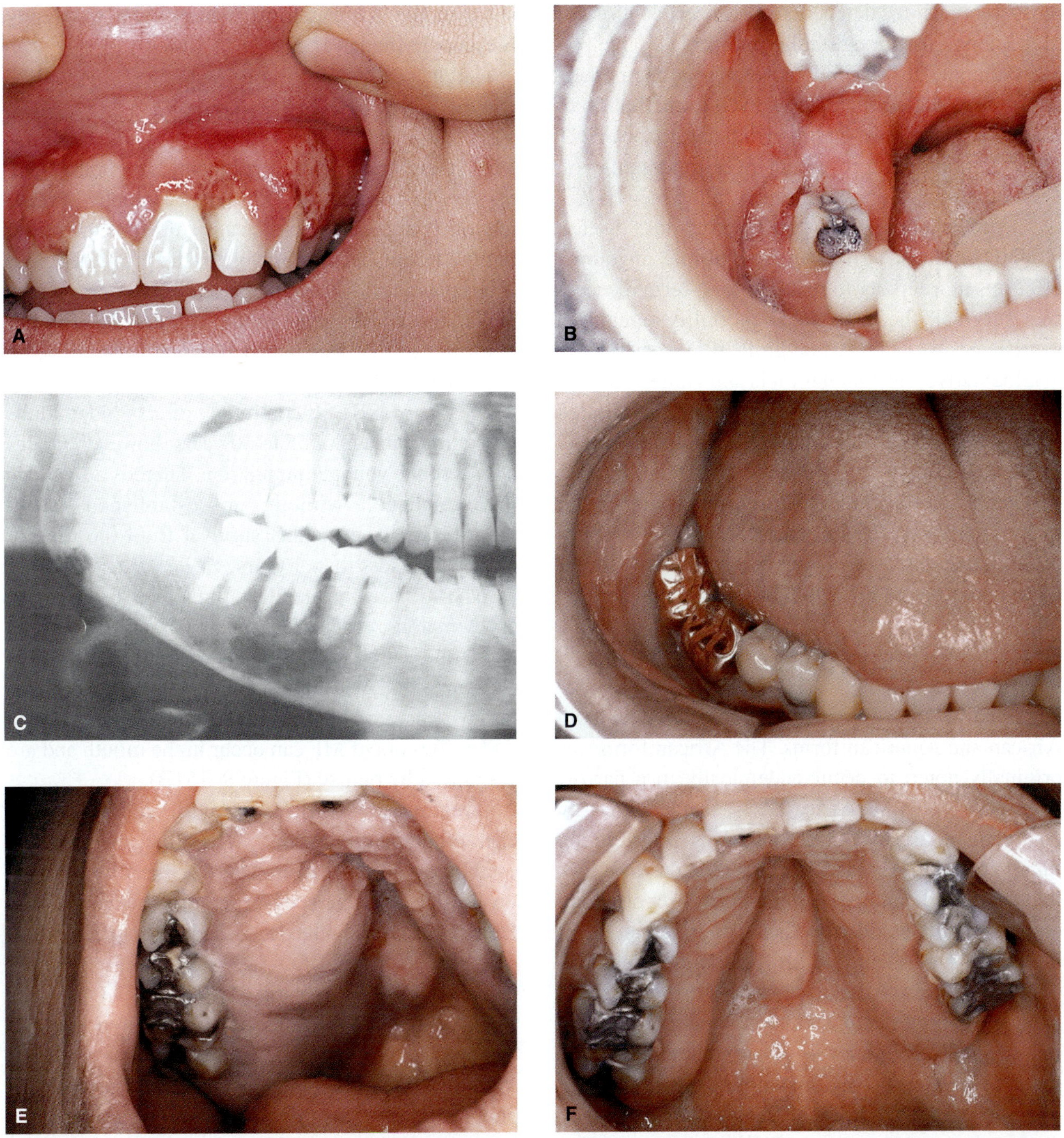

Figure 9–14. Extranodal lymphoproliferative disease in the mouth. *A*, This 20-year-old woman had a 3-month history of progressive, painful, necrotic gingivitis. Biopsy revealed a cellular infiltrate that was diagnosed as atypical lymphoreticular proliferation consistent with a variant of malignant lymphoma. The patient was successfully treated by local irradiation. *B*, This 26-year-old, human immunodeficiency virus (HIV)-positive patient had a painful swelling adjacent to his lower carious molar. Biopsy revealed a Burkitt's-type lymphoma ("starry-sky" pattern of B-cell proliferation). He died 4 months later from widespread lymphoma. *C*, A mildly painful mandibular lesion of multiple myeloma (courtesy of University of the Pacific, Oral Pathology Service). *D*, Gross tongue enlargement that had been noticed by this myeloma patient for almost 1 year. Biopsy confirmed amyloidosis. Note the displacement of the lower posterior teeth from the tongue pressure. The patient expired 6 months later. *E*, Localized non-Hodgkin's lymphoma of the palate. Mild discomfort was associated with the increasing mass of the palate. *F*, Complete resolution following 5,500 cGy radiation given over a 5-week period.

measurements to detect excessive production of monoclonal immunoglobulin molecules. The primary therapy for multiple myeloma is chemotherapy, with radiation therapy reserved for palliation of painful bony lesions. Results from autologous HCT show a modest improvement over treatment with chemotherapy alone. Although allogeneic HCT (with the potential for a graft-versus-host disease [GVHD]-induced graft-versus-multiple myeloma effect) is more likely to result in long-term disease-free survival, therapy-related mortality remains a significant obstacle. Although it is still early, non-myeloablative transplantation is showing encouraging results, especially for older or more debilitated patients who are not candidates for allogeneic transplantation.

Dental complications and precautions are similar to those encountered in other myelo- and lymphoproliferative diseases. These are related to diminished resistance to infection, bleeding, and anemia.

BURKITT'S LYMPHOMA

BL is an unusual type of NHL that includes both African and American forms. The African form was originally noted to occur endemically in a narrow zone across central Africa. It is characterized by enlargement of jaw bones caused by proliferating tumor cells. This disease was first thought to be limited to African children, but subsequent reports have emphasized its worldwide distribution.

Studies have identified EBV particles in cells cultured from most African cases, but EBV particles have rarely been demonstrated in American cases of BL. In addition, high levels of antibodies to EBV are found in all African children with BL but in only half of normal African children. BL is routinely associated with cytogenetic abnormalities demonstrating several characteristic chromosome translocations.

Diagnosis is based on a characteristic microscopic pattern of small, noncleaved B-cell lymphoid proliferation with a high mitotic count and a "starry-sky" pattern. Treatment consists of radiation and chemotherapy. The prognosis varies, depending on stage and type of disease. The American type, which demonstrates more frequent initial involvement of lymph nodes and bone marrow, has a worse prognosis than the African form, which most frequently presents in the jaws.

MYCOSIS FUNGOIDES

MF is an uncommon malignant lymphoma. MF appears to arise in the skin and eventually spreads into other organs. The basic cause of MF is unknown, but the lesions are attributable to the proliferation of T lymphocytes. Although MF may develop in young adults, most cases begin in the fifth decade of life. It is estimated that less than 1,000 new cases develop each year in the United States and represent 2% of new cases of NHL. It commonly affects older adults with a median age of 55 to 60 years; however, it does not spare the younger population. There is a 2:1 male predominance, without an established racial predilection. The median survival from the time of diagnosis is less than 5 years.[14]

The initial skin manifestations of MF appear as erythematous, eczematous, and psoriasiform patches or plaques, usually associated with intense pruritus (Figure 9–15, A). Subsequently, MF progresses to a tumor phase infiltrating plaques and remote lymph nodes. Tumors of MF can occur in the mouth and are diagnosed by biopsy (Figure 9–15, B).

Treatment is primarily with radiation and chemotherapeutic agents. When the diagnosis is established in the early phases of the disease, survival time and chances of control are improved. Pain, infection, cachexia, and despair often minimize the quality of life.

MIDLINE "NONHEALING" GRANULOMA

Midline granuloma (MG) is considered under lymphoproliferative disorders because, occasionally, a lesion transforms into a lymphoma or is associated with a lymphomatous process. This painful lesion of sudden onset is frequently manifested initially as a necrotic, progressive ulceration of the palatal or oropharyngeal mucosa (Figure 9–16). MG can affect alveolar bone and lead to destruction of bone and roots of teeth, leading to nonpainful increased mobility. Palatal bone and nasal cartilage are often involved. Although this lesion mimics a malignancy or acute infection, biopsy specimens characteristi-

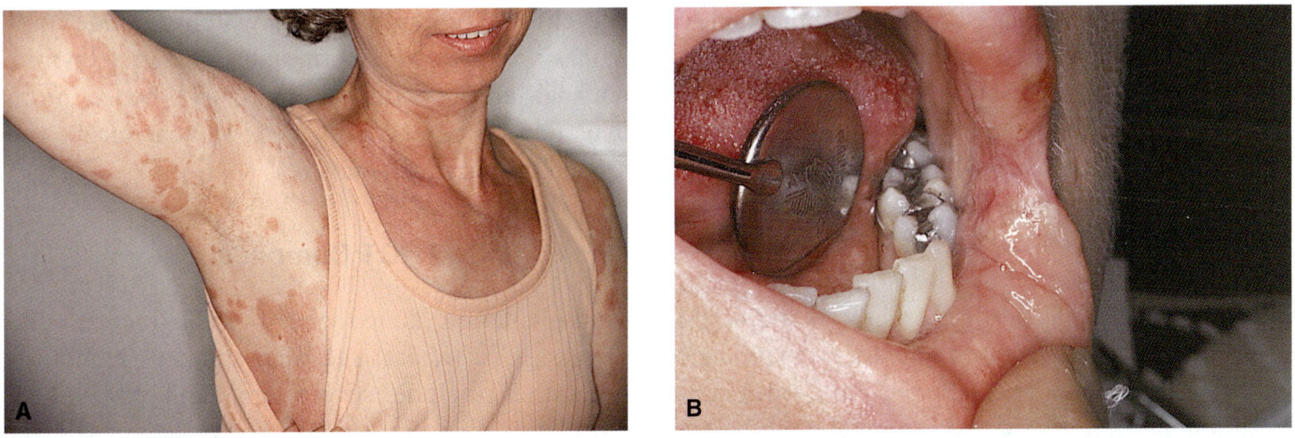

Figure 9–15. Manifestations of mycosis fungoides. The patient was referred for evaluation of painful oral lesions. *A*, Widespread skin manifestations. *B*, A painful nodule on the labial mucosa. Biopsy confirmed that this was a lymphomatous infiltrate of mycosis fungoides, and the lesion was treated successfully by irradiation. The patient eventually died of her disease.

cally show nonspecific, benign inflammation and ulceration. These lesions are not self-limiting, and low-dose radiation is used for control. Clinically, it is difficult at times to differentiate MG from Wegener's granulomatosis, a more generalized disease that responds to immunosuppressive chemotherapy.

HEMATOPOIETIC CELL TRANSPLANTATION

The use of high-dose chemotherapy with or without TBI followed by transplantation of hematopoietic stem cells is an intense form of cancer therapy that is a reasonable therapeutic option for leukemias and lymphomas in many instances, especially where it is difficult to establish durable remissions with chemotherapy alone. Transplantation is used primarily to treat diseases that involve the marrow or where survival following intense cancer therapy depends on establishing a new healthy marrow.[15–17] Hematopoietic stem cells can be harvested from bone marrow (bone marrow transplantation), from peripheral circulation using apheresis machines (peripheral blood stem cell transplantation), or from cells harvested from umbilical cords and are generally referred to as HCT.

Transplantation phases include (1) pretransplantation patient assessment and donor identification, (2) conditioning of the patient to receive the transplant, (3) hematopoietic stem cell infusion and early engraftment phases, (4) engraftment and recovery of circulating counts, and (5) immune reconstitution and long-term survival:

> Phase 1: Prior to undergoing transplantation, the patient must be carefully and thoroughly evaluated and a suitable marrow or stem cell donor identified. Donors are classified as (a) autologous (using stem cells collected from the patient), (b) syngeneic (using stem cells obtained from an identical twin), and (c) allogeneic (using stem cells from siblings, parents, or unrelated individuals who carry the same HLAs, for example, HLA-DR antigens; based on the degree of HLA matching, the terms "matched" or "mismatched" are applied).

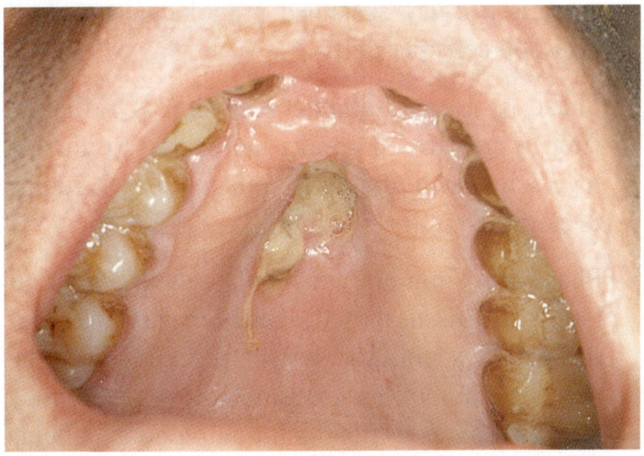

Figure 9–16. Large, necrotic, foul-smelling ulcer observed in the hard palate. A biopsy showed this to be consistent with a midline granuloma (MG). Moderate-dose irradiation controlled the lesion. MG occasionally transforms into or is associated with lymphoma.

Phase 2: Conditioning includes (a) eradication of the underlying disease or condition when necessary and (b) immunosuppression of the patient to prevent rejection of the transplanted cells. Conditioning regimens include high-dose chemotherapy with or without TBI. In certain instances, localized radiation can be used to further augment killing of tumor cells. Conditioning regimens totally eradicate all vestiges of marrow and would be inherently fatal without a transplant to produce a new, healthy marrow. After a 1- to 2-week conditioning period, the hematopoietic cells are infused into the bloodstream, and the cells home to the empty marrow spaces and begin to proliferate and repopulate the marrow.

Phase 3: During this neutropenic phase, marrow engraftment occurs and circulating counts begin to slowly increase. Neutrophil counts can be less than 100 per mm^3, platelet transfusions are used to try to keep counts above 20,000 mm^3, and hematocrits are often in the high 20% range. Trilineage marrow engraftment (evidence on bone marrow biopsy of production of white cells, RBCs, and platelets) is noted around 2 weeks post-transplantation for autologous transplants and 19 to 20 days for allogeneic transplants. Patients are at significant risk for infections and bleeding complications. Acute toxicities occur, which include oropharyngeal and gastrointestinal mucositis, nausea and vomiting, fevers of unknown origin, and veno-occlusive disease. Early evidence of engraftment is a 2-day sustained granulocyte count of over 500 cells per mm^3.

Phase 4: Hematopoietic recovery is reflected first by neutrophil counts increasing to normal levels and with platelet counts tending to return to normal.

Phase 5: As immune cells repopulate (both circulating and tissue based), functional recovery of the patient's immune system proceeds over the next several months. Immunologic recovery may take as long as 6 months for autologous patients and as long as 12 months for allogeneic patients.

Following phase 5, most patients are able to resume normal lives. However, patients can develop late-chronic complications, which include pulmonary fibrosis, endocrine dysfunction (thyroid, gonadal, and hypothalamic-pituitary), ocular problems (keratoconjunctivitis sicca and cataracts), and second primary malignancies.

Oral HCT Complications

Transplantation is associated with frequent and often significant oral and head and neck complications that include severe oral and pharyngeal mucositis, pain, infections, hemorrhage, salivary hypofunction, and dysgeusia.[1] The development of new agents to prevent and/or treat bacterial and fungal infections has drastically improved the short-term survival rates for transplantation, and the use of prophylactic acyclovir/valacyclovir has essentially eliminated the risk of reactivation of HSV.

GVHD is a major complication of allogeneic HCT. When immunocompetent T lymphocytes are included in the grafted stem cells, a reaction can occur. The grafted cells may not develop immunologic tolerance toward host tissues, and a cascade of immunologic reactions occurs wherein the "grafted" immune system attacks the host tissues as being "foreign." Two clinical forms of GVHD exist: (a) acute GVHD, which occurs between 14 and 100 days post-transplantation, primarily involving skin, liver, and gut (including the oral cavity), and (b) the more severe chronic GVHD, which occurs more than 100 days post-transplantation and involves multiple organ systems. Because GVHD causes immune dysregulation and immunosuppressive therapies are used for management, patients with GVHD are at significant risk for infection. Infection is the leading cause of death for patients with GVHD.

Allogeneic HCT recipients are given immunosuppressive drugs to prevent acute GVHD, with most protocols using a variety of agents including cyclosporine, methotrexate, prednisone, mycophenolate, or tacrolimus. These drugs can be used alone or in combination. Prophylactic therapy is started shortly after the transplantation and continued as necessary up to 100 days post-transplantation. Methotrexate contributes to the severity and duration of oral mucositis. Oral complications of cyclosporine (gingival hypertrophy) are usually not encountered with prophylactic doses. However, prophylaxis is generally not effective at preventing chronic GVHD. As already indicated, treatment of GVHD uses the same agents as those used to prevent acute GVHD but at much higher doses. GVHD treatment continues until the graft-versus-host reaction subsides and graft tolerance occurs, which can take up to many years.

The most common presentations of oral GVHD are mucosal erythema, atrophy, ulcerations, xerostomia, and hyperkeratotic lichenoid changes (hyperkeratotic striae, papules, and plaques). GVHD can also produce a Sjögren's-like syndrome with oral-ocular sicca; in addition to xerostomia, patients can also suffer from mucoceles. Depending on the severity of the oral involvement, patients can have varying degrees of oral pain and dryness. Diagnosis can generally be established by clinical assessment of oral signs and symptoms, with biopsy providing confirmatory evidence of oral mucosal and minor salivary gland involvement (Figure 9–17).

The primary management of oral GVHD depends on successful systemic therapy management. However, topical immunosuppressive agents (eg, steroids, azathioprine, cyclosporine) can reduce the severity of mucosal reactions, reduce oral symptoms, and improve oral function. Patients are encouraged to continue careful oral hygiene; any infection, including gingivitis, periodontitis, or odontogenic infections, can result in a flare of

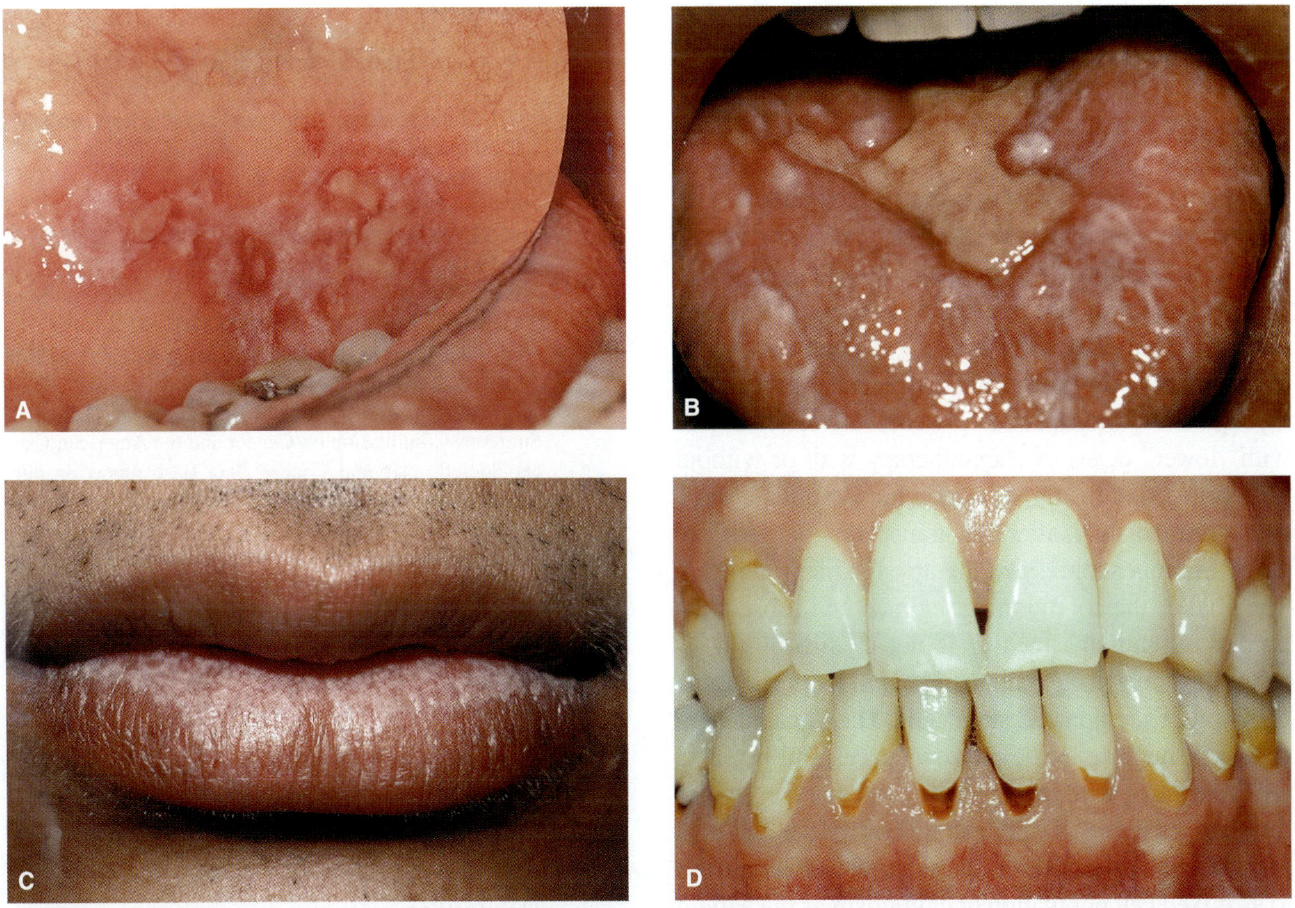

Figure 9–17. *A*, Heavy lichenoid changes interspersed with several pseudomembranous ulcerations in a patient with extensive chronic graft-versus-host disease (GVHD) 4 1/2 years post-transplantation (mirror view of left buccal mucosa). *B*, Severe, chronic GVHD tongue manifestations 5 years following bone marrow transplantation for acute myelogenous leukemia. Note the lichenoid hyperkeratotic and pseudomembranous ulcerative lesions. *C*, Acute GVHD lichenoid keratotic lesion of the lower lip in a 22-year-old patient with chronic myelogenous leukemia 51 days post–allogeneic transplantation. *D*, Advanced cervical caries resulting from severe xerostomia 1 year following hematopoietic cell transplantation for acute myelogenous leukemia. The patient had been conditioned with high-dose chemotherapy and single-dose total-body irradiation (1,000 cGy).

GVHD and make management more difficult. Viral, fungal, and bacterial infections can be difficult to recognize in patients with oral GVHD because of atypical appearances; thus, increased use of laboratory tests to detect potential infections is an important consideration for effective care.

Donor Lymphocyte Infusions and Nonmyeloablative Transplantation

Although GVHD is realistically considered a potentially serious complication of allogeneic HCT, a potential graft-versus-leukemia (GVL) reaction has become evident: patients who develop acute and/or chronic GVHD are at a statistically lower risk of relapse of their primary disease. Although first recognized for patients transplanted for leukemia, the same benefit has been noted for a number of malignancies (eg, lymphomas, multiple myeloma). Building on this finding, protocols have been developed to exploit the ability of the GVL reaction. One protocol involves administering a donor lymphocyte infusion that contains immunocompetent T lymphocytes to specifically induce a GVHD/GVL response that can attack and eliminate recurrent or residual disease.

A second protocol referred to as a nonmyeloablative transplant uses a dramatically different approach to treatment of the underlying malignancy.[18] With nonmyeloablative transplants, patients are conditioned with "lower" doses of chemotherapy with or without TBI prior to infusion of donor hematopoietic stem cells. Immediately after the transplant, patients are given immunosuppressive therapy for many months. The goal of the conditioning regimen and subsequent immunosuppressive therapy is not to directly eliminate the underlying malignancy but to prevent the rejection of the donated stem cells. The donated stem cells will migrate to the marrow spaces and begin to replicate along with host marrow cells. For a period of time, the patient will demonstrate both donor and host hematologically derived cells—a state that is referred to as mixed cell population or chimerism as the patient simultaneously has blood and immune cells of different genetic origin. Over time, the grafted donor cells come to dominate and will eliminate the original host hematopoietically derived cells, along with the underlying malignant cells. Thus, the GVHD/GVL response provides the cure for malignant disease. Although still under intense study, early results are very encouraging for this technique.

With the use of less aggressive conditioning regimens, early toxicity is dramatically reduced, and the complications and fatality related to serious infections and organ failure are significantly lower.[19] A significant reduction in the cost of care can often be appreciated. There is virtually no oral mucositis, xerostomia, or taste dysfunction. Oral infections and neutropenic ulcerations have been noted early posttransplantation but are not severe and respond quickly to therapy with no or minimal systemic sequelae. Oral GVHD is still a potential complication, and the diagnostic and management strategies are similar to those employed for oral GVHD occurring in standard allogeneic transplant patients.

REFERENCES

1. Antin JH. Clinical practice. Long-term care after hematopoietic-cell transplantation in adults. N Engl J Med 2002;347:36–42.
2. Cline MJ. The molecular basis of leukemia. N Engl J Med 1994;330:328–36.
3. Pagano JS. Viruses and lymphomas. N Engl J Med 2002; 347:78–9.
4. Lowenberg B, Downing JR, Burnett A. Acute myeloid leukemia. N Engl J Med 1999;341:1051–62.
5. Sawyers CL. Chronic myeloid leukemia. N Engl J Med 1999;340:1330–40.
6. Diehl LF, Karnell LH, Menck HR. The American College of Surgeons Commission on Cancer and the American Cancer Society. National Cancer Data Base report on age, gender, treatment, and outcomes of patients with chronic lymphocytic leukemia. Cancer 1999;86:2684–92.
7. Clarkson JE, Worthington HV, Eden OB. Interventions for treating oral candidiasis for patients with cancer receiving treatment. Cochrane Database Syst Rev 2002;(1): CD001972.
8. Lefebvre JL, Domenge C. A comparative study of the efficacy and safety of fluconazole oral suspension and amphotericin B oral suspension in cancer patients with mucositis. Oral Oncol 2002;38:337–42.
9. Raut A, Huryn JM, Hwang FR, Zlotolow IM. Sequelae and complications related to dental extractions in patients with hematologic malignancies and the impact on medical outcome. Oral Surg Oral Med Oral Pathol Oral Radiol Endod 2001;92:49–55.
10. Silverman S Jr, Kramer AM. Drugs for neoplastic disorders. In: Ciancio S, editor. ADA guide to dental therapeutics. 2nd ed. Chicago: ADA Publishing; 2000:481–93.
11. Sonis ST. Mucositis as a biologic process: a new hypothesis for the development of chemotherapy-induced stomatotoxicity. Oral Oncol 1998;34:39–43.

12. Epstein JB, Epstein JD, Le ND, Gorsky M. Characteristics of oral and paraoral malignant lymphoma: a population-based review of 361 cases. Oral Surg Oral Med Oral Pathol Oral Radiol Endod 2001;92:519–25.
13. Meurman JH, Laine P, Keinanen S, et al. Five-year follow-up of saliva in patients treated for lymphomas. Oral Surg Oral Med Oral Pathol Oral Radiol Endod 1997;83:447–52.
14. Weinstock MA, Reynes JF. The changing survival of patients with mycosis fungoides. A populaton-based assessment of trends in the United States. Cancer 1999;85:208–12.
15. Appelbaum FR. Hematopoietic cell transplantation as a form of immunotherapy. Int J Hematol 2002;75:222–7.
16. Singhal S, Powles R, Mehta J. Hematopoietic reconstitution by transplantation of stem cells from bone marrow or blood. N Engl J Med 2001;344:1641–2.
17. Witherspoon RP, Deeg HJ, Storer B, et al. Hematopoietic stem-cell transplantation for treatment-related leukemia or myelodysplasia. J Clin Oncol 2001;19:2134–41.
18. Shimoni A, Nagler A. Non-myeloablative stem-cell transplantation in the treatment of malignant and non-malignant disorders. Isr Med Assoc J 2002;4:272–9.
19. Peterson DE, Schubert MM. Oral toxicity. In: Perry MC, editor. The chemotherapy sourcebook. 3rd ed. Philadelphia: Lippincott, Williams and Wilkins; 2001. p. 406–23.

10

Malignant Salivary Gland Tumors

JOSEPH A. REGEZI, MS, DDS
SOL SILVERMAN JR., MA, DDS
DAVID W. EISELE, MD

Salivary gland cancers account for about 0.5% of all malignancies (approximately 5,000 new cases each year in the United States). Most of these cancers occur in the major salivary glands (parotid, submandibular, and sublingual) as opposed to the minor salivary glands, which are distributed throughout the oral mucosa.

The National Cancer Institute's SEER (Surveillance, Epidemiology, and End Results) Program recorded data on 5,374 patients with salivary gland malignancies from 9 different geographic and population centers in the United States between 1973 and 1996. The profile indicated that 84% of the patients were over the age of 40, reflecting that salivary gland malignancies are strongly associated with aging. Over 90% of the tumors occurred in white men and women. There was a slight male predominance, with 54% of the tumors occurring in men. Fourteen percent of salivary gland cancers were squamous cell carcinomas and 86% were adenocarcinomas. The most common histologic subtypes were adeno-, mucoepidermoid, and adenoid cystic carcinomas. Only 54% of salivary gland malignancies were diagnosed in early, localized stages, resulting in an overall 5-year survival rate of 57%. In comparing the periods 1973 to 1984 and 1985 to 1996, there was a slight 2% increase in reported cases of salivary gland malignancies. In the latter period (1985 to 1996), the 5-year survival rate increased to 69%, probably owing to more aggressive surgical and/or radiation approaches.

DIAGNOSIS

The initial sign is usually a lump, which is usually asymptomatic but may be painful. These lumps may resemble benign growths, cysts, inflammations, or infections, making the differential diagnosis challenging (Figure 10–1). The diffuse enlargement of salivary glands caused by systemic disease is seldom mistaken for tumor.

There is an extremely important difference in the approach to salivary tumor diagnosis relative to minor and major glands. Early or even immediate biopsy of minor salivary gland lesions is in order, whereas biopsy of major salivary glands should be avoided in favor of less invasive diagnostic approaches. Biopsy of the major glands (prior to definitive treatment) may "seed" tumor cells into adjacent tissues; may cause nerve injury owing to the intimate relationship of the glands to the facial, hypoglossal, and lingual nerves; or may cause scar formation and inflammation, which might complicate definitive surgical resection.

For major salivary gland tumors, fine-needle aspiration biopsy (FNAB) is accurate and has become an acceptable diagnostic modality to distinguish neoplasia from inflammatory disease before definitive surgical resection (Figure 10–2).[1] Equipment for FNAB consists of a 22- to 25-gauge needle, a 20 mL syringe, and a special syringe holder that provides a good vacuum. The aspirated contents are prepared by cytologic techniques.

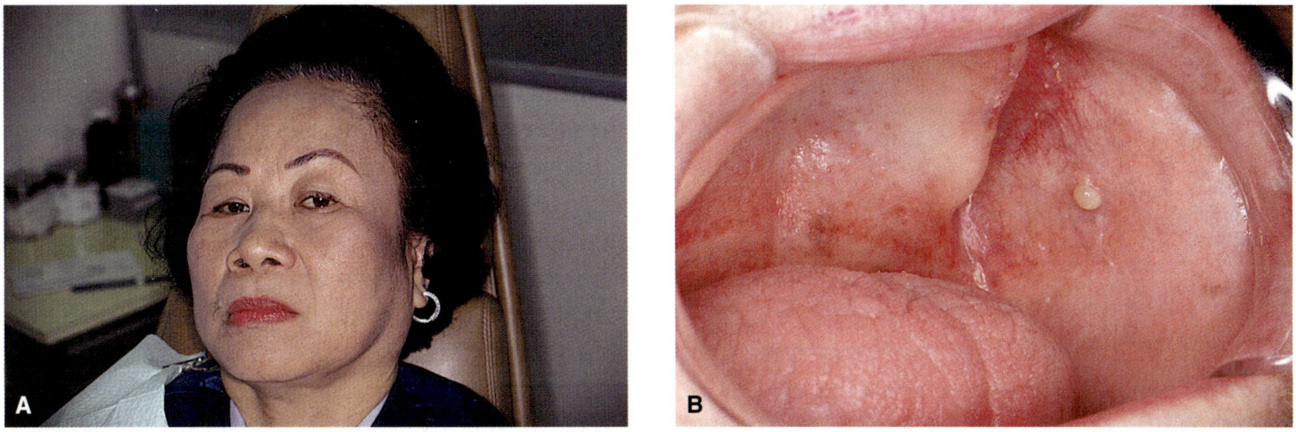

Figure 10–1. A 58-year-old woman with sialadenitis. *A*, Painful swelling first noticed 2 weeks before photograph was taken. *B*, Suppurative exudates from left parotid and orifice of Stensen's duct. The swelling and pain responded to antibiotics. A sialogram revealed idiopathic sialectasia.

Magnetic resonance imaging (MRI) and computed tomography (CT) have proved to be extremely helpful in assessing the extent of salivary gland disease. Accurate differentiation of benign tumors from malignant tumors, however, is difficult with MRIs and CT scans. At the present time, positron emission tomography (PET) appears to have no added advantage over CT or MRI in the evaluation of salivary gland neoplasms.

MAJOR SALIVARY GLANDS

By far the most frequently involved major salivary gland is the parotid. It accounts for about 85% of all major salivary gland tumors. About 20% of all parotid tumors are malignant. The relative incidence of tumors in the three types of major salivary glands and the percentage of these tumors that are malignant are shown in Table 10–1.

These tumors are infrequent in individuals under the age of 40, and both sexes and all ethnic groups share essentially the same risk. Mucoepidermoid cancers and adenoid cystic carcinomas are the most frequent histologic types.[2] Carcinomas occasionally develop from long-standing benign mixed tumors. Primary lymphomas arising in salivary glands are very uncommon (see Chapter 9, "Leukemia and Lymphoma").

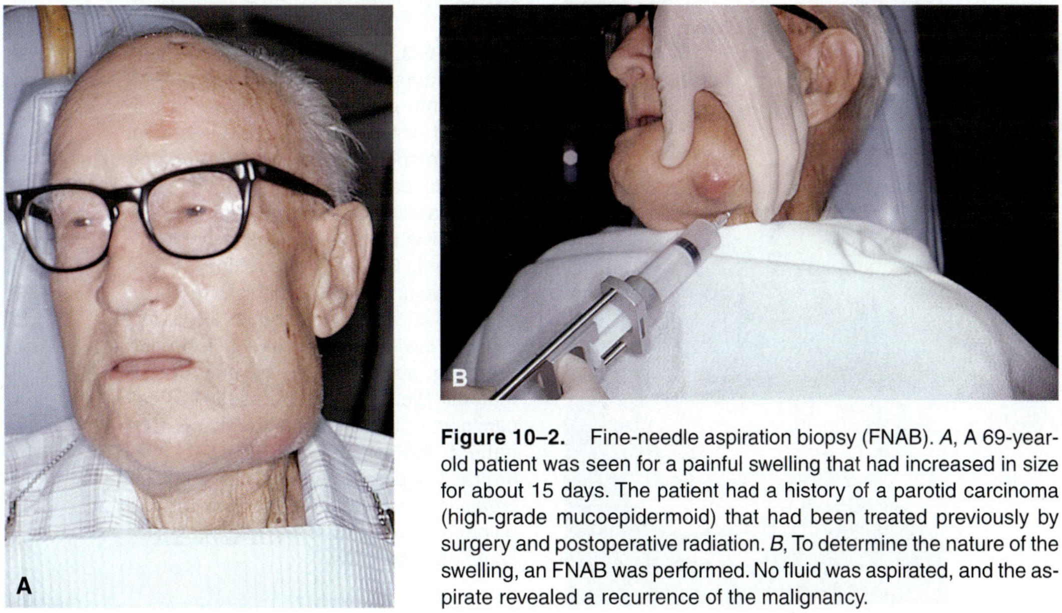

Figure 10–2. Fine-needle aspiration biopsy (FNAB). *A*, A 69-year-old patient was seen for a painful swelling that had increased in size for about 15 days. The patient had a history of a parotid carcinoma (high-grade mucoepidermoid) that had been treated previously by surgery and postoperative radiation. *B*, To determine the nature of the swelling, an FNAB was performed. No fluid was aspirated, and the aspirate revealed a recurrence of the malignancy.

Table 10–1. MAJOR SALIVARY GLAND TUMORS

Gland	Approximate Distribution of Tumors (%)	Approximate Distribution of Malignancy (%)
Parotid	85–90	25
Submaxillary	10–15	50
Sublingual	1	75

The most common first sign of a malignant tumor is an asymptomatic mass (Figure 10–3). Growth is often moderately rapid, with occasional pain at the onset. Sometimes enlargement is slow, however, which may diminish a patient's concern and delay diagnosis. Facial paralysis may be an early sign of malignant parotid lesions resulting from involvement of the facial nerve (Figure 10–4). The differential diagnosis must include conditions such as infections, stones, adenomas, or inflammatory/autoimmune gland enlargement. For selected cases of major salivary gland lesions, radiography and response to antibiotics prior to tissue diagnosis can be helpful both in management and as diagnostic approaches. If a lesion persists, the diagnosis of a malignancy can be determined only by tissue analysis. FNAB serves this purpose and has been extremely useful in differentiating benign and malignant tumors and often in classifying lesions. MRI is useful in differentiating neoplastic from other tissue changes and delineating the extent of the lesion (see Chapter 4, "Diagnosis"). Sialography and radionuclide scans are of little help in evaluating malignant salivary gland tumors.

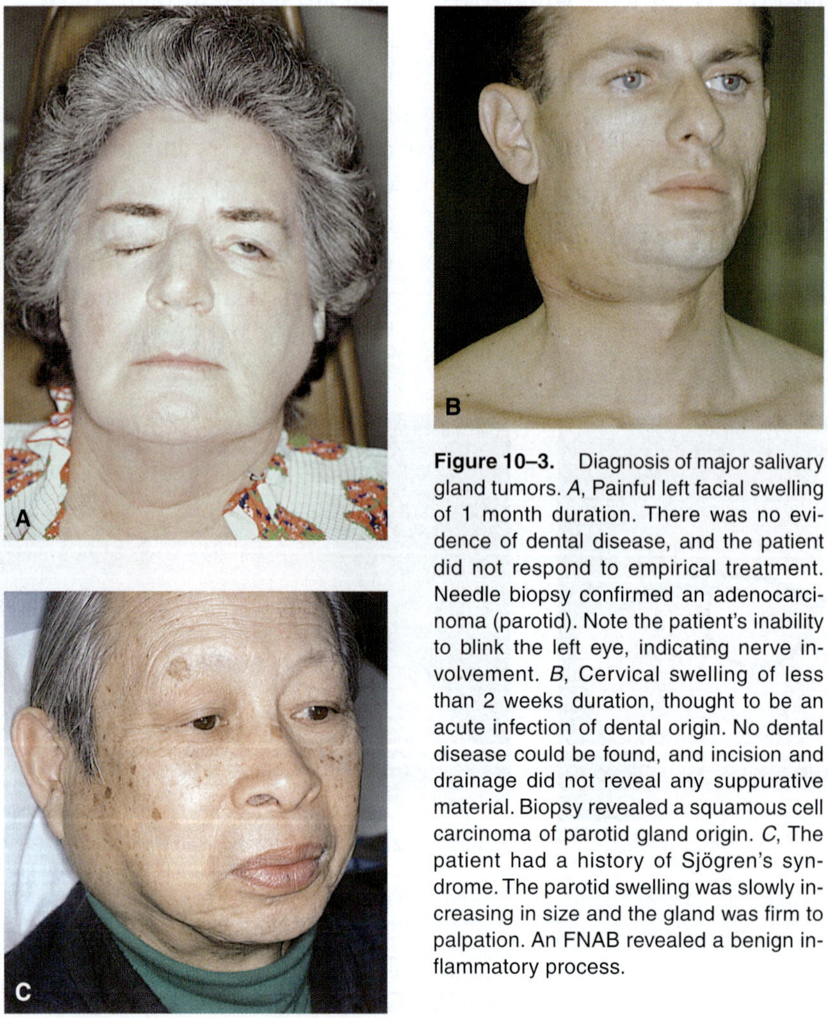

Figure 10–3. Diagnosis of major salivary gland tumors. *A*, Painful left facial swelling of 1 month duration. There was no evidence of dental disease, and the patient did not respond to empirical treatment. Needle biopsy confirmed an adenocarcinoma (parotid). Note the patient's inability to blink the left eye, indicating nerve involvement. *B*, Cervical swelling of less than 2 weeks duration, thought to be an acute infection of dental origin. No dental disease could be found, and incision and drainage did not reveal any suppurative material. Biopsy revealed a squamous cell carcinoma of parotid gland origin. *C*, The patient had a history of Sjögren's syndrome. The parotid swelling was slowly increasing in size and the gland was firm to palpation. An FNAB revealed a benign inflammatory process.

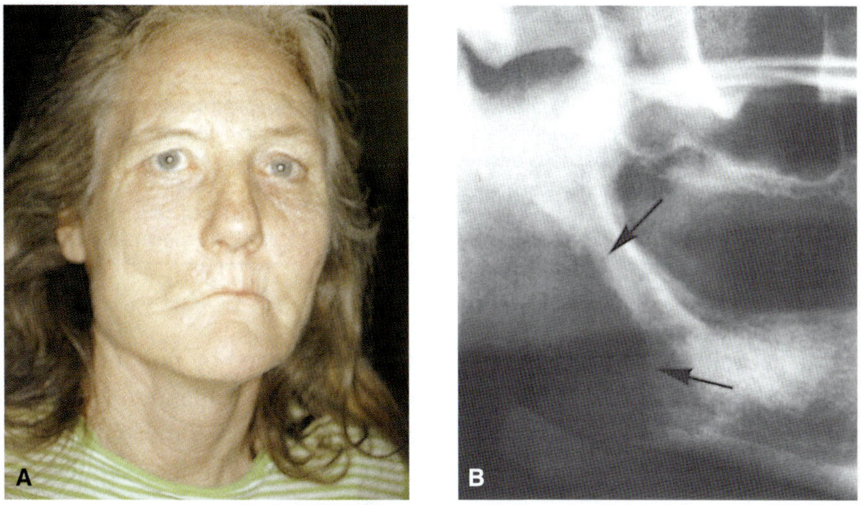

Figure 10–4. Right facial paralysis (Bell's palsy) of 3 months duration. *A*, Lip drooping and inability to close the eyelid (loss of blink reflex) are characteristic of facial nerve involvement. *B*, Radiograph revealed a destructive lesion in the posterior mandible, which was diagnosed as an extention of a parotid mucoepidermoid carcinoma.

TREATMENT OF MAJOR SALIVARY GLAND MALIGNANCIES

Complete surgical resection is the treatment of choice for malignant major salivary gland neoplasms.[3] The amount of resection is dictated by the degree of tumor extension. The facial nerve or other nerves are preserved provided that they are functional preoperatively and a surgical plane of dissection between the tumor and nerve is present. A neck dissection is indicated for cervical metastases identified preoperatively or intraoperatively. Radiation therapy is used as an adjunct to surgery in selected cases. Usual indications for postoperative radiation therapy include high-grade malignancies, large malignancies, close or positive surgical margins, perineural or perilymphatic invasion, or nodal metastases. Chemotherapy is used for the palliative treatment of recurrent unresectable tumors and metastatic, symptomatic salivary gland malignancies.

With notable exceptions, most cancers of salivary gland origin have a good prognosis if they are diagnosed at an early stage and treated properly (Table 10–2).[4,5] Poorer prognosis and outcome are generally associated with high-grade lesions (Table 10–3).[6] Treatment results appear to be best for the low-grade malignancies, mucoepidermoid and acinic cell carcinoma, and worst for the high-grade malignancies, such as undifferentiated carcinoma, adenoid cystic carcinoma, high-grade mucoepidermoid carcinoma, and carcinoma ex-pleomorphic adenoma. Malignant tumors of major salivary glands occasionally can represent metastases from other primary sites including head and neck cutaneous primaries or infraclavicular primaries. In these cases, the diagnostic approaches and treatments are variable and the prognosis is poor.

MINOR SALIVARY GLANDS

Minor salivary gland carcinomas occur infrequently, usually after age 30. Like major salivary gland tumors, they show diversity in histologic appearance, anatomic site, and clinical course (Figures 10–5 to 10–10). Their usual location is the palate,

Table 10–2. STAGE AND RELATIVE 5-YEAR SURVIVAL RATES OF 923 PATIENTS WITH MAJOR SALIVARY GLAND MALIGNANCIES (SEER,* 1973–1984)

Stage	Distribution (%)	5-Year Survival (%)
Localized	52.8	91
Regional spread	36.5	56
Distant metastasis	10.7	25

*Surveillance, Epidemiology, and End Results Program of the National Cancer Institute.

Table 10–3. SALIVARY GLAND MALIGNANCIES CLASSIFIED ACCORDING TO BIOLOGIC BEHAVIOR

Low Grade	Intermediate Grade	High Grade
Mucoepidermoid carcinoma	Mucoepidermoid carcinoma	Mucoepidermoid carcinoma
Acinic cell carcinoma	Epimyoepithelial carcinoma	Adenoid cystic carcinoma
Polymorphous low-grade adenocarcinoma	Sebaceous adenocarcinoma	Carcinoma ex mixed tumor and malignant mixed tumor
Basal cell carcinoma		Salivary duct carcinoma
		Squamous cell carcinoma
		Oncocytic adenocarcinoma

followed by the lip, buccal mucosa, and, occasionally, the tongue. A painless mass, often resembling a cyst, a fibroma, or even a vascular growth, is the most common initial sign. The diagnosis is established by incisional biopsy.

Tumors of minor oral salivary glands account for about 20% of all salivary gland neoplasms; about half of them are malignant. The most common histologic type appears to be mucoepidermoid carcinoma, followed by polymorphous low-grade adenocarcinoma and adenoid cystic carcinoma.[7] Benign mixed tumors (pleomorphic adenomas) are the most common benign minor salivary gland tumors.

Necrotizing sialometaplasia, a non-neoplastic, inflammatory disease of minor salivary glands, can be confused with a malignant process (squamous cell carcinoma or mucoepidermoid carcinoma) both clinically and microscopically. It most commonly

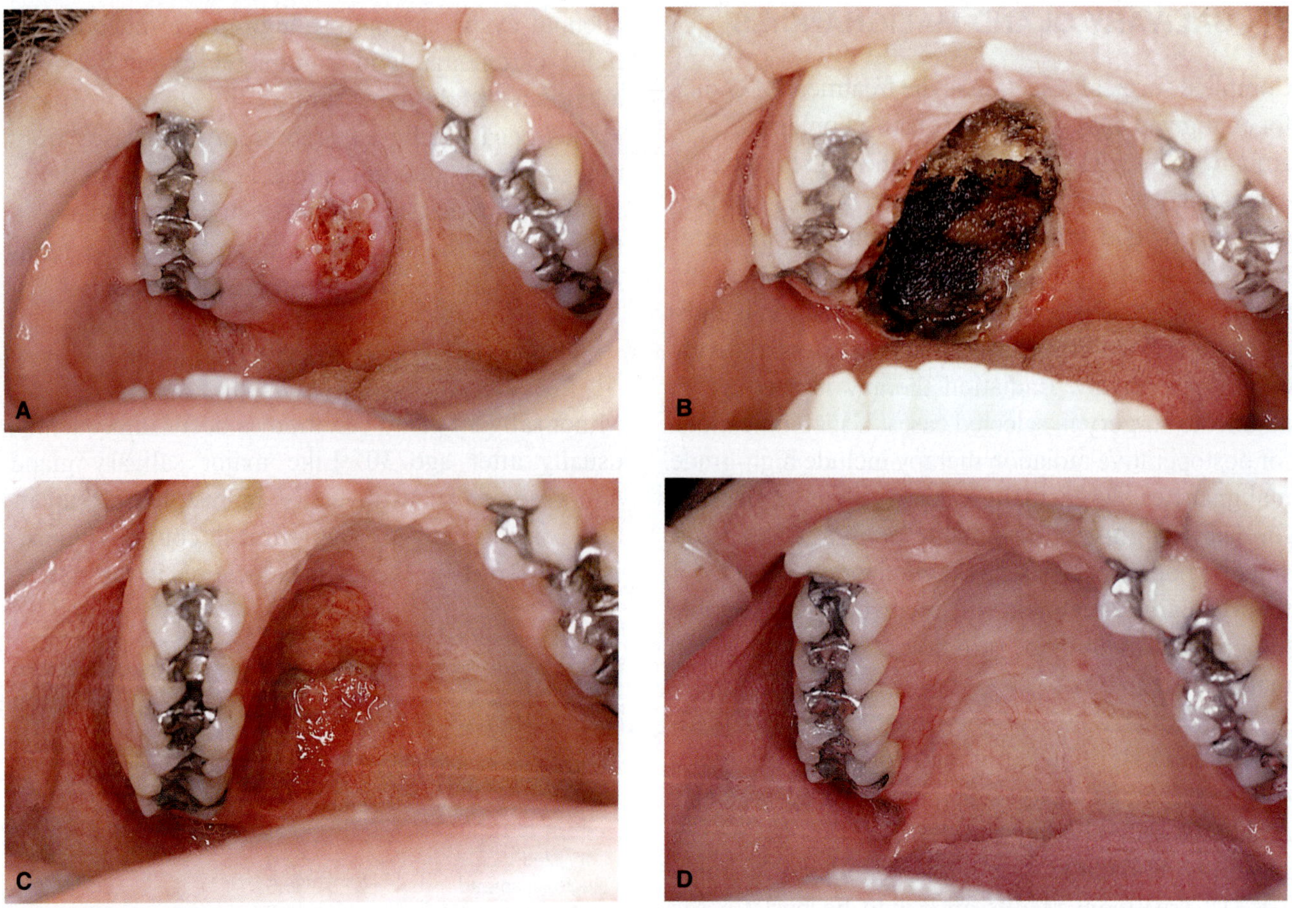

Figure 10–5. Laser excision of a mixed tumor of a minor salivary gland in the palate. *A*, Growth before surgery. *B*, Immediately after laser excision. Note excision site and laser charring of intact maxillary bone. *C*, Two weeks after surgery, granulation tissue is filling the defect. *D*, Three months after surgery, the patient is asymptomatic and without evidence of tumor. In long-term follow-up, there was no recurrence.

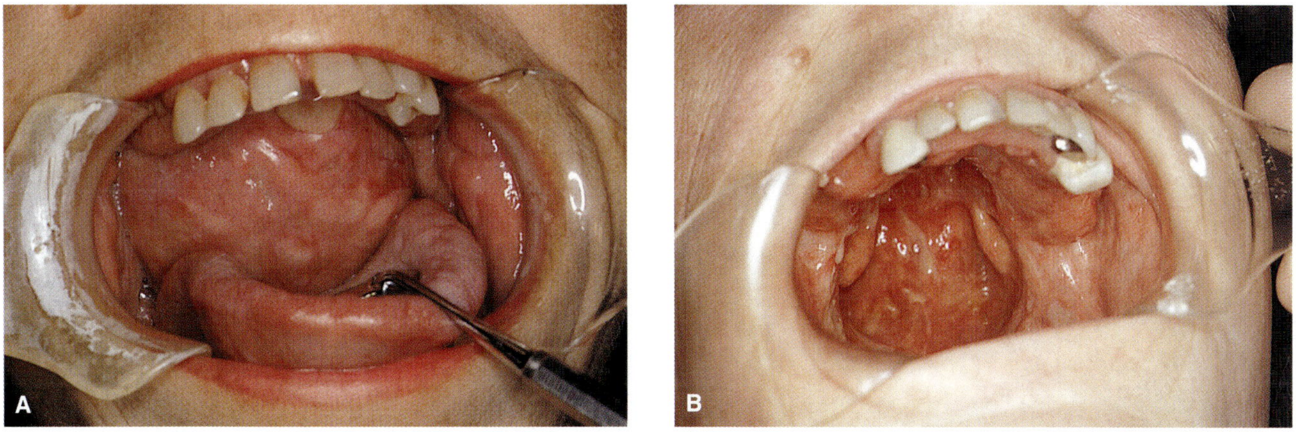

Figure 10–6. *A*, Mixed tumor, primary in the hard palate, that had been slowly enlarging for "over a year." The patient sought emergency help because of difficulty in breathing as well as food intake. *B*, Treatment required a partial maxillectomy.

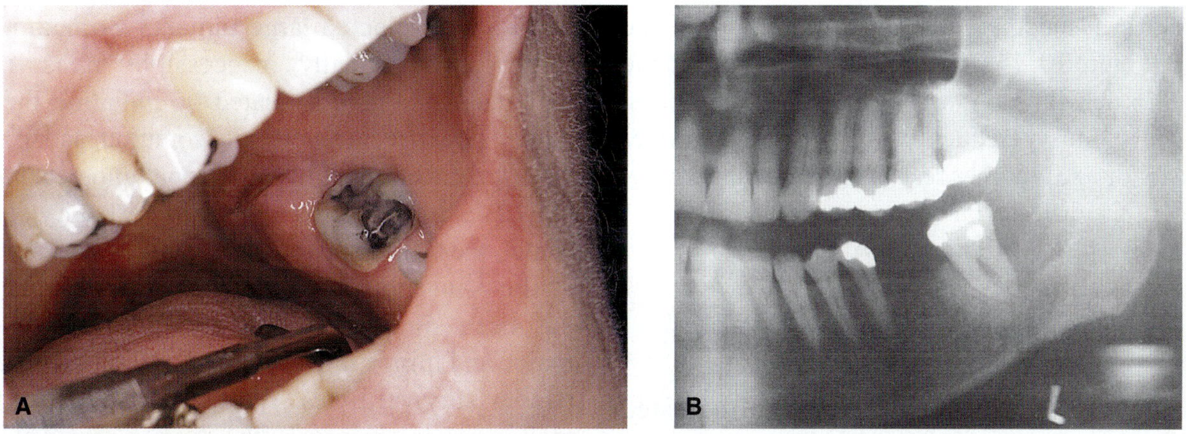

Figure 10–7. *A*, This patient was referred because of a retromolar mandibular swelling that had first been noticed 3 months earlier and did not respond to antibiotics. *B*, A panograph revealed a large retromolar bone defect. An incisional biopsy revealed a polymorphous adenocarcinoma of minor salivary gland origin that was controlled by surgery and postoperative radiotherapy.

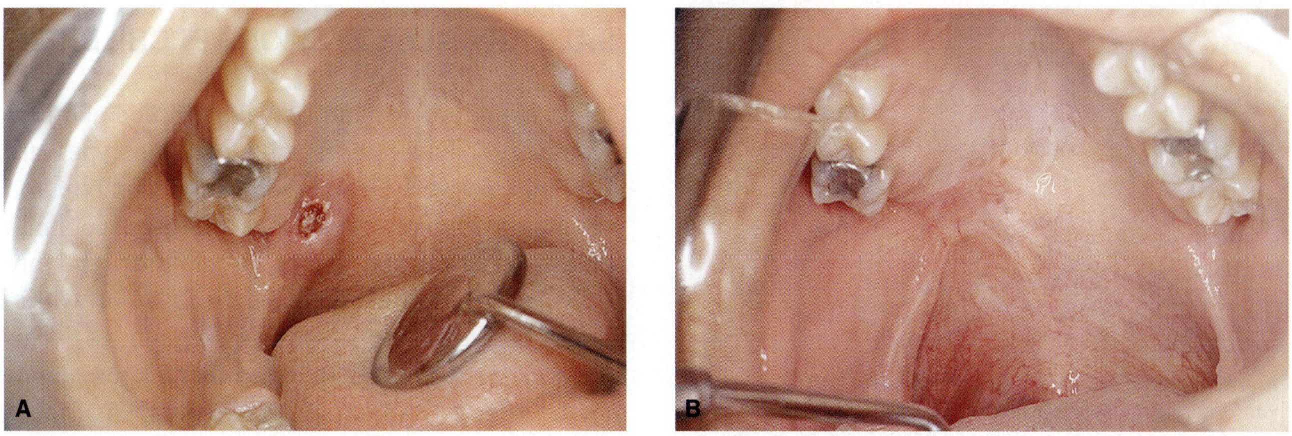

Figure 10–8. *A*, A 15-year-old boy complained of a lump in the right soft palate that had persisted for over a month. An incisional biopsy revealed a polymorphous adenocarcinoma of minor salivary gland origin. *B*, Treatment was accomplished by a local excision.

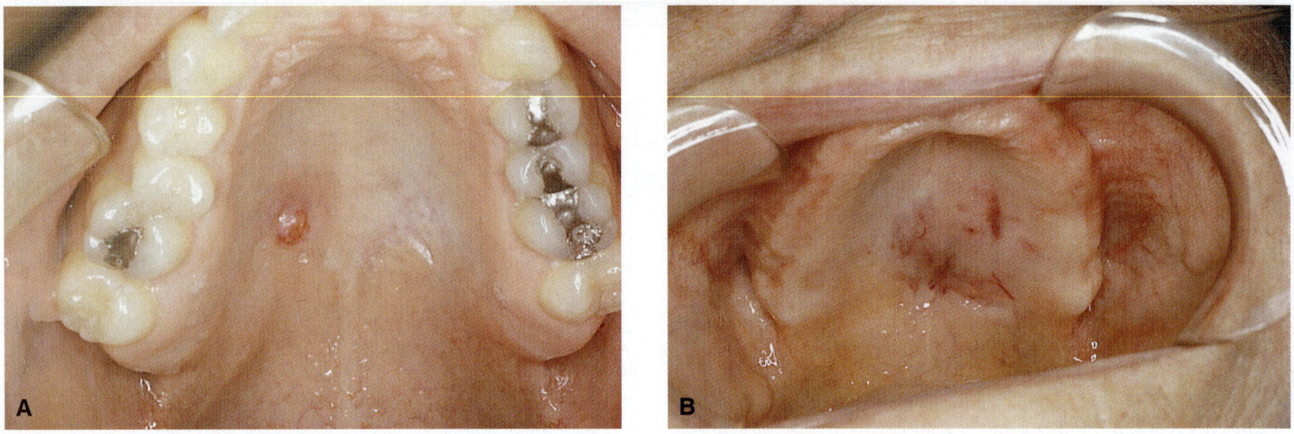

Figure 10–9. Varying appearances of mucoepidermoid carcinomas. *A*, The patient had noticed a palatal swelling for about a month. Although mucocele was suspected, aspiration revealed no fluid. A biopsy showed a low-grade mucoepidermoid carcinoma. *B*, Another patient noticed a sessile growth in her palate that was interfering with seating of the denture. Aspiration showed no fluid (blood or mucus), and an incisional biopsy revealed a mucoepidermoid carcinoma.

occurs as a sudden progressive ulceration of the palate (Figure 10–11). The cause is unknown and the disease is self-limiting, usually lasting 4 to 6 weeks. It occurs most frequently in individuals over 40 years of age, another reason for including malignancy in the differential diagnosis.

TREATMENT OF MINOR SALIVARY GLAND MALIGNANCIES

Minor salivary gland malignancies are also treated by complete surgical excision. Postoperative radiation therapy is recommended for high-grade tumors and selected large tumors.[8] Sometimes in critical or surgically inaccessible areas, these malignant tumors are treated by radiation therapy alone. Local recurrences are common and metastases are uncommon. In a clinicopathologic study of 492 cases treated at a major New York City cancer center, the 5-year survival rate was 42%. Experience at the University of California at San Francisco has been similar and has also pointed out that major and minor salivary gland malignancies have similar survival times. With minor salivary gland malignancies, however, the 5-year survival rate should not be considered the cure rate because many patients die of their disease more than 5 years after diagnosis, especially those with adenoid cystic carcinomas.

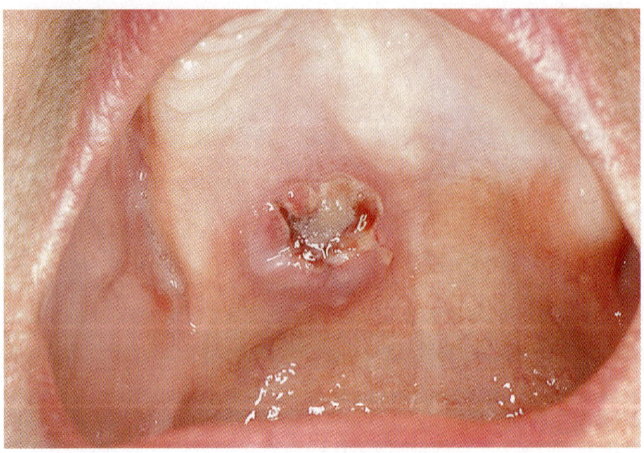

Figure 10–10. This patient complained of a palatal mass of 3 months duration that was increasing in size and causing discomfort. An incisional biopsy revealed an adenocystic carcinoma. Because this histologic type is always considered "high grade," treatment included surgical excision followed by radiotherapy.

SALIVARY GLAND TUMORS IN CHILDREN

Children and young adults develop limited numbers of salivary gland tumors, although the types are fairly distinctive.[9] Hemangioma and combination hemangioma/lymphangioma are the most common "tumors" in salivary glands of children and are rarely seen in adulthood. Occurring at or within months of birth, these lesions are seen almost exclusively in the parotid, although other major glands may be affected. An unpredictable number of these lesions will involute if left untreated. Large lesions and rapidly growing lesions are justifiably treated by

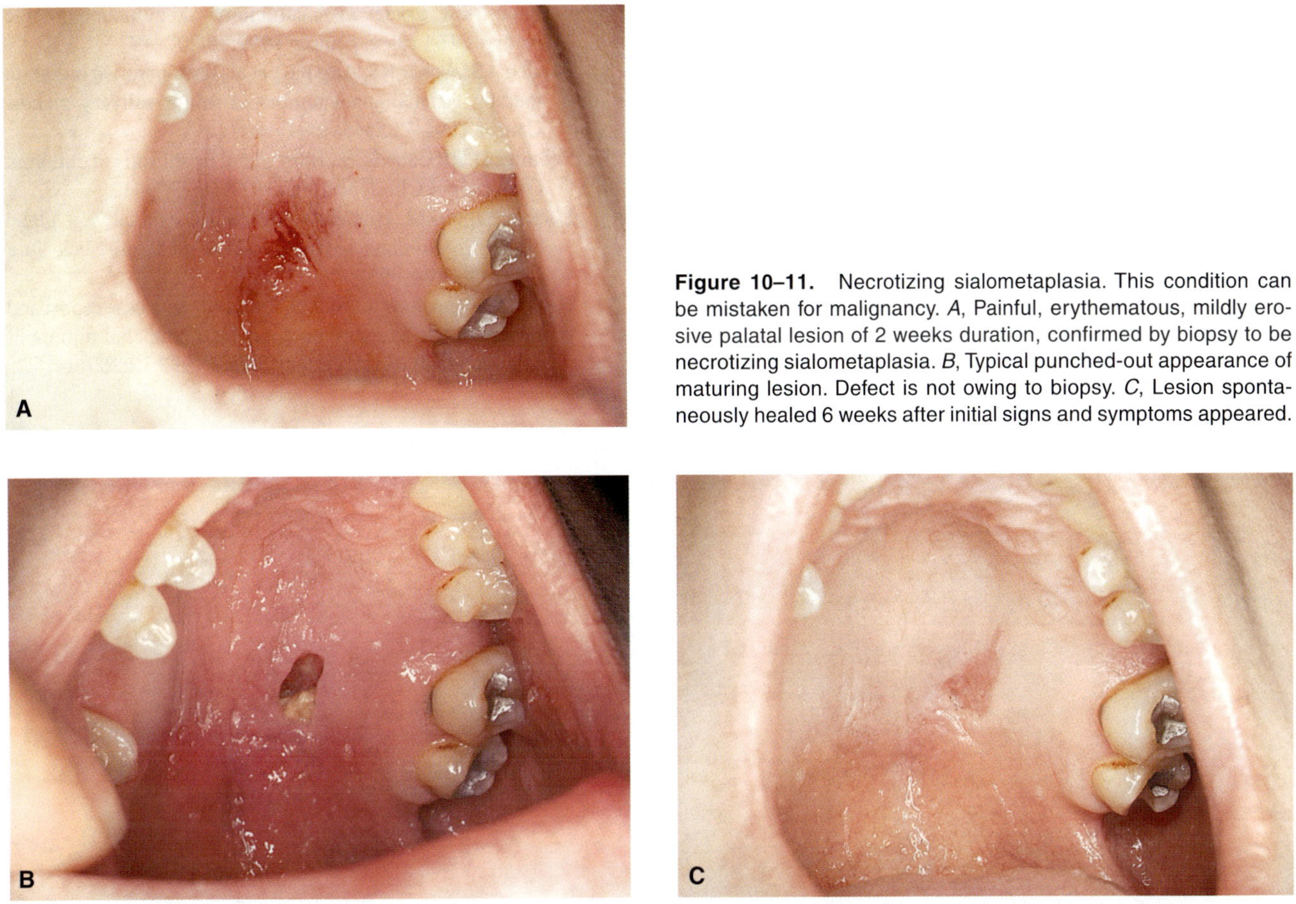

Figure 10–11. Necrotizing sialometaplasia. This condition can be mistaken for malignancy. *A*, Painful, erythematous, mildly erosive palatal lesion of 2 weeks duration, confirmed by biopsy to be necrotizing sialometaplasia. *B*, Typical punched-out appearance of maturing lesion. Defect is not owing to biopsy. *C*, Lesion spontaneously healed 6 weeks after initial signs and symptoms appeared.

surgical excision. Radiation therapy should be reserved only for special circumstances when surgery is contraindicated or the prognosis with surgery alone is extremely poor.

In children, the number of malignant salivary gland neoplasms exceeds the number of benign neoplasms.[10] The large majority are found in the parotid. Mucoepidermoid carcinoma is the most common malignancy, typically exhibiting a low- or intermediate-grade microscopic pattern. Acinic cell carcinoma is less commonly seen, and adenoid cystic carcinoma is rarely reported. These malignancies exhibit biologic behaviors similar to those in adults and are generally treated by complete surgical resection with or without postoperative radiation therapy.

Of all of the neoplasms of salivary gland origin in children, mixed tumors are the most frequently seen neoplasm (excluding hemangiomas and lymphangiomas), and these most commonly occur in the parotid gland. Their presenting appearance and biologic behavior appear to be similar to their adult counterparts. Complete surgical resection is recommended. For the parotid gland, parotidectomy is indicated. Submandibular and sublingual tumors require gland extirpation.

The term sialoblastoma has recently been applied to a rare congenital neoplasm of major salivary glands.[11] It presents at or around the time of birth as a firm, unilateral mass (up to 1.5 cm in diameter) almost exclusively in the parotid. Microscopically, it resembles a monomorphic adenoma, but it is composed of both epithelial and myoepithelial cells. Because recurrences have been documented for this tumor, excision is the recommended treatment.

REFERENCES

1. Zurrida S, Alasio L, Tradati N, et al. Fine-needle aspiration of parotid masses. Cancer 1993;72:2306–11.
2. Goode RK, Auclair PL, Ellis GL. Mucoepidermoid carcinoma of the major salivary glands. Cancer 1998;82:1217–24.
3. North CA, Lee DJ, Piantadosi S, et al. Carcinoma of the

major salivary glands treated by surgery or surgery plus postoperative radiotherapy. Int J Radiat Oncol Biol Phys 1990;18:1319–26.

4. Frankenthaler RA, Luna MA, Lee SS, et al. Prognostic variables in parotid gland cancer. Arch Otolaryngol Head Neck Surg 1991;117:1251–6.
5. Gallo O, Franchi A, Bianchi S, et al. p53 oncoprotein expression in parotid gland carcinoma is associated with clinical outcome. Cancer 1995;75:2037–44.
6. Seifert G, Sobin LH. The World Health Organization's histological classification of salivary gland tumors. Cancer 1992;70:379–85.
7. Castle JT, Thompson LDR, Frommelt RA, et al. Polymorphous low grade adenocarcinoma: a clinicopathologic study of 164 cases. Cancer 1999;86:207–19.
8. Garden AS, Weber RS, Ang KK, et al. Postoperative radiation therapy for malignant tumors of minor salivary glands. Cancer 1994;73:2563–9.
9. Schuller D, McCabe B. Salivary gland neoplasms in children. Otolaryngol Clin North Am 1977;10:399–412.
10. Lack E, Upton M. Histopathologic review of salivary gland tumors in childhood. Arch Otolaryngol Head Neck Surg 1988;114:898–906.
11. Hsueh C, Gonzalez-Crussi F. Sialoblastoma: a case report and review of the literature on congenital epithelial tumors of salivary gland origin. Pediatr Pathol 1992;12:205–14.

11

Other Malignancies and Oral Oncology

SOL SILVERMAN JR., MA, DDS
NANCY LEE, MD (Nasopharyngeal Carcinoma)
JOSEPH A. REGEZI, MS, DDS (Oral Mucosal Melanomas)
CATHERINE M. FLAITZ, DDS, MS (Cancer in Children and Adolescents)
MICHAEL J. KAPLAN, MD (Malignancies Involving Jawbones)
HERBERT DEDO, MD (Laryngeal Carcinoma)

MALIGNANCIES INVOLVING THE JAWBONES

Squamous Cell Carcinoma involving the Mandibular Alveolar Ridge

The most common malignancy affecting the mandible and the maxillary alveolar ridge and hard palate is squamous cell carcinoma (SCC) that has arisen from a mucosal surface and invaded deeply to involve bone (see Chapter 5, "Spread of Tumor, Staging, and Survival"). Patients with oral cavity SCC usually have a history of alcohol or tobacco use or both. At times, there may be only minimal mandibular cortical erosion along the alveolar ridge. When there has been no prior radiation therapy, a marginal rim mandibulectomy may be sufficient as part of the surgical resection, preserving the inferior cortex. When the marrow space is involved, however, a segmental resection is required. Reconstruction of a segmental defect may be accomplished with an osseocutaneous microvascular free flap (such as fibula) or with a titanium plate beneath a pectoralis major myocutaneous flap. A free flap is preferred, especially in anterior defects, when the patient's overall health allows such a procedure to be done.

Detecting subtle bone destruction radiographically may be difficult. Computed tomographic (CT) scans may fail to detect subtle cortical erosion and will often underestimate the extent of bone involvement. A panorex is even less sensitive. Magnetic resonance imaging (MRI) is best in detecting the extent of marrow space involvement but may overestimate the extent if there are also inflammatory changes in the marrow. Cortical invasion may be detected on MRI by soft tissue changes along the mucosa that extend into the cortical bone, interrupting the normally linear appearance at this interface.

In addition to extension from mucosa, SCC may, on rare occasions, occur in the epithelial lining of odontogenic cysts. This may be suspected when there is a large cystic mass within the mandible and little or no apparent mucosal involvement. The diagnosis in this setting is often made when unsuspected SCC is found at the time of a tooth extraction.

Primary intraosseous carcinoma (PIOC) within the mandible (sometimes referred to as odontogenic carcinoma) is rarer still, with fewer than 50 cases reported in the literature.[1–4]

MAXILLARY SINUS AND HARD PALATE MALIGNANCIES

SCC may involve the maxillary alveolar ridge either as an oral cavity tumor, similar to involvement of the mandible, or from inferior extension of a maxillary sinus malignancy. Among primary maxillary sinus malignancies, SCC represents about 80%, with salivary gland malignancies (mucoepidermoid carcinoma [low grade and high grade], adenocarcinoma, adenoid cystic carcinoma, and acinic cell carcinoma) the next most common, and other histologies including lymphomas and sarcomas also possible. In addition, salivary gland malignancies may arise directly from the minor salivary glands of the hard palate. Adenoid cystic carcinoma, mucoepidermoid carcinoma, and low-grade adenocarcinomas are the most common non-SCCs of the minor salivary glands of the oral cavity.

Maxillary sinus malignancies may mimic the symptoms of chronic sinusitis or allergic rhinitis, but unilaterality of symptoms and the lack of prior nasal-sinus symptoms should arouse suspicion in the physician or dentist listening to a patient (Figure 11–1). The presence of bleeding, numbness in V2 distribution, proptosis, loose teeth, and cheek or palate swelling should prompt further evaluation. If tumor is suspected, MRI is key in defining its extent and planning intervention. CT may at times supplement MRI evaluation, but MRI is almost always superior and usually sufficient. Because about 20% of SCCs of the maxillary sinus may spread to neck nodes, the neck should be evaluated carefully, clinically and radiographically.

Treatment of hard palate malignancies depends heavily on the specific histology and on the extent of involvement. Low-grade malignancies may often be treated with surgery alone and may or may not require removal of the underlying bone. High-grade lesions likely will require resection and postoperative irradiation, with a prosthesis usually the best reconstruction.

Treatment of maxillary sinus malignancies also depends on histology on extent of involvement. For instance, for lymphoma, the only surgery generally required is an initial biopsy as treatment will be by chemotherapy and possibly radiation. Most SCCs of the maxillary sinus are best treated with a combination of surgery and postoperative irradiation. The extent of surgery and recommended reconstruction will be determined by preoperative evaluation of the orbit, skull base, and neck. When resectable with clear surgical margins, cure rates for SCC may be as high as 40 to 60%. Poorer prognoses are seen when there is skull base dural involvement, orbit involvement, extension posteriorly into the pterygomaxillary space, and spread to neck nodes.

Sarcoma

Primary sarcomas of the mandible and maxilla are rare, with an incidence of less than 1 in 1,000,000. Osteosarcoma is the most common sarcoma seen in this region, with about 775 cases reported in the English literature in the past 30 years, representing about 0.5 to 1% of all osteosarcomas. The mandible is involved in more than two-thirds of cases (Figures 11–2 and 11–3). In those patients with a prior history of irradiation, the incidence of sarcomas is more frequent, and these tumors appear to be more

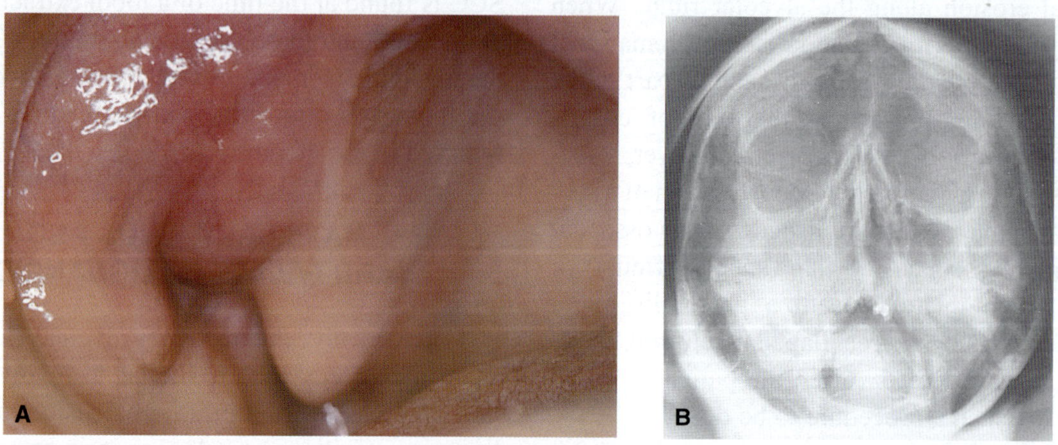

Figure 11–1. Maxillary sinus cancer. *A*, An increasing mass in the right maxillary reflex prevented the patient's denture from seating. The patient also complained of nasal stuffiness and sinusitis. *B*, An anteroposterior head film revealed opacity of the right maxillary sinus, which was obliterated by tumor. Reflex mass was an extension of tumor, a low-grade adenocarcinoma, which had eroded sinus walls and invaded adjacent tissues.

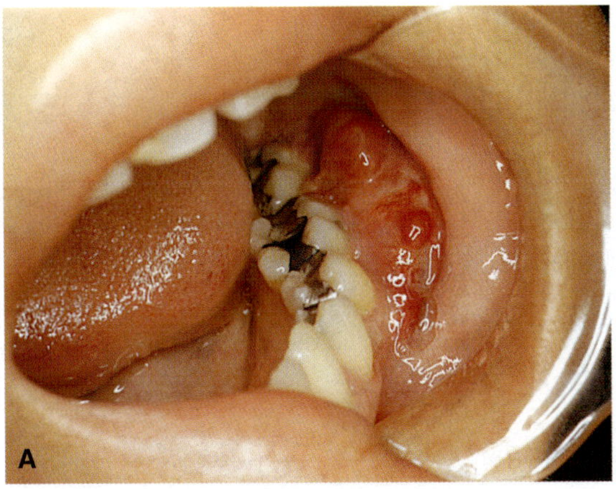

Figure 11–2. Osteogenic sarcoma of the mandible in a 25-year-old woman who had noticed this "growing lump" for 2 months. *A*, Clinical view of the osteogenic sarcoma at the initial examination and prior to the confirmatory biopsy. *B*, Radiograph of the osteogenic sarcoma illustrating bone destruction by tumor. *C*, Surgical resection specimen.

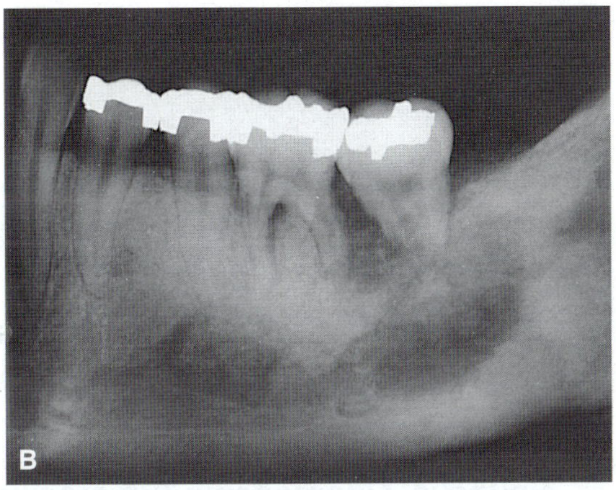

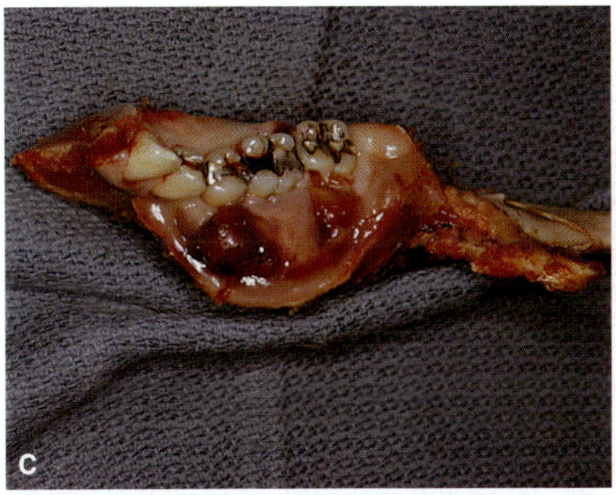

aggressive. Unlike the 95% of osteosarcomas that occur elsewhere in the body, predominantly in children and young adults, the mean age of patients with osteosarcomas of the mandible and maxilla is 32 to 40 years, a decade later than the usual presentation in long bones. Tumors have been reported, however, in infants as well as octogenarians. Symptoms are nonspecific: swelling with or without pain, with less frequent dental problems, ulceration, or V3 numbness. Radiographically, they may appear as osteolytic, osteoblastic, or mixed lesions. Compared with other sites, jaw osteosarcomas have a better prognosis, and only about a third develop metastases, predominantly to the lung. It is likely that histologic grade, as in other sites, correlates with prognosis. Five-year cure rates of about 60% are often reported in patients without initial metastatic disease. This rate appears to have improved in recent years, presumably associated with chemotherapy, and is better than the 30 to 40% cure rate seen in osteosarcomas of long bones. In the absence of metastases, most authors agree that the best treatment involves adequate resection (with reconstruction) and chemotherapy.[5,6] The role of radiation therapy in patients with adequate surgical margins is unclear.

Among children under 18 years of age, osteosarcomas of the head and neck are even rarer, with a review of the Armed Forces Institute of Pathology (AFIP) Tumor Registry between 1970 and 1997 reporting only 22 cases, less than 1% of all head and neck primary tumors in children and less than 3% of all pediatric osteosarcomas. Primary surgery is indicated, as it is with adults. Consideration of adjuvant chemotherapy is recommended. In the AFIP series, there were no metastases (although lung and bone metastases have been reported), and there was a 32% recurrence rate.[7] Chondrosarcomas are equally rare in children, present similarly, and should be treated similarly. Given their rarity, it is difficult to interpret survival data that are accumulated over several decades of changing treatment from different

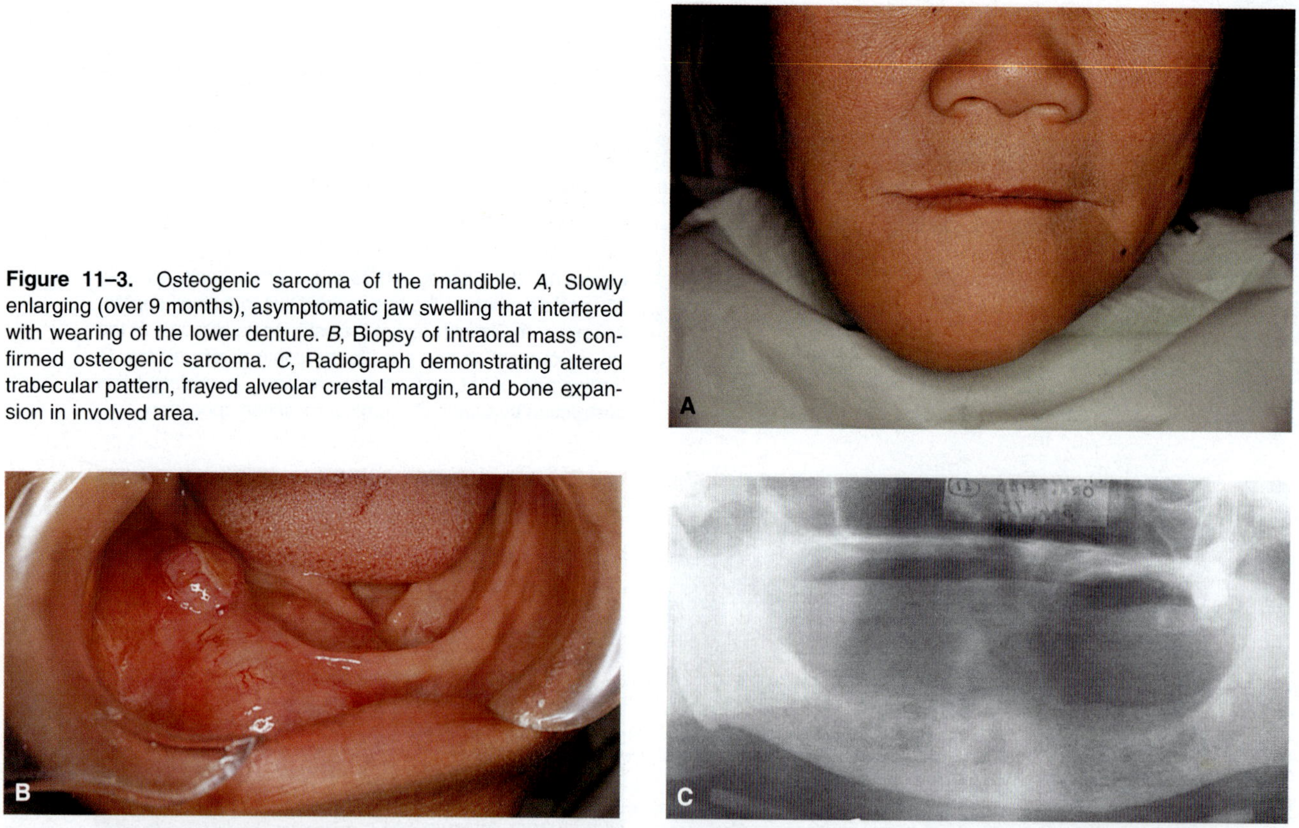

Figure 11–3. Osteogenic sarcoma of the mandible. *A*, Slowly enlarging (over 9 months), asymptomatic jaw swelling that interfered with wearing of the lower denture. *B*, Biopsy of intraoral mass confirmed osteogenic sarcoma. *C*, Radiograph demonstrating altered trabecular pattern, frayed alveolar crestal margin, and bone expansion in involved area.

institutions. It would appear, however, that chondrosarcomas are usually low grade, and survival with adequate surgery should be expected, with survival rates reported in the recent literature in excess of 67% and the 2000 AFIP report of 14 cases reporting a 90% 5-year disease-free survival.

Metastases

Metastases to the mouth are uncommon, with bony metastases (usually to the mandible) more common than soft tissue metastases. Sources of metastases include breast, lung, renal, other bone, colon, and melanoma. Certainly, in a patient with a known prior malignancy, signs or symptoms of a local dental process should lead the clinician to at least consider the possibility of a metastasis in the differential diagnosis of more common inflammatory or infectious entities. Frequently, however, a mandibular metastasis presenting as a destructive ill-marginated radiolucency is the first manifestation of disease, with the diagnosis made by biopsy and subsequent evaluation clarifying the total picture.

Epithelial Odontogenic Tumors with Malignant Potential: Ameloblastoma, Odontogenic Ghost Cell Tumor, and Clear Cell Odontogenic Tumor

Distinguishing one apparently cystic mandibular lesion from another requires histopathologic examination. Although a number of cystic lesions and tumors may behave aggressively locally when inadequately resected, a few may exhibit true malignant features.[8,9] This section reviews these three lesions; a fourth odontogenic tumor with malignant features (PIOC) was reviewed earlier in this section.

Ameloblastoma

Ameloblastomas are epithelial tumors of odontogenic origin that occur most commonly in the posterior mandible (more anteriorly in black patients), with over 80% of tumors presenting in the mandible (Figure 11–4).[10,11] The usual age of patients at presentation is 30 to 40 years, with unicystic variants presenting somewhat earlier. The

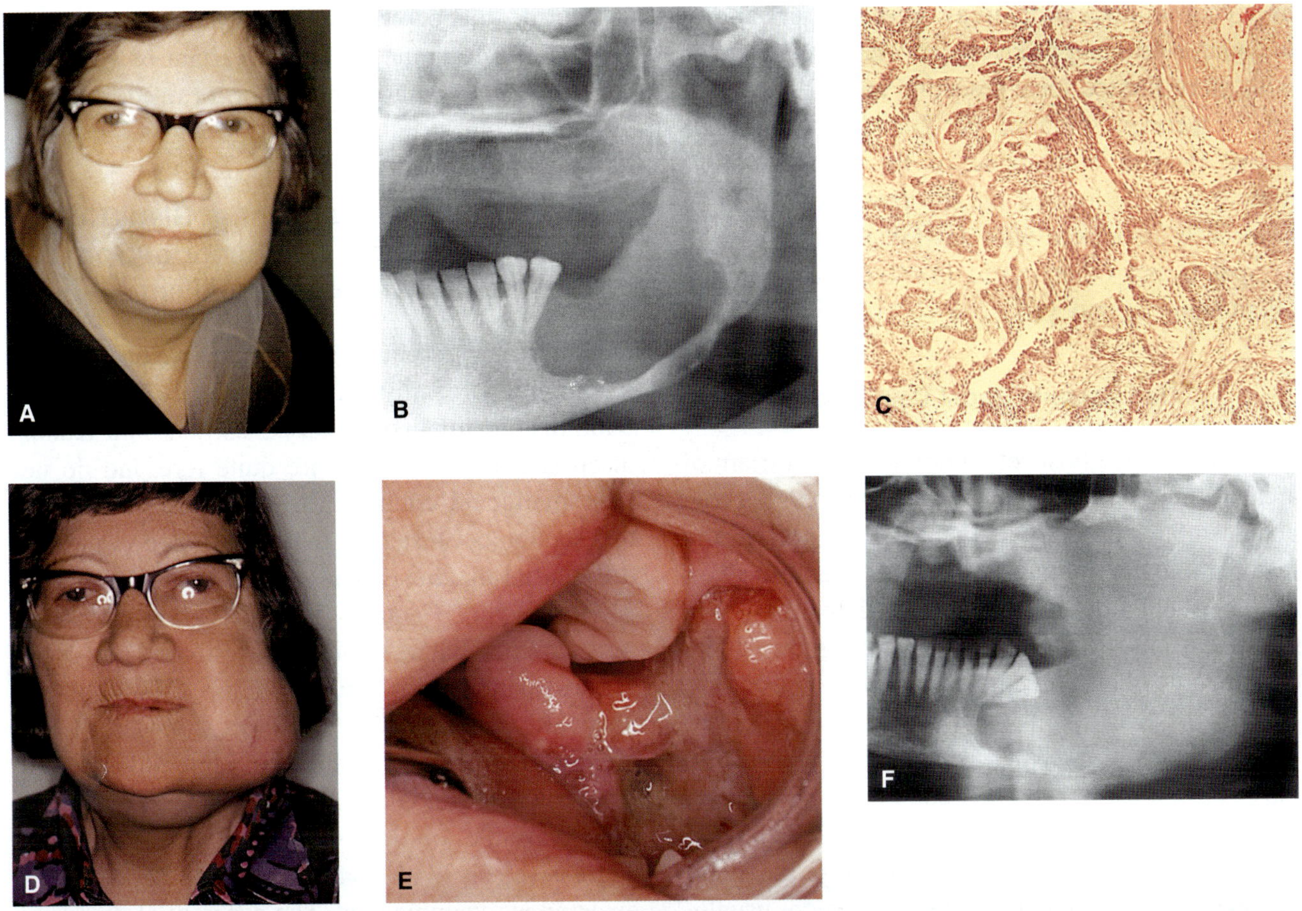

Figure 11–4. Ameloblastoma. *A*, The patient had noticed left mandibular swelling and pain for more than a year. *B*, Radiograph showed massive mandibular destruction. *C*, Biopsy confirmed the diagnosis of ameloblastoma. *D*, The patient refused treatment and returned 2 years later because of marked pain and inability to chew and swallow. *E*, Extensive intraoral proliferation of tumor. *F*, Radiograph reflects massive local extension of the tumor, which did not respond to an attempt at control by radiation therapy.

usual presentation is painless swelling. Radiographically, over 50% appear as multiloculated, sharply delineated radiolucencies. The different microscopic patterns of ameloblastoma (plexiform, follicular and its variant acanthomatous, desmoplastic) share common features, such as peripheral palisading and budding, and clinically behave similarly.[12] Ameloblastomas may recur locally when inadequately resected and, on very rare occasion, metastasize.[13] They may also dedifferentiate to a true ameloblastic carcinoma locally, with metastases to neck nodes and the lungs.[14]

The extent of surgical treatment of ameloblastomas is controversial. The two options are radical resection (rim mandibulectomy, if possible; segmental resection, if needed) or conservative therapy, such as enucleation, curettage, or marsupialization. The choice may depend in part on the location of the tumor, whether it is unicystic or multicystic, and how extensive "radical" surgery would need to be. Higher recurrence rates (33% versus 7%) have been reported with conservative treatment than with more extensive resection.[15] If segmental resection is the alternative, especially in anterior lesions or in those in whom a fibula free flap would be contraindicated, then conservative initial treatment may, in fact, be more acceptable to some patients. A thorough discussion of the alternatives is clearly indicated for each individual situation. If the tumor is unilocular, then it is more likely that local curettage may be able to remove all parts of the cyst. Close follow-up is important given the significant rate of recurrence with conservative treatment.

Peripheral ameloblastomas, representing about 2% of all ameloblastomas, are ameloblastomas that are not intraosseous; they occur in the soft tissue overlying tooth-bearing areas. These tumors appear to behave less aggressively and can be managed with more limited local resection and close follow-up.[16] Overexpression of bcl-2 and the oncogene *mdm2* (human homologue of the murine double minute type 2) located on chromosome 12q13–15 have been associated with ameloblastomas, as well as with some other cystic jaw lesions, including odontogenic keratocysts.

Odontogenic Ghost Cell Tumor

An odontogenic ghost cell tumor is a solid variant of a calcifying odontogenic cyst and considered a true neoplasm (as opposed to a cyst). Its noteworthy histopathologic finding is ghost cell keratinization of the epithelial lining. It can be malignant on very rare occasions, in which case it is referred to as an odontogenic ghost cell carcinoma.

Clear Cell Odontogenic Tumor

Another rare tumor that has been reported to metastasize is a clear cell odontogenic tumor or clear cell odontogenic carcinoma (CCOT),[16] which usually occurs in women over age 60. Unlike ameloblastoma, CCOTs are more frequently seen in the anterior mandible. Because of the clear cells seen histologically, it is important to distinguish this from a low-grade mucoepidermoid carcinoma, metastatic renal cell carcinoma, clear cell variant of a calcifying epithelial odontogenic tumor, or a poorly fixed ameloblastoma.

Giant Cell Lesions: Central Giant Cell Granuloma, Giant Cell Tumor of Bone, and Hyperparathyroidism

Other lesions presenting in the mandible and maxilla may mimic clinically and radiologically some of the odontogenic tumors discussed earlier. The lesions discussed in this section are quite rare and do not have malignant counterparts. They are included in this section because they may at times enter into the differential diagnosis, and at least some familiarity is worthwhile. Central giant cell granulomas are rare, multiloculated, radiolucent lesions. They occur in the mandible in young adults. CD68-positive giant cells are seen within a fibroblastic field. These are not granulomas despite their name, nor are they reparative. Histologic appearance does not predict their variable clinical behavior, which may be aggressive. As with many cysts and jaw lesions, excision is recommended. The differential diagnosis includes true giant cell tumors of bone (Figure 11–5), which are usually found in long bones and are clinically more aggressive, as well as the brown tumor/osteoclastoma of hyperparathyroidism and

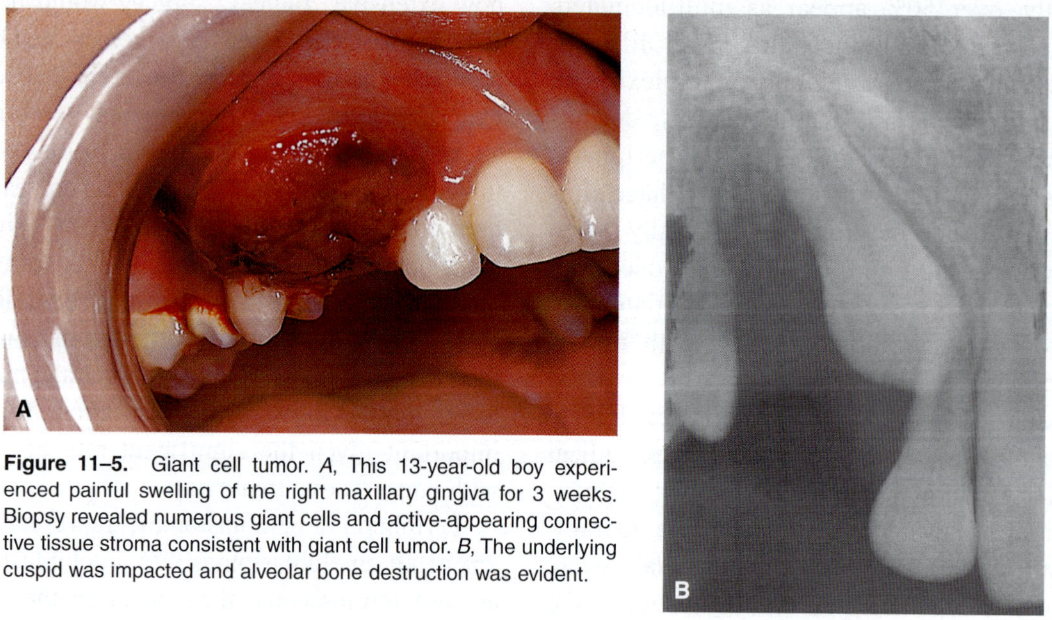

Figure 11–5. Giant cell tumor. *A*, This 13-year-old boy experienced painful swelling of the right maxillary gingiva for 3 weeks. Biopsy revealed numerous giant cells and active-appearing connective tissue stroma consistent with giant cell tumor. *B*, The underlying cuspid was impacted and alveolar bone destruction was evident.

cherubism, and aneurysmal bone cyst. Regezi reviewed the above lesions and additional myxoid and cystic lesions that may also mimic tumors with locally aggressive behavior.[10]

ORAL MUCOSAL MELANOMAS

Pigmented lesions of oral mucous membranes range from physiologic to neoplastic. Fortunately, oral melanomas are rare. However, in early, potentially curable stages, melanomas often mimic benign processes, such as ethnic pigmentation, smoking-associated pigmentation, drug-induced pigmentation, nevi, melanotic macule, and amalgam tattoo (Figures 11–6 and 11–7). It is important, therefore, for the clinician to identify and biopsy any newly acquired, unexplained pigmented lesion or any pigmented lesion showing changes in size and shape. Likewise, it is important for the pathologist to be aware of the subtle microscopic features associated with many melanomas that have an in situ growth phase (see below).[17]

Etiology

No etiologic factors have been identified for oral melanomas.[18] Risk factors have also remained elusive. There appear to be no geographic differences and possibly only slight ethnic and gender differences.[19] The previously reported phenomenon of melanosis preceding the appearance of oral melanoma is now believed to be an event that represents an early in situ growth phase of melanoma prior to the penetration or invasion of the submucosa.[20] Malignant transformation of a benign oral nevus seems to be highly unlikely.

Clinical Features

Oral melanomas are much less common than their cutaneous counterparts and probably represent less than 5% of all melanomas.[21] It should be recalled that more than 40,000 skin melanomas are reported annually in the United States, and that number has

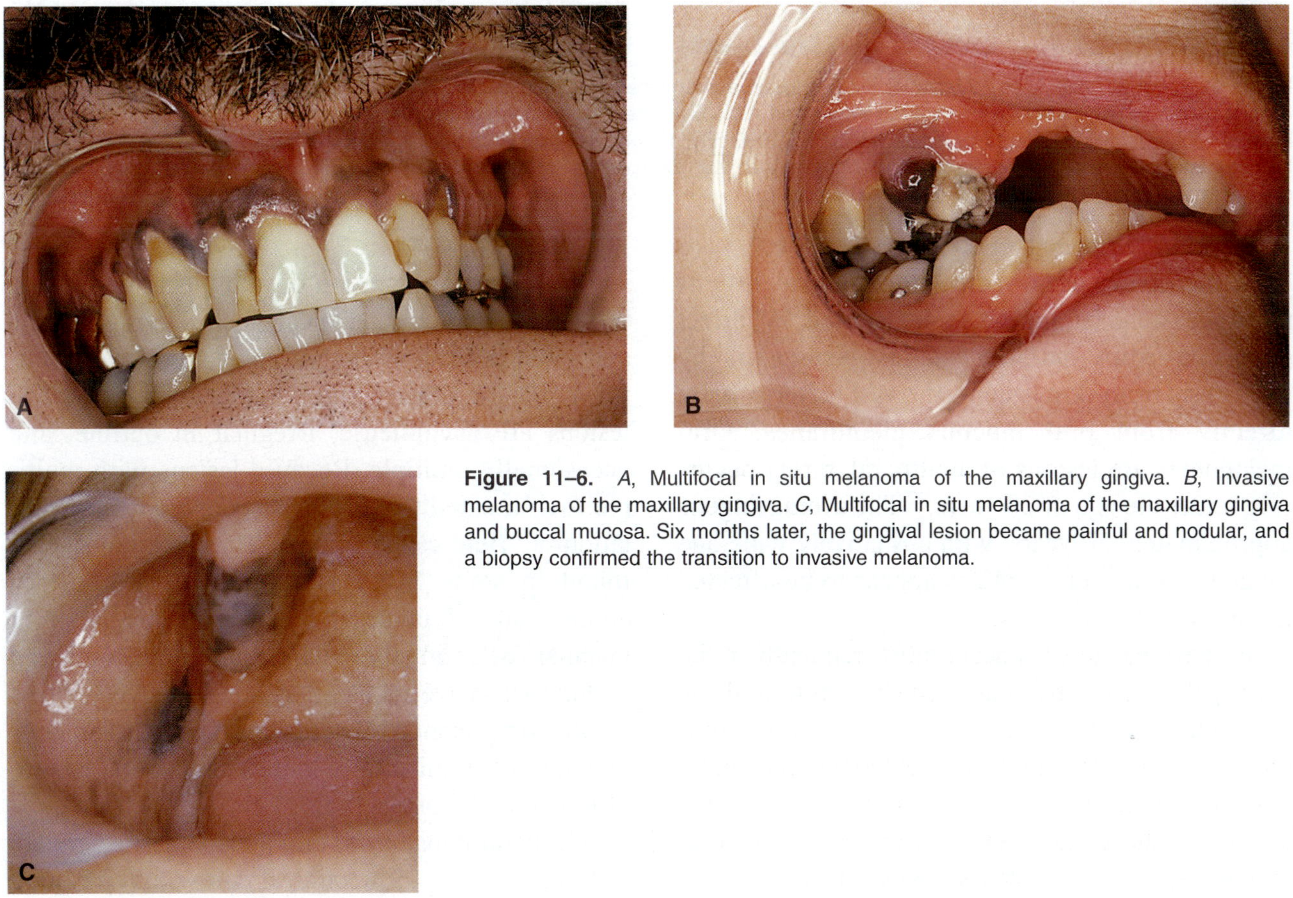

Figure 11–6. *A*, Multifocal in situ melanoma of the maxillary gingiva. *B*, Invasive melanoma of the maxillary gingiva. *C*, Multifocal in situ melanoma of the maxillary gingiva and buccal mucosa. Six months later, the gingival lesion became painful and nodular, and a biopsy confirmed the transition to invasive melanoma.

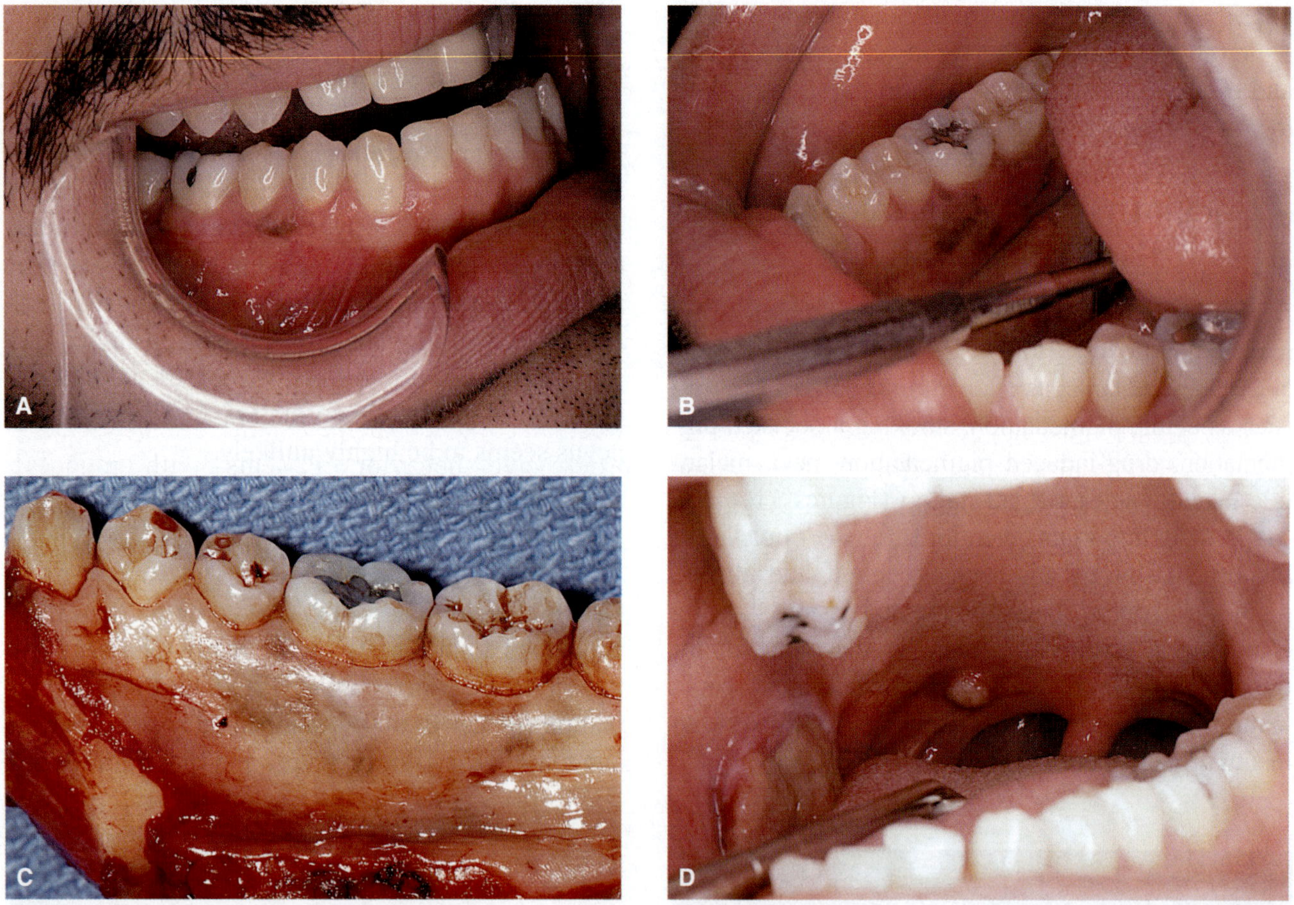

Figure 11–7. A 29-year-old asymptomatic man with invasive melanoma of the mandibular gingiva. On a routine examination, flat pigmentations of the buccal (*A*) and lingual (*B*) gingivae were noted. A biopsy of the lingual gingiva revealed invasive melanoma. Management included hemimandibulectomy (*C*) followed by radiation therapy (3,000 cGy in six treatments). Note diffuse, multifocal pigmentation that could be mistaken for benign melanosis. Five years later, the patient was seen for acute pain. Note lesions on buccal mucosa and palate that were both diagnosed as recurrent melanoma by biopsies (*D*).

been increasing each year. Although oral lesions may occasionally appear to be caused by direct extension from maxillary sinus lesions or by metastasis from skin lesions, the vast majority arise directly from oral mucous membranes. Oral melanomas are lesions of adulthood, rarely occurring under the age of 20 years.[22] The average age is approximately 50 years, with a relatively wide age range (2 to 80 years). Males appear to be affected more often than females.

Primary melanomas occur most frequently in the hard palate and maxillary gingiva, followed by mandibular gingiva. In these sites, clinical differential diagnosis may include melanoma, melanotic macule, smoking-associated melanosis, nevus, amalgam tattoo, and Kaposi's sarcoma. Other oral mucosal sites are only occasionally affected.

The clinical coloration of oral melanomas has a wide range, which can appear as black, gray, purple, and even reddish. Whereas some lesions are uniform in color, others exhibit marked variations. The lesions are asymmetric, irregular in outline, and occasionally multiple. Because lesions with multiple foci or satellites exhibit discontinuous pigmentation, a "field cancerization" effect similar to that found in some SCCs is suggested. The surface architecture of mucosal melanomas ranges from macular (often in situ melanomas) to ulcerated and nodular (invasive melanomas and invasive with an in situ component). Most lesions are heterogeneous in color and architecture. Induration is not a feature of in situ melanomas.

The natural history of oral melanomas is variable and unpredictable. The clinical course may be quite rapid or remarkably protracted (in situ lesions), lasting as long as 10 years. Clinically, oral melanomas may present as multiple lesions or with synchronous onset and may give the erroneous impression of physiologic pigmentation.

Histopathology

Microscopically, one of two basic patterns may be seen with mucosal melanomas: an in situ pattern in which the neoplasm is limited to the epithelial-connective tissue interface and an invasive pattern in which the neoplasm is found within the supporting connective tissue (Figure 11–8). A combined pattern of invasive melanoma with an in situ component is seen in most advanced lesions.

In melanomas, an increased density of atypical melanocytes is found, with individual or nested cells irregularly distributed at the epithelial–connective tissue interface. Neoplastic cells in invasive melanomas exhibit a wide variety of shapes, including spindled, plasmacytoid, and epithelioid. Correlation of microscopic patterns (tumor thickness and depth of invasion) with clinical behavior or patient outcome has generally been ineffective because of the advanced stage of most oral melanomas when biopsied.

Diagnostic Problems

Diagnosis of oral mucosal melanomas may be difficult for several reasons, including (1) small biopsy size, (2) unrepresentative sampling, (3) insufficient clinical information, and (4) lack of recognition of early in situ lesions by both clinician and pathologist. It appears that many in situ lesions have initially been underdiagnosed (and consequently undertreated). Hesitation to perform an incisional biopsy because of theoretical "cell seeding" is unfounded and without merit.

Prognosis and Treatment

Most mucosal melanomas exhibit an unrelenting progressive behavior. Patients with mucosal melanomas (both in situ and invasive lesions) generally have had a poor disease course. The poor prognosis associated with oral melanomas is believed to be attributable in large part to the advanced nature of these melanomas at the time of definitive diagnosis and treatment. However, a biologic propensity for spread and field cancerization probably play significant roles.

To improve prognosis, aggressive treatment must be initiated early in the natural history of oral melanomas. Surgery remains the primary treatment modality, and radiation and/or chemotherapy may serve as adjuncts. Even when the lesion presents as an in situ proliferation, wide excision is mandatory, especially in the presence of multiple or satellite lesions. Because of the high recurrence rate associated with oral lesions, combination therapy may be advantageous during primary treatment. Vaccines

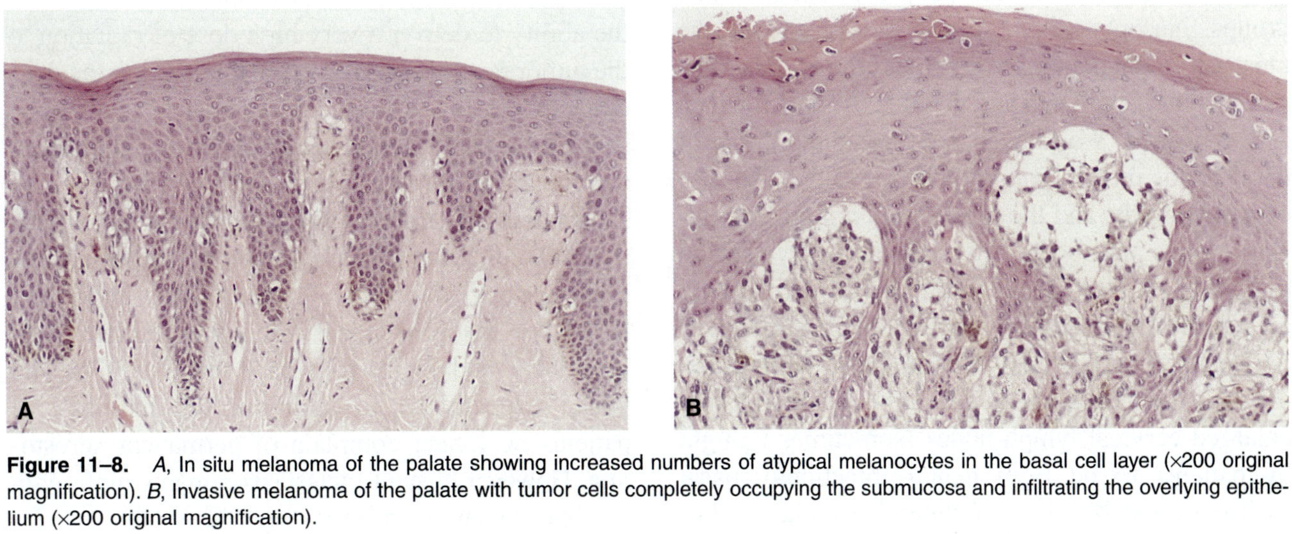

Figure 11–8. *A*, In situ melanoma of the palate showing increased numbers of atypical melanocytes in the basal cell layer (×200 original magnification). *B*, Invasive melanoma of the palate with tumor cells completely occupying the submucosa and infiltrating the overlying epithelium (×200 original magnification).

derived from a patient's own tumor cells are being evaluated.

Classification

It is somewhat difficult to apply the traditional cutaneous melanoma classification (nodular, superficial spreading, lentigo maligna, acral lentiginous) to oral melanomas.[17,23] One of the problems is that most oral melanomas are discovered and biopsied in an advanced stage, contributing to heterogeneous microscopic patterns. Another difference between oral and cutaneous melanomas is the particularly poor prognosis for oral melanomas in contrast to the fairly good control of most cutaneous lesions. Until more is known about oral melanomas, it remains difficult to explain the biologic differences between oral and cutaneous lesions. However, a simple subclassification of oral melanomas into in situ and invasive types would be valid and helpful.

NASOPHARYNGEAL CARCINOMA

Cancers of the nasopharynx represent less than 1% of all head and neck cancers in the United States. Between 1975 and 1998, there were 2,120 cases of nasopharyngeal carcinoma according to the SEER data (1,424 men and 696 women). The main histologic type is SCC. Chinese people from the southern province of Canton are known to have a genetic predisposition to this disease; their risk is up to 30 times greater (depending on the population used for comparison) than the risk for people of other ethnic groups. Nasopharyngeal carcinoma is one of the most common malignancies in southern Asia. The risk increases with age and is twice as great for men as for women. Working in poor ventilation, use of nasal balms or oils, consumption of salted fish, use of herbal drugs, and the presence of a high Epstein-Barr virus antibody titer (specifically serum immunoglobulin A against viral capsid antigen) are all statistically associated predisposing risk factors.[24]

Dental clinicians may become involved in either diagnosis or management. Often the initial signs are enlarged cervical lymph nodes (sometimes thought by patients to be from dental infections), nasal stuffiness and bleeding, unilateral earache, and/or hearing loss (Figure 11–9, A).[25] Early diagnosis and aggressive treatment help to increase survival.

Because therapy requires aggressive irradiation (including the major salivary glands, oropharynx, and neck), xerostomia, dental caries, and osteonecrosis are major problems (see Chapter 7, "Complications of Treatment"). Pretreatment dental planning is extremely important. Furthermore, although mortality from nasopharyngeal carcinoma exceeds 50%, the survival time is often prolonged, and most patients require preventive and therapeutic oral care before, during, and after treatment. Chinese patients with nasopharyngeal carcinoma treated in China have shown similarly poor long-term survival. However, recently, a randomized trial by the Head and Neck Intergroup in the United States and Canada showed a significantly improved 3-year disease-free survival (69% versus 24%; $p < .001$) and overall survival (78% versus 47%; $p = .002$) with combined chemotherapy and radiotherapy compared with radiotherapy alone for patients with stage III or IV nasopharyngeal carcinoma.[26] For carcinoma of the nasopharynx, the incidence of distant metastasis is relatively high, especially in patients with lymphoepitheliomas. The overall incidence of distant metastasis has been reported in the range of 18 to 34% and 50% in patients with stage N2 and N3 disease. Overall, the most common metastatic sites have been lung and bone.

Recently, with the advent of a highly conformal three-dimensional radiation treatment, namely intensity-modulated radiation therapy (IMRT), the results of treatment have improved tremendously. IMRT has the ability to deliver a very high dose of radiation to the tumor target precisely, while minimizing the dose delivered to the surrounding critical normal tissue (Figure 11–9, B).[27] As a result, the local and regional control rates for nasopharyngeal carcinoma have substantially increased when compared with conventional radiotherapy. The University of California-San Francisco experience of 67 patients who underwent IMRT for nasopharyngeal carcinoma resulted in 4-year local and regional control rates of 97% and 98%, respectively. In addition, the majority of patients no longer complain of permanent xerostomia. However, distant metastasis remains high, with a 4-year distant metastases–free rate of 66%.

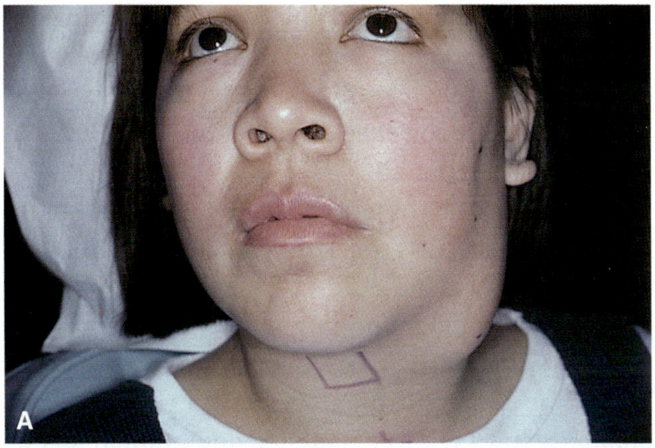

Figure 11–9. *A*, This 28-year-old woman was seen because of the mass in her neck. She also complained of headaches and nasal stuffiness. There was no evidence of dental pathology. A fine-needle aspiration biopsy revealed carcinoma in lymphoid tissue. Imaging and biopsy showed this to be a metastatic node from a nasopharyngeal carcinoma. The tumor responded to a combination of radiation and chemotherapy. *B*, Isodose curves of an inverse intensity-modulated radiotherapy plan delivered using MIMiC for a patient with T4N1 carcinoma of the nasopharynx displayed on the axial (a), coronal (b), and sagittal (c) planes through the centroid of the primary tumor and the dose-volume histograms for the relevant structures (d). The gross tumor volume is shown in red and the clinical target volume is shown in orange.

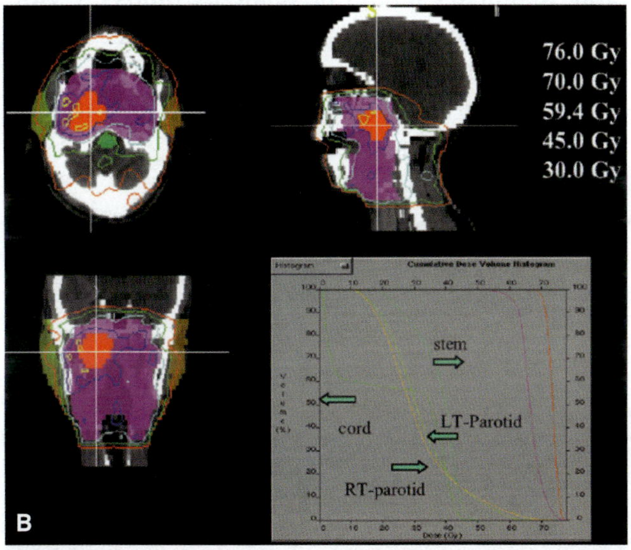

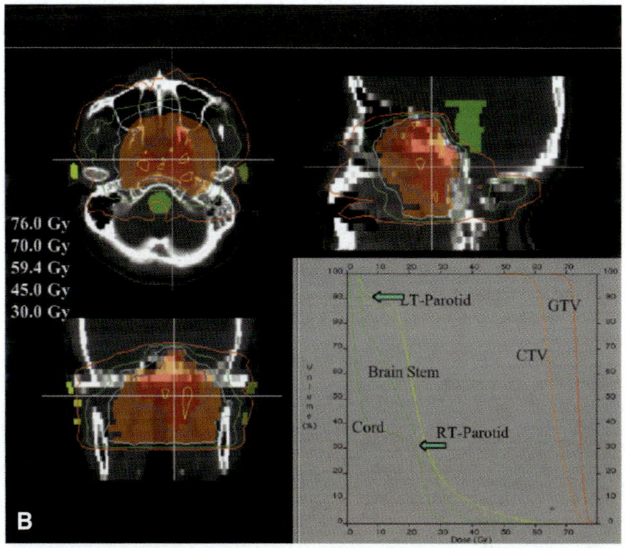

LARYNGEAL CARCINOMA

Carcinoma of the larynx accounts for about 11,000 new cases in the United States each year. More than 80% of cases occur in men. As with oral cancer patients, most laryngeal cancer victims are heavy users of tobacco and alcohol, and leukoplakia is a common precancerous lesion of the larynx. Early signs and symptoms include a chronic sore throat, hoarseness, change in voice, and blood spotting in saliva. These complaints should alert the clinician to suspect tumor and minimize delays in diagnosis.

Early diagnosis and treatment greatly improve survival and curability. The overall 5-year patient survival rate is about 65%. However, when the lesions are localized, the 5-year survival rate for patients in this group exceeds 80%. Radiation therapy has been effective by itself or in combination with surgery in extending survival, increasing curability, and decreasing morbidity by avoiding some laryngectomies, thus saving speech. These tumors can usually be seen well by indirect laryngoscopy, and diagnosis is confirmed by biopsy.

Pretreatment dental planning and post-treatment care are important. Because the radiation field is often extended to major salivary gland tissue (to include regional lymph nodes), as well as portions of the mandible, alteration in saliva and subsequent radiation caries may become rehabilitation problems (see Chapter 7).

SKIN AND LIP CANCERS

Skin cancer is important because it is by far the most common form of cancer and its most frequent site is the head and neck. Yearly, new cases in the United

States probably approximate a million. Predisposing factors include light complexion, exposure to actinic rays, and age. Fortunately, these cancers seldom metastasize and respond well to treatment. Five-year cure rates are in excess of 95%. Initial signs may not arouse the patient's concern for many months, or even years, because these malignancies are usually slow growing and are not painful (Figure 11–10).

Basal cell carcinoma is the most prevalent skin cancer. The early lesion may appear as a small ulcer, scab, or waxy pearl-like formation and may be mistaken for a benign skin condition. Therefore, persistent skin lesions should be referred for diagnosis and management.

The nevoid basal cell carcinoma syndrome is a rare condition that involves oral care because multiple jaw cysts are often found. This syndrome includes multiple nevi and basal cell carcinomas of the skin, rib anomalies, epidermal pits of the hands and feet, and a variety of other defects. The prognosis is good, but constant examination and continual treatment are required.

Lip cancer is often preceded by a premalignant change of cheilitis or keratosis (Figure 11–11; also see Figures 4–19 to 4–21). Chronic outdoor exposure and pipe smoking appear to be causally related. Protective or therapeutic ointments should be initiated in an attempt to reverse these changes. In case of persistence and clinical suspicion, diagnosis should be made by biopsy. Cytology and toluidine blue staining in this area are not accurate and are difficult to interpret because of the high degree of squamous cell differentiation and keratinization.

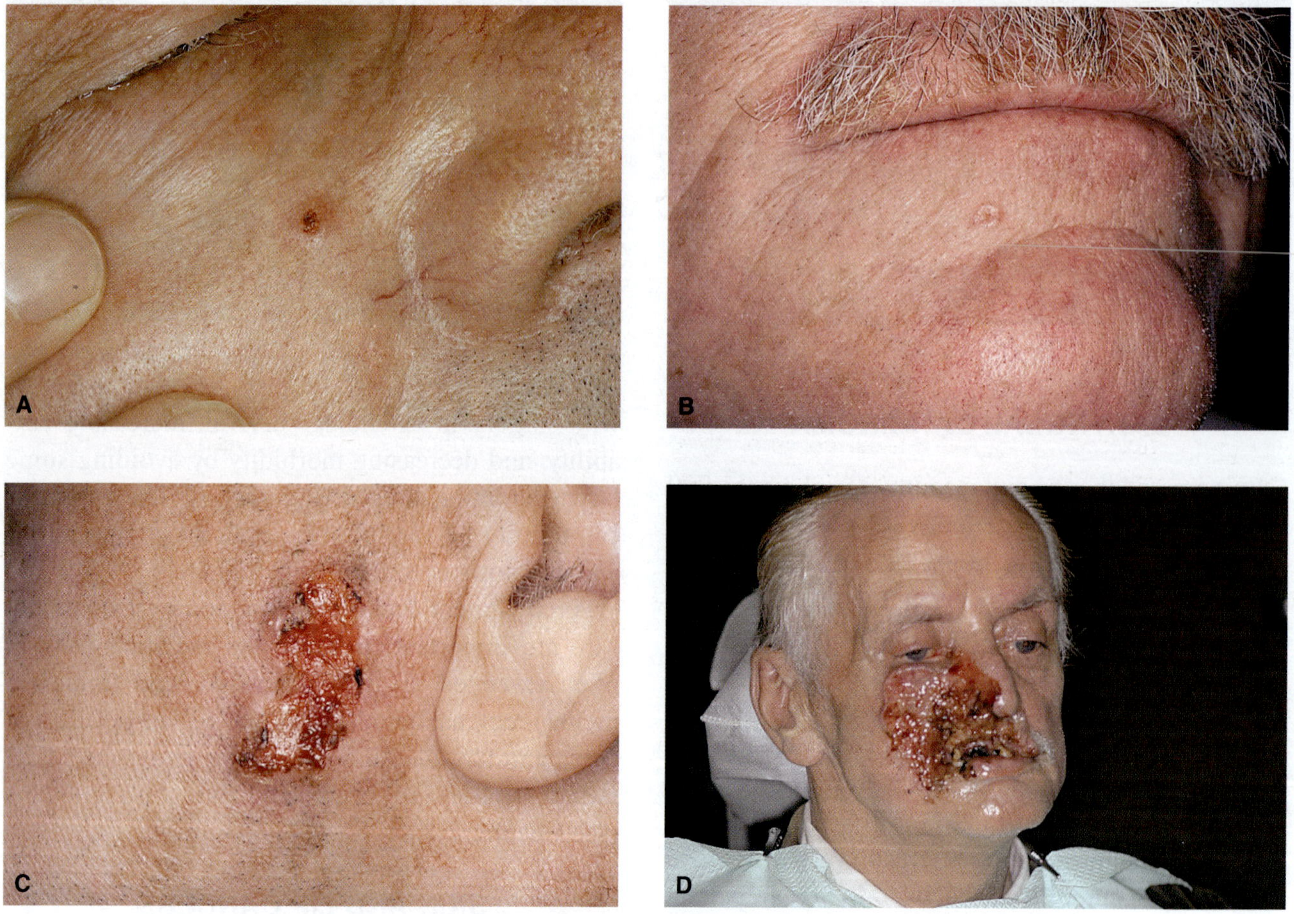

Figure 11–10. Skin cancers. *A*, A slowly growing lesion of the cheek noticed for 1 year. The only complaint was itchiness. A biopsy revealed basal cell carcinoma. *B*, A basal cell carcinoma below the lower lip (right chin area) noticed by the patient for 6 months. *C*, Moderately advanced basal cell carcinoma of the cheek anterior to the tragus of the ear. It had been ignored for over 2 years. *D*, An advanced, long-standing basal cell carcinoma that originated on the cheek and was left untreated by the patient. Although locally invasive and destructive, basal cell carcinomas rarely metastasize.

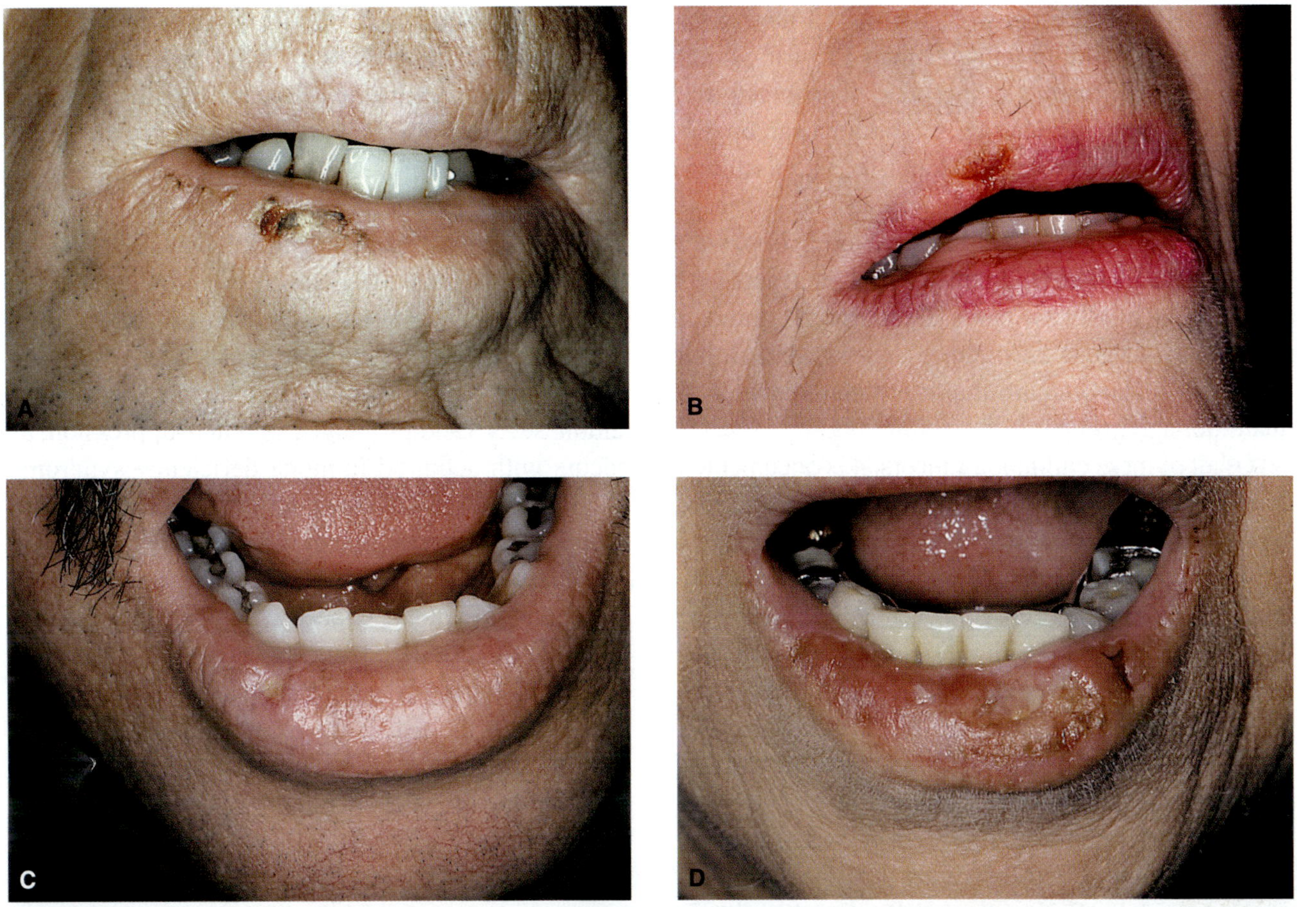

Figure 11–11. Cancers of the lips. *A*, Chronic cheilitis with areas of microscopic epithelial dysplasia. *B*, Basal cell carcinoma of the upper lip. *C*, Early squamous cell carcinoma of the lower lip noticed for only 3 weeks. *D*, Moderately advanced squamous cell carcinoma of the lower lip. This painful ulcer had been bothering the patient for over 3 months.

The lower vermilion border is by far the most common site, and SCC is the most common type. Because most of these lesions remain localized, cure rates are extremely good. This is the only oral cancer that is decreasing in incidence.

CANCER IN CHILDREN AND ADOLESCENTS

More than 8,000 cases of cancer are diagnosed annually in children younger than 15 years of age in the United States, and this risk continues to increase each year at an annual rate of 1 to 2%.[28,29] Despite these numbers, it is considered to be a rare disease, with only 1 to 2 children developing cancer for every 10,000 children. The risk for developing childhood cancer is greatest in the first 3 years of life and then declines until the age of 9, after which time there is a steady increase throughout adolescence. For most forms of childhood cancer, there is a higher male predominance, except for thyroid cancer, which has a marked predilection for females. When evaluating the role of race and ethnicity, it is the white child who has the highest incidence rates for most cancers, whereas the Native American child has a much lower risk than all of the other groups. Although significant strides in treating childhood cancers have been made, this disease still claims more than 1,600 lives each year. Surpassed only by accidental trauma, cancer is the second leading cause of death in children under the age of 15, accounting for 11% of the total deaths in this age group.

In contrast to adult malignancies, there is a predominance of sarcomas in the pediatric population. The two most frequently diagnosed childhood cancers are leukemia and central nervous system (CNS) tumors, which represent over 50% of all new cases each year. In children younger than 15 years, other common malignancies include neuroblastoma, Wilms' tumor, lymphoma, rhabdomyosarcoma,[30] germ cell tumors, retinoblastoma, hepatoblastoma, osteosarcoma, and Ewing's sarcoma. This disease pattern changes in the 15- to 19-year age group, with Hodgkin's and non-Hodgkin's lymphoma accounting for 25% of all new cases. Besides CNS tumors, germ cell and gonadal tumors, thyroid cancer, and malignant melanoma are important malignancies in this older age group.

Of all of these childhood cancers, it is documented that 12% occur in the head and neck region and that approximately 1% represent a second malignancy. Furthermore, it is estimated that 25% of all primary malignancies in children will eventually involve the head and neck site. Over time, an increase in head and neck cancer incidence among children has been noted, which is greater than the overall increase in the malignancy rate for this age group. The most commonly diagnosed malignancies to develop at this location are lymphomas, followed by neural tumors, thyroid carcinoma, and soft tissue sarcomas. In sharp contrast to adults, SCC in the head and neck region is rare in children, accounting for less than 2% of the malignancies. Regarding specific locations, the neck is the most frequently involved site, whereas only 4% are diagnosed in the oropharyngeal region.

Although the causes of childhood cancers are unknown, chromosomal and genetic aberrations are identified in many of these malignancies. Certain syndromes such as Down's syndrome, Beckwith-Wiedemann syndrome, Bloom syndrome, Li-Fraumeni syndrome, neurofibromatosis, and multiple endocrine neoplasia syndrome are examples with well-defined cancer risks. Environmental carcinogens that are associated with an increased risk of childhood cancer are high levels of ionizing radiation or radiotherapy, excessive sun exposure, and certain chemotherapeutic agents, in particular alkylating agents and topoisomerase II inhibitors. Similar to adults, severe and prolonged immunosuppression, as occurs with acquired immune deficiency syndrome (AIDS) and organ transplantation, increases the risk for developing certain cancers, especially lymphoma. Suspected, but unproven, risk factors include environmental pollutants, exposure to pesticides and toxins, and infectious agents. Owing to the rarity of childhood cancers, the heterogeneous nature of these tumors, and the difficulty in obtaining an accurate prenatal and postnatal history, the identification of etiologic factors is challenging.

Diagnosis

Because this group of malignancies represents a variety of entities, their clinical presentation and symptoms differ. In the child, most solid tumors present as a progressively enlarging mass that may be painful. In contrast, hematopoietic diseases frequently cause lymphadenopathy, bleeding problems,

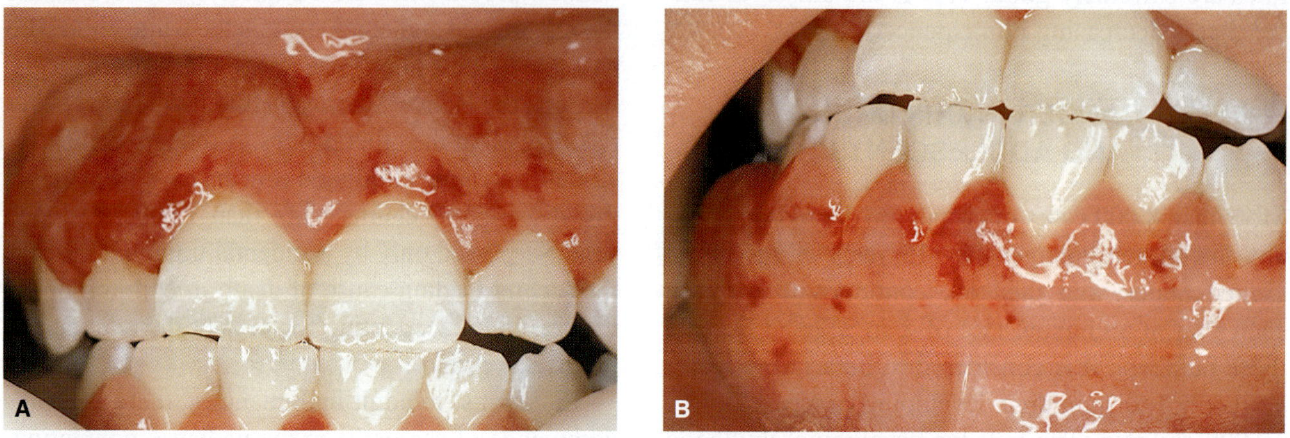

Figure 11–12. This lethargic 8-year-old Hispanic girl presented with generalized gingival enlargements involving both the maxilla (*A*) and the mandible (*B*) of 3 weeks duration. For the past 3 months, the child had been treated for multiple ear and sinus infections and vague abdominal problems. The purpuric gingival enlargements were the result of leukemic infiltrates in a child with acute myelogenous leukemia.

bruising, fatigue, fever, joint pain, and increased susceptibility to infections (Figure 11–12). When the head and neck region is the site of involvement, the early signs and symptoms include lymphadenopathy, otalgia, otorrhea, rhinorrhea, nasal congestion, sinusitis, and headache. These are problems that often mimic common, benign illnesses in this age group.

Because malignancies of the oral cavity are very rare, a definitive diagnosis is often delayed because early signs and symptoms can be confused with inflammatory and benign reactive lesions.[31] Typically, malignancies of soft tissue origin present as tender, asymmetric enlargements with a red, ulcerated surface. These rapidly growing lesions are firm and fixed to the underlying tissues, often destroying alveolar bone and displacing adjacent teeth. Although soft tissue sarcomas can occur at any site in the oral cavity, the gingiva, palate, and tongue are the most frequently involved. Rhabdomyosarcoma, fibrosarcoma, leukemic infiltrates, and metastatic disease are examples of intraoral soft tissue malignancies in this age group. Although SCC and its variants have been diagnosed in the pediatric population, this form of oral cancer is a distinct rarity unless there is direct extension of a nasopharyngeal carcinoma into this site.

Sarcomas of the jawbones in children cause diffuse enlargements with facial asymmetry, extrusion and premature loss of vital teeth, and trismus. Although paresthesia or dysesthesia can be present, it is not easy for a young child to communicate this aberrant sensation. Important radiographic findings include a radiolucent or mixed radiolucent and radiopaque lesion with poorly defined borders, loss of the dental lamina and dental crypt, and occasional proliferative periostitis. An ominous radiographic finding is the "floating tooth phenomenon," when there is no evidence of pulpal disease. Irregular external root resorption and atypical widening of the pulpal canal and chamber are additional dental findings. Langerhans' cell histiocytosis, Burkitt's lymphoma, Ewing's sarcoma, osteosarcoma, and mesenchymal chondrosarcoma have a predilection for children and can involve the jaws (Figure 11–13).

Definitive diagnosis requires surgical biopsy, in addition to complete blood count, blood chemistry analysis, liver profile, and advanced imaging studies. Depending on the cancer type and site, CT, MRI, plain films, and isotope scans, in addition to lumbar puncture and bone marrow aspirate, are often necessary to detect metastatic disease.

Treatment and Prognosis

Over 90% of children younger than 15 years of age receive multimodality treatments to manage their malignancies, including multiagent chemotherapy, total-body or localized irradiation, and aggressive surgery. Overall, the 5-year survival rate exceeds 75% for the most common cancers.[32] Using DNA microarrays to assess the entire expressed gene profile of these pediatric cancers, the potential exists for identifying tumor subsets and, subsequently, tailoring treatment to the individual for improved outcomes.[33] A serious complication associated with

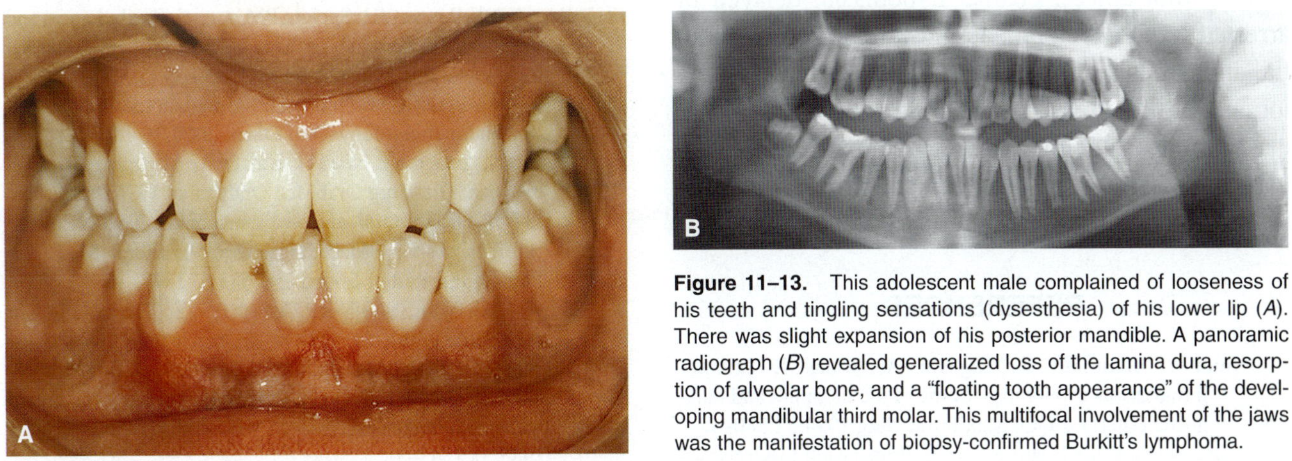

Figure 11–13. This adolescent male complained of looseness of his teeth and tingling sensations (dysesthesia) of his lower lip (*A*). There was slight expansion of his posterior mandible. A panoramic radiograph (*B*) revealed generalized loss of the lamina dura, resorption of alveolar bone, and a "floating tooth appearance" of the developing mandibular third molar. This multifocal involvement of the jaws was the manifestation of biopsy-confirmed Burkitt's lymphoma.

increased survival from intensive multimodality therapy is the risk of developing a second malignancy.[34] The cumulative incidence of second cancers appears to be 3 to 12% within 20 years following the initial cancer. Second cancers are the most common cause of death in long-term survivors if recurrent primary disease is excluded. Children who are at greatest risk for a subsequent malignancy include survivors with a primary diagnosis of Hodgkin's disease, retinoblastoma, or the genetic form of Wilms' tumor or children with a genetic disease that makes them susceptible to cancer. Therapeutic radiation, exposure to alkylating agents, female gender, and young age are all risk factors that increase the likelihood for a second malignancy. The most common hematopoietic second malignancy is acute nonlymphoblastic leukemia, whereas solid tumors are associated with radiation, especially within the therapeutic ports. It is not uncommon for the second malignancy to develop in the head and neck region, especially when patients receive cranial irradiation for the treatment of solid tumors. These second malignancies usually occur within the first 15 years following treatment and include brain tumors and thyroid and parotid gland cancers.

Late effects of cancer treatment can be devastating because of neurologic, physical, and psychologic problems.[35] Maxillofacial abnormalities are observed in the majority of children who receive radiotherapy to this region.[36] These complications can affect facial appearance and quality of speech. Depending on the age of the child during treatment, the side effects can include hypoplasia of the maxilla and mandible, abnormal occlusal relationship, nasal voice, short or blunted root apices, enamel hypoplasia, delayed or arrested tooth development and eruption, microdontia, and caries secondary to radiation-induced xerostomia. For these reasons, the child who survives cancer becomes a lifelong patient, requiring a sensitive team approach for the management of post-treatment sequelae and the early diagnosis of second cancers.

REFERENCES

1. Suei Y, Tanimoto K, Taguchi A, Wada T. Primary intraosseous carcinoma: review of the literature and diagnostic criteria. J Oral Maxillofac Surg 1994;52:580–3.
2. Shimoyama T, Ide F, Horie N, et al. Primary intraosseous carcinoma associated with impacted third molar of the mandible: review of the literature and report of a new case. J Oral Sci 2001;43:287–92.
3. Thomas G, Pandey M, Mathew A, et al. Primary intraosseous carcinoma of the jaw: pooled analysis of world literature and report of two new cases. Int J Oral Maxillofac Surg 2001;30:349–55.
4. Zwetyenga N, Pinsolle J, Rivel J, et al. Primary intraosseous carcinoma of the jaws. Arch Otolaryngol Head Neck Surg 2001;127:794–7.
5. Chindia ML. Osteosarcoma of the jaw bones. Oral Oncol 2001;37:545–7.
6. Bennett JH, Thomas G, Evans AW, Speight PM. Osteosarcoma of the jaws: a 30-year retrospective review. Oral Surg Oral Med Oral Pathol Oral Radiol Endod 2000;90:323–32.
7. Gadwal SR, Gannon FH, Fanburg-Smith JC, et al. Primary osteosarcoma of the head and neck in pediatric patients: a clinicopathologic study of 22 cases with a review of the literature. Cancer 2001;91:598–605.
8. Eversole LR. Malignant epithelial odontogenic tumors. Semin Diagn Pathol 1999;16:317–24.
9. Reichart PA, Philipsen HP, Sonner S. Ameloblastoma: biologic profile of 3,677 cases. Eur J Cancer B Oral Oncol 1995;31B:86–9.
10. Regezi JA. Odontogenic cysts, odontogenic tumors, fibro-osseous, and giant cell lesions of the jaws. Mod Pathol 2002;15:331–41.
11. Verneuil A, Sapp P, Huang C, Abemayor E. Malignant ameloblastoma: classification, diagnostic, and therapeutic challenges. Am J Otolaryngol 2002;23:44–8.
12. Simko EJ, Brannon RB, Eibling DE. Ameloblastic carcinoma of the mandible. Head Neck 1998;20:654–9.
13. Nakamura N, Higuchi Y, Mitsuyasu T, et al. Comparison of long-term results between different approaches to ameloblastoma. Oral Surg Oral Med Oral Pathol Oral Radiol Endod 2002;93:13–20.
14. Philipsen HP, Reichart PA, Nikai H, et al. Peripheral ameloblastoma: biological profile based on 160 cases from the literature. Oral Oncol 2001;37:17–27.
15. Maiorano E, Altini M, Viale G, et al. Clear cell odontogenic carcinoma. Report of two cases and review of the literature. Am J Clin Pathol 2001;116:107–14.
16. Iezzi G, Rubini C, Fioroni M, Piattilli A. Clear cell odontogenic carcinoma. Oral Oncol 2002;38:209–13.
17. Barrett AW, Bennett JH, Speight PM. A clinicopathological and immunohistochemical analysis of primary oral mucosal melanoma. Eur J Cancer B Oral Oncol 1995;31B:100–5.
18. Hicks MJ, Flaitz CM. Oral mucosal melanoma: epidemiology and pathobiology. Oral Oncol 2000;36:152–69.
19. Tanaka N, Amagasa T, Iwaki H, et al. Oral malignant melanoma in Japan. Oral Surg Oral Med Oral Pathol 1994;78:81–90.
20. WESTOP Group. Oral mucosal melanomas: The WESTOP Banff workshop proceedings. Oral Surg Oral Med Oral Pathol Oral Radiol Endod 1997;83:672–9.
21. Smyth AG, Ward-Booth RP, Avery BS, To EW. Malignant melanoma of the oral cavity—an increasing clinical diagnosis? Br J Oral Maxillofac Surg 1993;31:230–5.
22. Rapini RP, Golitz LE, Greer RO, et al. Primary malignant melanoma of the oral cavity: A review of 177 cases. Cancer 1985;55:1543–51.

23. Perkocha LA. Classification of melanoma in adults and children. In: LeBoit PE, editor. Malignant melanoma and melanocytic neoplasms, pathology: state of the art reviews. Vol 2. Philadelphia: Hanley & Belfus; 1994. p. 299–338.
24. Zong YS, Sham JS, Ng MH, et al. Immunoglobulin A against viral capsid antigen of Epstein-Barr virus and indirect mirror examination of the nasopharynx in the detection of asymptomatic nasopharyngeal carcinoma. Cancer 1992; 69:3–7.
25. Epstein JB, Jones CK. Presenting signs and symptoms of nasopharyngeal carcinoma. Oral Surg Oral Med Oral Pathol 1993;75:32–6.
26. Al-Sarraf M, LeBlanc M, Giri PG, et al. Chemoradiotherapy vs. radiotherapy in patients with locally advanced nasopharyngeal cancer: phase III randomized intergroup study 0099. J Clin Oncol 1998;16:1310–7.
27. Lee N, Xia, Quivey JM, et al. Intensity-modulated radiation therapy in the treatment of nasopharyngeal carcinoma: an update of the UCSF experience. Int Radiat Oncol Biol Phys 2002;53:12–22.
28. Albright JT, Topham AK, Reilly JS. Pediatric head and neck malignancies. US incidence and trends over 2 decades. Arch Otolaryngol Head Neck Surg 2002;128:655–9.
29. Reis LAG, Smith MA, Gurney JG, et al. Cancer incidence and survival among children and adolescents: United States SEER Program 1975–1995. Bethesda (MD): National Cancer Institute, SEER Program; 1999. NIH Publication No.: 99-4649.
30. Hicks J, Flaitz CM. Rhabdomyosarcoma of the head and neck in children. Oral Oncol 2002;38:450–9.
31. Flaitz CM. Differential diagnosis of oral mucosal lesions in children and adolescents. Adv Dermatol 2000;16:39–79.
32. Mertens AC, Yasui Y, Neglia JP, et al. Late mortality experience in five-year survivors of childhood and adolescent cancer: the Childhood Cancer Survival Study. J Clin Oncol 2001;19:3163–72.
33. Triche TJ, Schofield D, Buckley J. DNA microarrays in pediatric cancer. Cancer J 2001;7:2–15.
34. Neglia JP, Friedman DL, Yasui Y, et al. Second malignant neoplasms in five-year survivors of childhood cancer: childhood cancer survivor study. J Natl Cancer Inst 2001;93:618–29.
35. Gleeson HK, Shalet SM. Endocrine complications of neoplastic diseases in children and adolescents. Curr Opin Pediatr 2001;13:346–51.
36. Dahllof G. Craniofacial growth in children treated for malignant diseases. Acta Odontol Scand 1998;56:378–82.

12

Human Immunodeficiency Virus–Associated Malignancies

CATHERINE M. FLAITZ, DDS, MS
SOL SILVERMAN JR., MA, DDS

For decades, it has been known that immunocompromised persons are at increased risk for developing specific types of cancers. Therefore, it is not surprising that individuals infected with the human immunodeficiency virus (HIV), who have been immunocompromised for a prolonged period, have an increased likelihood of developing a malignancy during the course of their disease.[1,2] In fact, increased survival with highly active antiretroviral therapy (HAART) extends that window of opportunity for HIV-associated malignancies to develop. Kaposi's sarcoma (KS)[3] and non-Hodgkin's lymphoma (NHL) demonstrate the strongest link to HIV infection, representing the majority of all cancers in patients infected with HIV. Until recently, it was estimated that these two malignancies affected between 20 and 40% of HIV-infected individuals during the course of their disease.[4] These numbers, however, have declined with the widespread use of HAART in industrialized countries.[5–7] There also appears to be a greater risk of developing Hodgkin's lymphoma and squamous cell carcinoma, although these malignancies are not as convincingly associated with HIV infection.[8] Even HIV-infected children experience a higher incidence of cancers, in particular, unusual smooth muscle tumors and NHL.[9]

The oral cavity provides important visual clues to the overall health status of an HIV-infected person. The mouth may reflect the first signs and symptoms of the disease and may be a site of a major complaint after HIV seroconversion. In addition, the frequency, chronicity, and severity of a wide range of oral lesions may indicate disease progression and further deterioration of the immune system. Included in this group of oral manifestations are several malignancies.

KAPOSI'S SARCOMA

KS is the most common malignancy associated with acquired immune deficiency syndrome (AIDS), although the number of new cases has declined significantly with widespread use of HAART regimens in industrialized countries.[10,11] This controversial entity, which has been defined as a multicentric angioproliferative disease, represents both an inflammatory hyperplasia and a neoplastic process.[12] It appears to be triggered by cellular factors, such as cytokines, growth factors, and HIV–tat gene product, acting in concert with the human herpesvirus 8 (HHV-8), that induce the formation of tumors in widespread tissues and organs.[13] A prominent feature of this tumor is the high secretion levels of angiogenic growth factors, which produce the characteristic vascular appearance of KS.

Although there has been a well-known endemic form of KS occurring mainly in Africa and the northern Mediterranean area, epidemic KS associated with HIV immunodeficiency is more aggressive. Besides immunosuppression and possible genetic factors, it is presently acknowledged that all forms of KS are associated with HHV-8. Of interest, this B-lymphotrophic gamma herpesvirus is found in many tissue sites and body fluids, but saliva contains the highest viral titers. The oropharyngeal tonsils, including the tonsillar epithelium and B lymphocytes, appear to be the major site of latent HHV-8 and, occasionally, lytic or replicating virus. Periodically, this virus is shed into the mouth and is found in whole saliva.[14] Sexual transmission of this virus is the most likely mode of infection in HIV-infected adults, whereas premastication of food by the mother is thought to be a possible route of infection to children in developing countries.

KS is one of the 27 AIDS-defining conditions and is characteristically associated with low CD4 lymphocyte counts. Before the HAART era, about 10 to 15% of all AIDS cases reported to the Centers for Disease Control and Prevention had KS as one of their initial AIDS-defining diseases in the United States. During this same period, approximately half of the patients with KS were diagnosed without a prior history of other opportunistic infections or systemic symptoms. At the present time, KS has decreased by 30 to 50% with the new HIV drug protocols. Of importance, in the early part of the HIV epidemic, up to 40% of HIV-infected individuals were diagnosed with oral KS, but this number has declined to 1% in the post-HAART era. Although KS occurs in all AIDS groups, it is more frequent in homosexual and bisexual males, indicating that HHV-8 appears to be preferentially transmitted through sexual behaviors. Men between the ages of 30 and 39 years have the highest incidence of this malignancy, and then it declines with age. An interesting geographic difference is observed in HIV-infected children regarding the incidence of KS. Although this tumor is rarely found in HIV-infected children of industrialized countries, KS has become the most common pediatric cancer in parts of Africa, with the number of new cases actually increasing.

Until recently, the mean time of survival after the diagnosis of KS was less than 2 years. However, with the initiation of HAART regimens, survival time has improved significantly. In fact, the use of these medications has reduced the risk of death among KS patients by over 80%. Although KS can involve multiple organs and be the primary cause of death, most KS patients succumb to opportunistic infections, other malignancies, especially NHL, and progressive wasting syndrome.

Diagnosis

Skin is the most common site of KS, but in about half of the patients with this disease, an oral presentation is observed (Figure 12–1). In many of these patients, oral KS is the first and sometimes

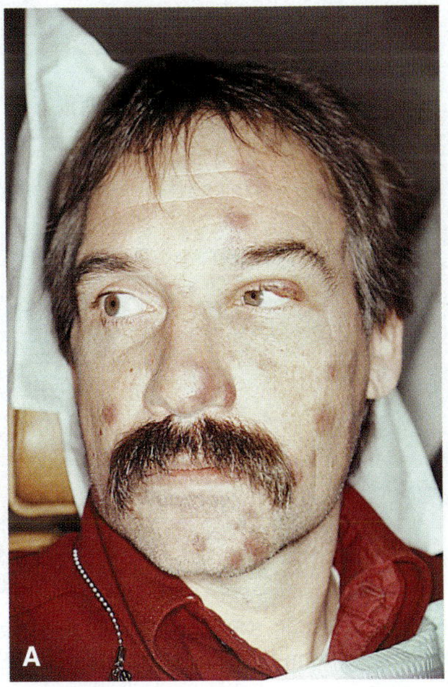

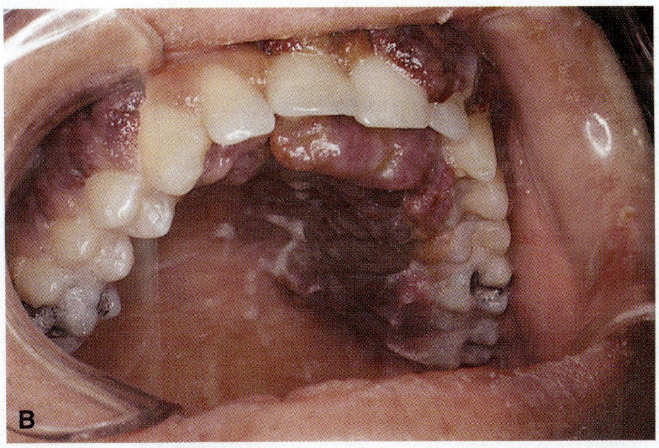

Figure 12–1. Kaposi's sarcoma (KS) in a patient with a rapidly falling CD4 count and increasing viral load. *A*, Multiple, progressive facial skin lesions. *B*, Rapidly increasing and painful hemorrhagic KS involving gingiva and palate. There was also associated oral candidiasis and flaring hepatitis. The patient died 2 weeks later.

the only tumor manifestation. Although any oral mucosal site can be affected, the palate is the most frequently involved site, followed by the gingiva. In rare instances, intraosseous lesions of the jaws have been diagnosed.

Initial manifestations appear as flat, red or purple, asymptomatic lesions (Figure 12–2). Owing to local cellular growth factors, these lesions increase in number and size, becoming nodular and symptomatic. Large palatal lesions may exhibit a yellow or amber

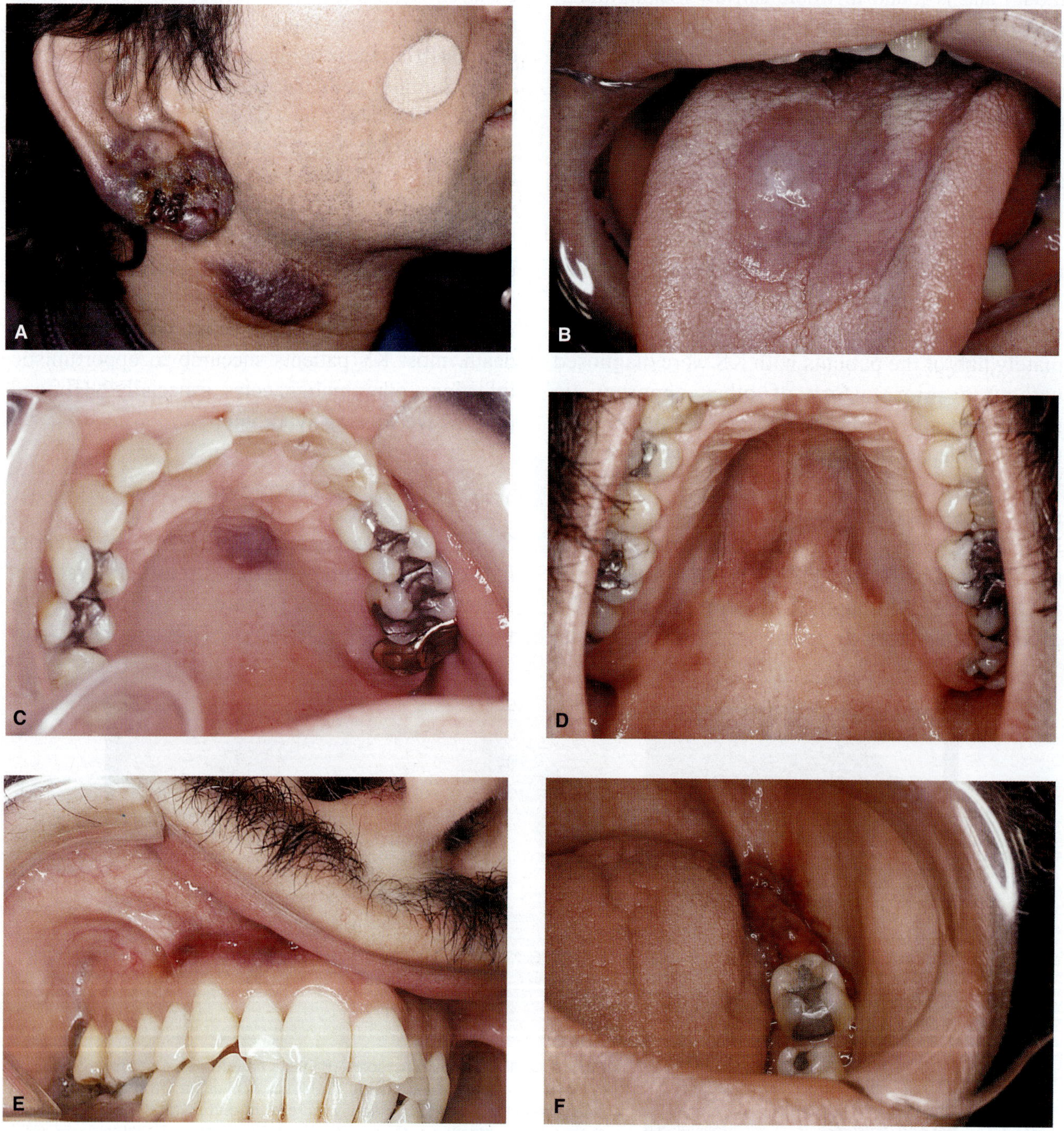

Figure 12–2. Kaposi's sarcoma (KS) in HIV-positive/AIDS patients. *A*, Progressive nodular skin KS. *B*, KS of tongue that is slightly symptomatic. *C*, Early asymptomatic KS of palate. *D*, Advanced KS of palate with mild symptoms. *E*, Flat, asymptomatic KS of gingiva. *F*, Nodular, symptomatic KS of retromolar area.

color at the posterior margin of the tumor, which is indicative of lymphedema. When KS lesions develop on the gingiva, erosion of bone, widening of the periodontal ligament spaces, and mobility of the teeth may occur in the late stage of tumor development. KS can dramatically affect the quality of life by causing esthetic problems, pain, bleeding, and interference with normal oral functions.

Because of the variable clinical features, the differential diagnosis of KS includes hemangioma, pyogenic granuloma, peripheral giant cell granuloma, purpuric lesions, and nonspecific inflammation. Bacillary angiomatosis is a bacterial infection that is characterized by proliferative vascular lesions that resemble KS. Bacillary angiomatosis is primarily a cutaneous infection that is caused by the *Bartonella* (*Rochalimaea*) bacteria, in particular, *B henselae* and *B. quintana*, and only rarely occurs in the oral cavity. To distinguish among this group of lesions that have a similar clinical presentation, a biopsy is needed for the definitive diagnosis of KS. The primary characteristic microscopic features include a proliferation of spindled tumor cells, angiogenesis, slit-like vascular spaces, extravasated red blood cells, and an inflammatory infiltrate. Most of the spindle-shaped tumor cells and endothelial cells within the KS lesions are latently infected with HHV-8, whereas only a few tumor cells, along with monocytes and lymphocytes, demonstrate lytic infection.

Treatment

Systemic chemotherapy is the most commonly used approach when KS lesions are widespread and disseminated to visceral organs or significantly interfere with normal function.[15] Several single and combination cytotoxic agents have been used to treat KS, although none of these chemotherapeutic protocols will cure the disease. For rapidly progressing and disseminated KS, the liposomal anthracyclines, such as doxorubicin and daunorubicin, are the initial treatment of choice. The principal combination chemotherapy that is used includes doxorubicin (Adriamycin), bleomycin, and vincristine (ABV) or bleomycin and vincristine (BV), which are administered every 2 to 4 weeks. Paclitaxel is another single agent that is used to treat advanced cases. Interferon-α, in combination with antiretroviral drugs or together with an anthracycline or paclitaxel, has been effective. Other treatment approaches include low-dose fractionated radiation therapy for difficult to treat sites, cryotherapy, intralesional chemotherapy, and topical retinoic acid for skin lesions. Novel treatment approaches for managing KS are being investigated including antiangiogenesis agents, cytokine inhibitors, immune modulators, and anti-HHV-8 medications. Of significant interest is the role that HAART appears to play in the treatment of KS. Tumor regression and complete remission have been documented in some patients who received HAART without chemotherapy. It is speculated that the improved immune function associated with taking these medications actually suppresses not only HIV but also HHV-8.

For oral lesions that are well localized, intralesional injection therapy with the cytotoxic drug vinblastine or the sclerosing agent sodium tetradecyl sulfate results in significant tumor regression (Figure 12–3, A and B).[16–18] Surgical excision is usually not recommended, except for tumor debulking or for obtaining diagnostic tissue (Figure 12–3, C and D). For more extensive oral involvement, systemic chemotherapy using the liposomal anthracyclines is the treatment of choice. Low-dose radiation has been effective in managing some tumors but has limited use because of inducing mucositis. When radiation treatment is administered, the total fractionated dose typically does not exceed 1,500 cGy; however, a useful alternative has been a single 800 cGy exposure (Figure 12–3, E and F).

In all of the management approaches, which are almost never curative, the treatment objective is to reduce both the signs and the symptoms. The choice of treatment is influenced by a number of factors, including the extent of the disease, the desires of the patient, the overall health status of the patient, and cost and compliance issues. Although treatment of KS, including oral lesions, improves the quality of life of an individual, there is no indication that it alters overall survival.

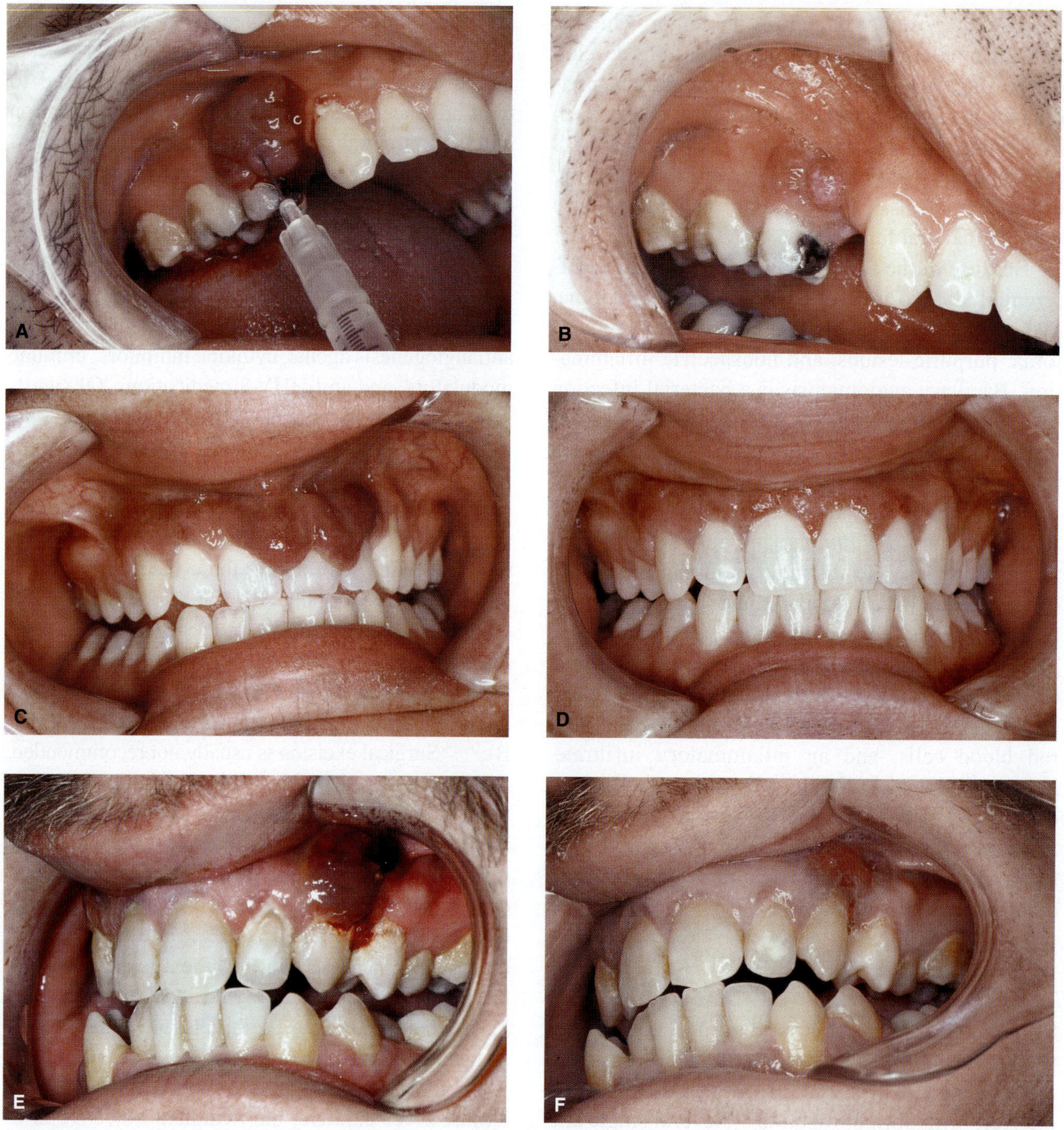

Figure 12–3. Treatment approaches for Kaposi's sarcoma (KS). *A*, Localized KS that was painful and bled easily. The patient's CD4 count was 130. Three percent sodium tetradecyl sulfate (a sclerosing agent) was injected using multiple "sticks" at one visit. *B*, Two weeks later, the KS was dramatically reduced and asymptomatic. There was no recurrence at 3 months, at which time the patient was lost to follow-up. *C*, Painful and esthetically undesirable gingival KS. *D*, Three weeks following removal by carbon-dioxide laser. Although not cured, the KS remained stable and acceptable to the patient during a 6-month follow-up. *E*, Painful hemorrhagic nodular gingival KS that was also increasing in size. *F*, Two weeks after radiation using 800 cGy in one treatment, the tumor flattened and was asymptomatic. Although not cured, the KS remained unchanged during the remaining 8 months that the patient lived.

NON-HODGKIN'S LYMPHOMA

The lifetime risk for HIV-associated lymphomas is expected to rise as the number of HIV-infected individuals increases and their life expectancy is extended without complete immune reconstitution.[19,20] Chronic hyperstimulation of B cells, infection with Epstein-Barr virus, persistent cytokine dysfunction, and loss of immune surveillance play a role in tumorigenesis. Genetic factors, such as mutations of the *c-myc* oncogene, *p53* tumor suppressor gene, and *bcl-6* oncogene, are also important. In addition, HHV-8 has been implicated in rare forms of HIV-associated lymphomas.

Approximately 3% of AIDS-defining diseases are NHL, and up to 10% of patients with AIDS are expected to develop this malignancy during the course of their HIV infection. Although NHL is declining with extended use of HAART regimens, the decrease has been modest in comparison with KS. Only central nervous system (CNS) lymphoma has declined significantly with the introduction of these new HIV drugs. Recently, NHL has become one of the most common AIDS-defining conditions among people taking HAART, accounting for about 9% of AIDS-related illnesses. If trends continue, it is predicted that NHL will become the most common cancer affecting HIV-infected individuals. Risk factors for developing NHL are also changing in the era of HAART. Besides CD4 counts of < 200 cells/mm^3, NHL has increased in HIV-infected older persons, women, Hispanic people, and those who acquired HIV through heterosexual contact. This change in disease pattern may be more of a reflection of the HIV-infected population than a real change in risk factors. In contrast to KS, the HIV exposure category does not influence significantly the development of NHL. It is generally agreed that prolonged suppression of the immune system is the primary risk factor for this malignancy.

Diagnosis

HIV-associated lymphomas usually present with widespread disease and demonstrate a predilection for the extranodal sites, including the oral cavity.[21] These tumors frequently involve the head and neck region in about 50% of cases. In some cases, oral NHL has been either the first or only evidence of this malignancy. The gingiva and palate are the most common sites of oral involvement. Oral manifestations can be either solitary or multifocal lesions that appear as rapidly growing, firm masses or persistent ulcerative lesions (Figure 12–4). Numbness of the lip, radiating jaw pain, and mobility of the teeth may precede the soft tissue findings in some instances. When the maxillary sinus is involved, a unilateral facial and lip swelling may mimic a cellulitis caused by an odontogenic infection. Occasionally, these lesions range from dark red to purple in color and are difficult to distinguish from oral KS. This diversity of signs and symptoms mandates a broad differential diagnosis so that important oral lesions are properly identified and managed.

Biopsy is necessary for definitive diagnosis and classification of NHL, but additional laboratory tests and imaging studies are required for staging and treatment.[22] Most of the tumors represent lymphomas of B-cell origin, with up to 60% representing high-grade tumors, followed by intermediate-grade disease. Although less frequently diagnosed, a 14-fold increase in low-grade lymphomas among HIV-infected individuals who had a previous AIDS-defining illness has been documented. The most common types of NHL are immunoblastic, small noncleaved cell Burkitt's-like, and diffuse large cell lymphomas. A recently recognized lymphoid malignancy is the plasmablastic lymphoma, which initially occurs in the oral cavity and has the propensity to infiltrate adjacent bone.[23] Molecular evidence of Epstein-Barr virus has been identified in about 60% of NHL and in nearly all cases of CNS lymphoma. In addition, HHV-8 has been identified in the rare HIV disease, primary effusion (body cavity) lymphoma.

Treatment

Aggressive chemotherapeutic regimens are required for optimal results but are often poorly tolerated by this group of patients (Figure 12–5).[24,25] Although positive trends exist, the use of HAART has not demonstrated a significant improvement in outcome

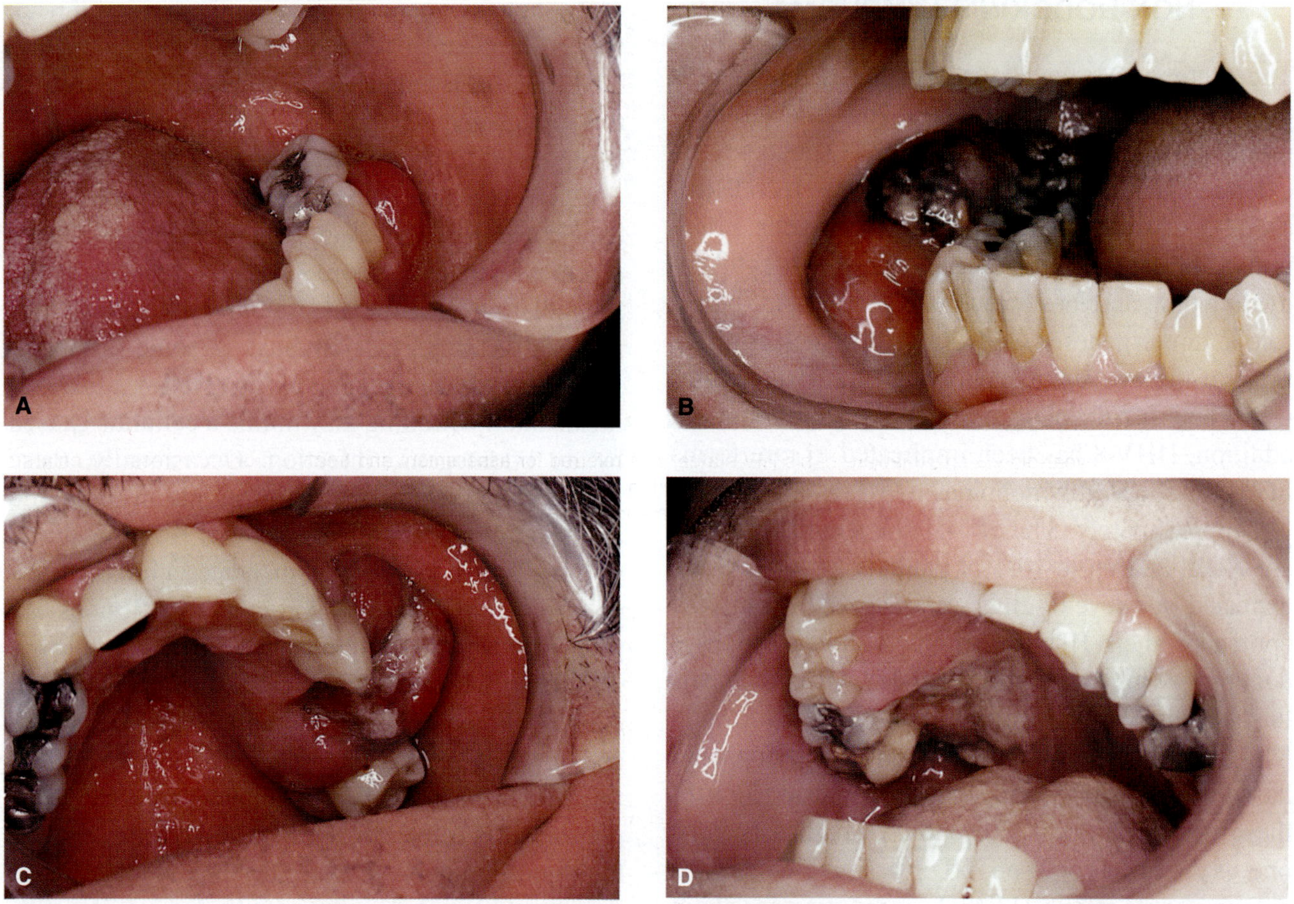

Figure 12–4. Non-Hodgkin's lymphoma (NHL) in HIV-positive patients. *A*, NHL at first mistaken for a periodontal abscess. *B*, Acute, painful swelling present for 2 months. A biopsy after no response to antibiotics showed NHL, which was the first evidence of both lymphoma and HIV disease. *C*, Maxillary swelling at first mistaken for a dental infection in an otherwise seemingly healthy patient. A biopsy showed NHL. This was the first sign of the patient's HIV disease. Aggressive chemotherapy led to temporary control for 4 months, at which time the lymphoma recurred, and the patient expired. *D*, A painful and progressive palatal-gingival ulceration noticed by the HIV-positive patient for about 1 month. The differential diagnosis included necrotizing stomatitis, fungal infection (histoplasmosis), and tumor. The biopsy revealed NHL.

or overall survival time for patients with NHL. Several multidrug protocols for managing AIDS-NHL are used, and individualization of the treatment is recommended. In the pre-HAART era, m-BACOD, which includes methotrexate, bleomycin, doxorubicin (Adriamycin®), cyclophosphamide, vincristine (Oncovin®), and dexamethasone, was a frequently used protocol. CHOP-HAART, which includes cyclophosphamide, hydroxydaunomycin (doxorubicin), vincristine, and prednisone, has been a successful combination in the post-HAART era. Infusional regimens with favorable response rates include a combination of etoposide, prednisone, vincristine, cyclophosphamide, and doxorubicin and CDE (cyclophosphamide, doxorubicin, and etoposide). This added immunosuppression obviously increases complications during and after therapy. Examples of oral diseases caused by these cytotoxic drugs include candidiasis, drug-induced mucositis, neutropenic and nonspecific ulcers, and lichenoid reactions (see Chapter 9).

Results from recent trials show that up to 20% of patients with NHL are cured and survive free from progression of their HIV disease. Furthermore, the overall risk of death decreases by 84% in patients who receive HAART. In the pre-HAART era, the median survival after diagnosis for NHL ranged from 4 to 7 months. With the use of HAART, the median survival rate is unknown for patients with NHL but appears to be greater than 28 months.

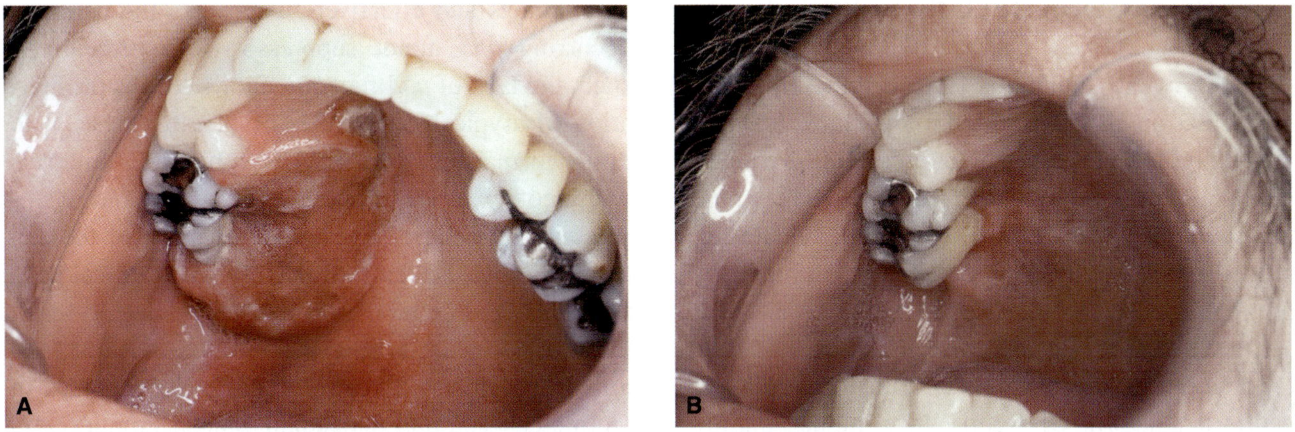

Figure 12–5. *A*, A 38-year-old patient, unaware of his HIV status, was referred for assessment and treatment of a progressively enlarging and painful ulceration. The biopsy showed non-Hodgkin's lymphoma. Serology confirmed his positive HIV status. *B*, An aggressive 12-week course of multicytotoxic drugs led to clinical remission of signs and symptoms. However, the patient survived less than 1 year.

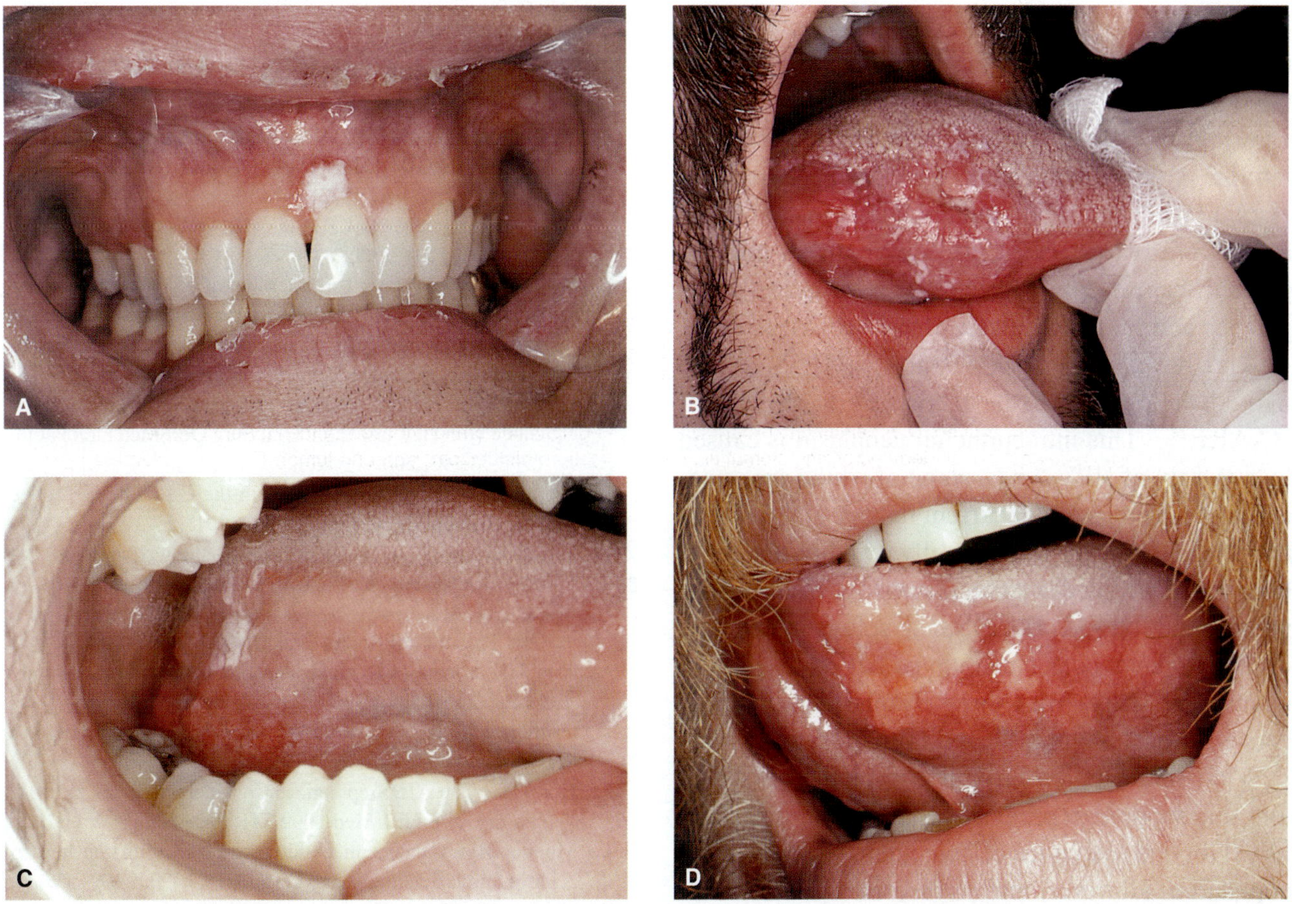

Figure 12–6. Squamous cell carcinoma (SCC). *A*, SCC of the gingiva at first mistaken for a gingival infection in a 40-year-old HIV-positive patient. The tumor responded to radiotherapy. The patient was a nonsmoker. *B*, SCC of the tongue in a 30-year-old HIV-positive patient who also had pseudomembranous oral candidiasis. The tumor did not respond to combined surgery and radiation. The patient was a smoker. *C*, Slightly painful erythroleukoplakia of the tongue in a 36-year-old homosexual HIV-positive man. Biopsy showed a squamous cell carcinoma. *D*, A 32-year-old heterosexual man had a 2-year history of nonspecific erosive lesions of the tongue. The patient had a history of venereal disease, hepatitis, and marijuana abuse. A biopsy showed squamous cell carcinoma.

SQUAMOUS CELL CARCINOMA

Oropharyngeal squamous cell carcinoma is not defined as an HIV-associated malignancy; however, this lesion has developed with increasing frequency in this group of individuals.[26] This malignancy tends to occur in men under the age of 45, but the age range is wide. In addition to persistent immunosuppression, well-established carcinogenic cofactors are associated with this malignancy and include cigarette smoking, alcohol abuse, and previous therapeutic irradiation. Of significance, human papillomavirus (HPV), including oncogenic genotypes, is identified in many of these oral cancers.[27] Rapid growth rate, early metastasis, and poor therapeutic response to radiation and surgery are characteristic findings of oropharyngeal carcinomas.

Most cases of carcinoma develop within preexisting lesions, such as leukoplakia or erythroplakia, but occasionally some tumors arise de novo (Figure 12–6). Although the tongue is the most common intraoral site of involvement, there has been no association with oral hairy leukoplakia. Most of these lesions present as persistent, tender ulcers that are greater than 2 cm in size; however, firm, warty plaques and fungating masses have been described.

The prevalence of oral warts in HIV-infected individuals appears to be increasing in the era of HAART.[28,29] This intraepithelial neoplasm is caused by a variety of HPV types, some of which are oncogenic. A previous or concurrent history of cutaneous and anogenital warts is frequently noted. When these lesions are biopsied, a small percentage of these oral warts exhibit mild to severe dysplasia. Although invasive squamous cell carcinoma has not been documented to arise from these dysplastic warts, the concern exists with prolonged immunosuppression.

Viral influence on proto-oncogenes, growth factors, and suppressor proteins has not been fully established for oral squamous cell carcinoma in this patient population. However, an increase in squamous cell carcinomas in the anorectal region of HIV-infected men and the uterine cervix of HIV-infected women has been associated with HPVs. In general, these squamous cell carcinomas have been associated with high-risk HPV types, including 16, 18, 31, 35, 53, and others. It is hypothesized that high-risk HPV protein E6 interacts and effectively inactivates the naturally occurring *p53* tumor suppressor gene protein. As such, the lack of *p53* function allows for the proliferation of atypical cells and promotes progression to tumor formation. Likewise, HPV protein E7 interacts with another tumor suppressor gene (*rb*) and inactivates it. This allows for the continuation of the cell cycle without the removal of defective atypical cells with damaged deoxyribonucleic acid. The end result is that normal tumor suppressor function is lost, and tumor surveillance is compromised. The increase in uterine-cervical and anogenital cancers implies sexual transmission as a key factor for squamous cell carcinomas at these sites.[30] As the life expectancy of an HIV-infected individual is extended and antiretroviral drugs are improved, this type of cancer may become a more significant oral malignancy.

REFERENCES

1. Flaitz CM, Nichols CM, Hicks MJ. Oral malignancies diagnosed in an HIV-dedicated dental clinic. Tex Dent J 1996; 113:49–57.
2. Smith C, Lilly S, Mann KP, et al. AIDS-related malignancies. Ann Med 1998;30:323–44.
3. Katano H, Sato Y, Sata T. Expression of p53 and human herpesvirus-8 (HHV-8)-encoded latency-associated nuclear antigen with inhibition of apoptosis in HHV-8-associated malignancies. Cancer 2001;92:3076–84.
4. Epstein J, Silverman S Jr. Head and neck malignancies associated with HIV infection. Oral Surg Oral Med Oral Pathol 1992;73:193–200.
5. Biggar RJ. AIDS-related cancers in the era of highly active antiretroviral therapy. Oncology 2001;15:439–49.
6. Patton LL, McKaig R, Strauss R. Changing prevalence of oral manifestations of human immunodeficiency virus in the era of protease inhibitor therapy. Oral Surg Oral Med Oral Pathol Oral Radiol Endod 2000;89:299–304.
7. Tam HK, Zhang Z-F, Jacobson LP, et al. Effect of highly active antiretroviral therapy on survival among HIV-infected men with Kaposi's sarcoma or non-Hodgkin's lymphoma. Int J Cancer 2002;98:916–22.
8. Fauci AS. The AIDS epidemic. Considerations for the 21st century. N Engl J Med 1999;341:1046–50.
9. Mueller BU. Cancers in children infected with the human immunodeficiency virus. Oncologist 1999;4:309–17.
10. Clarke CC, Glaser SL. Epidemiologic trends in HIV-associated lymphomas. Curr Opin Oncol 2001;13:354–9.
11. Jones JL, Hanson DL, Dworkin MS, Jaffe HW. Incidence and trends in Kaposi's sarcoma in the era of effective antiretroviral therapy. J Acquir Immune Defic Syndr Hum Retroviral 2000;24:270–4.
12. Antman K, Chang Y. Kaposi's sarcoma. N Engl J Med 2000; 342:1027–38.

13. Flaitz CM, Jin YT, Hicks MJ, et al. Kaposi's sarcoma-associated herpesvirus-like DNA sequences (KSHV/HHV8) in oral AIDS-Kaposi's sarcoma: a PCR and clinicopathologic study. Oral Surg Oral Med Oral Pathol Oral Radiol Endod 1997;83:259–64.
14. Pauk J, Huang M-I, Brodie SJ, et al. Mucosal shedding of human herpesvirus 8 in men. N Engl J Med 2000;343: 1369–77.
15. Mitsuyasu RT. Update on the pathogenesis and treatment of Kaposi sarcoma. Curr Opin Oncol 2000;12:174–80.
16. Flaitz CM, Nichols CM, Hicks MJ. Role of intralesional vinblastine administration in treatment of intraoral Kaposi's sarcoma in AIDS. Eur J Cancer B Oral Oncol 1995;31B: 280–5.
17. Lucatorto FM, Sapp JP. Treatment of oral Kaposi's sarcoma with a sclerosing agent in AIDS patients. A preliminary study. Oral Surg Oral Med Oral Pathol 1993;75:192–8.
18. Ramirez-Amador V, Esquivel-Pedraza L, Lozada-Nur F, et al. Intralesional vinblastine vs. 3% sodium tetradecyl sulfate for the treatment of oral Kaposi's sarcoma. A double blind, randomized clinical trial. Oral Oncol 2002;38:460–7.
19. Bower M, Fife K. Current issues in the biology of AIDS-related lymphoma. HIV Medicine 2001;2:141–5.
20. Carbone A, Vaccher E, Barzan L, et al. Head and neck lymphomas associated with human immunodeficiency virus infection. Arch Otolaryngol Head Neck Surg 1995;121: 210–8.
21. Lozada-Nur F, de Sanz S, Silverman S Jr, et al. Intraoral non-Hodgkin's lymphoma in seven patients with acquired immunodeficiency syndrome. Oral Surg Oral Med Oral Pathol Oral Radiol Endod 1996;82:173–8.
22. Finn DG. Lymphoma of the head and neck and acquired immunodeficiency syndrome. Clinical investigation and immunohistological study. Laryngoscope 1995;105:1–18.
23. Flaitz CM, Nichols CM, Walling DM, Hicks MJ. Plasmablastic lymphoma: an HIV-associated entity with primary oral manifestations. Oral Oncol 2002;38:96–102.
24. Levine AM, Sadeghi S, Espina B, et al. Characteristics of indolent non-Hodgkin lymphoma in patients with type 1 human immunodeficiency virus infection. Cancer 2002;94:1500–6.
25. Otieno MW, Banura C, Katongole-Mbidde E, et al. Therapeutic challenges of AIDS-related non-Hodgkin's lymphoma in the United States and East Africa. J Natl Cancer Inst 2002;94:718–32.
26. Flaitz CM, Nichols CM, Adler-Storthz K, et al. Intraoral squamous cell carcinoma in human immunodeficiency syndrome virus infection. A clinicopathologic study. Oral Surg Oral Med Oral Pathol Oral Radiol Endod 1995;80:55–62.
27. Frisch M, Biggar RJ, Goedert JJ. Human papillomavirus-associated cancers in patients with human immunodeficiency virus infection and acquired immunodeficiency syndrome. J Natl Cancer Inst 2000;92:1500–10.
28. Greenspan D, Canchola AJ, MacPhail LA, et al. Effect of highly active antiretroviral therapy on frequency of oral warts. Lancet 2001;357:1411–2.
29. King MD, Resnik DA, O'Daniels CM, et al. Human papillomavirus-associated oral warts among human immunodeficiency virus-seropositive patients in the era of highly active antiretroviral therapy: an emerging infection. Clin Infect Dis 2002;34:641–8.
30. Scully C. Oral squamous cell carcinoma: from an hypothesis about a virus, to concern about possible sexual transmission. Oral Oncol 2002;38:227–34.

Index

Page numbers followed by f indicate figure. Pages numbers followed by t indicate table.